AMERICAN JOURNAL of PUBLIC HEALTH
MAY 2026
Issue 5

AJPH

A PUBLICATION OF THE
AMERICAN PUBLIC HEALTH ASSOCIATION

250 Years of Race, Medicine, and Health in the United States

- "Scientific" Race Thinking
- Tragic Legacies of Slavery
- Separate and Unequal Facilities and Access
- Failures, Successes, and Retreats of Policies
- Service Principles vs. Demographic and Economic Realities

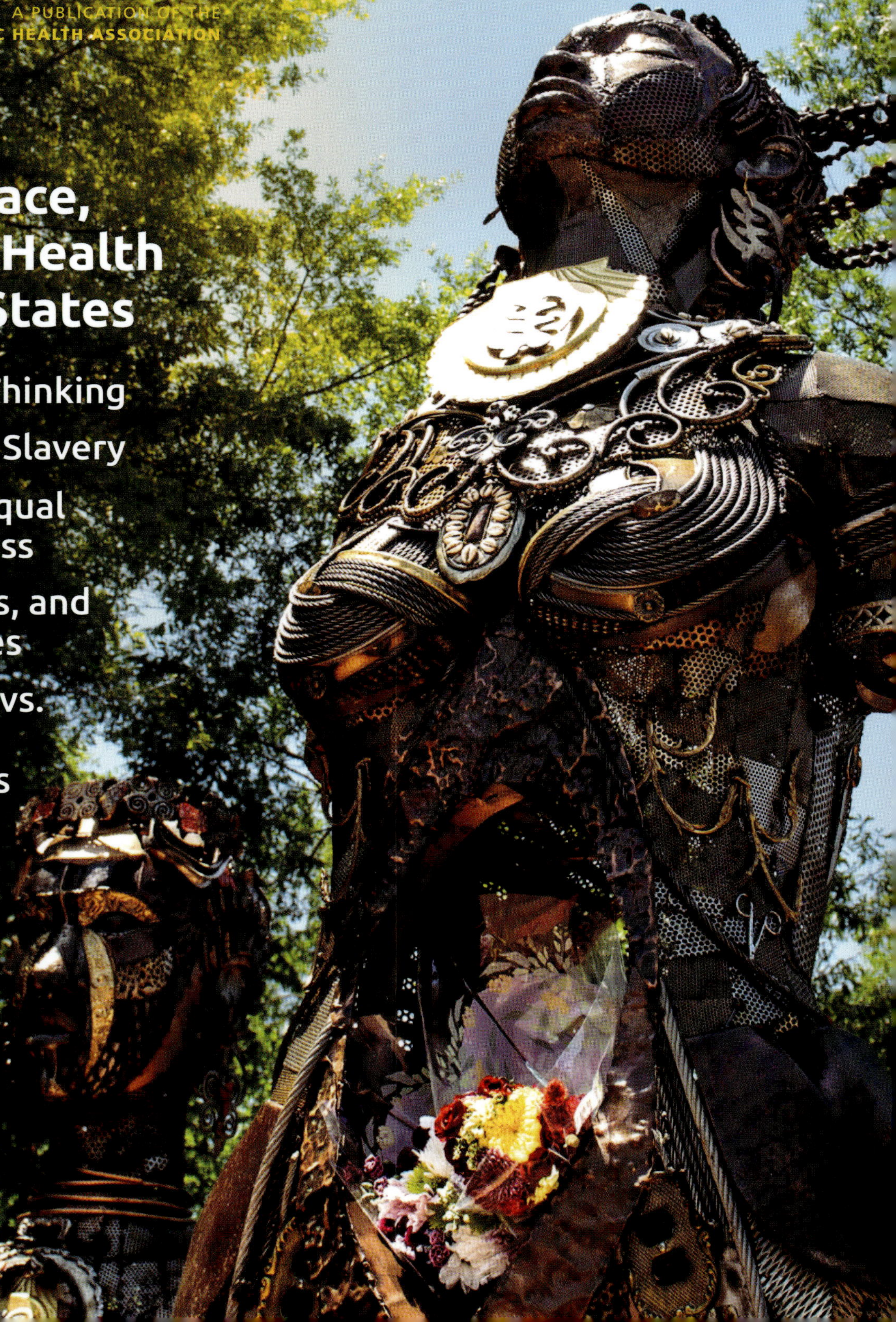

APHA
AMERICAN PUBLIC HEALTH ASSOCIATION
For science. For action. For health.

AJPH®, published monthly, is the official Journal of the American Public Health Association®, 800 I St NW, Washington, DC 20001-3710; (202) 777- APHA; TDD (202) 777-2500. APHA is a nongovernmental professional society founded in 1872, representing all disciplines and specialties in public health.

The *American Journal of Public Health*® (*AJPH*) (print ISSN: 0090-0036; electronic ISSN: 1541- 0048), first published in 1911, is the official journal of the American Public Health Association® (APHA). The oldest and largest organization of public health professionals in the world, APHA represents approximately 30 000 members from more than 50 occupations of public health.

Submissions: Visit www.editorialmanager.com/ajph for online manuscript preparation and submission guidelines. Contributions of original unpublished research, social science analyses, scholarly essays, critical commentaries, departments, and letters to the editor are welcome. Questions? Write ajph.submissions@apha.org or call APHA at (202) 777-2469.

Print plus online subscriptions: Institutional price (print copy with online access) for a single institution and all authorized users, regardless of geographic location varies by size of organization; multiple campuses not permitted without special arrangement. To order, write apha.subscriptions@apha.org.

Online-only subscriptions: Institutional price for one US federal institution and its authorized users is $1,015–$1,510. To order, write apha.subscriptions@apha.org. For academic, non-US federal consortia, or multisite subscriptions, contact apha.subscriptions@apha.org or visit http://research.ebsco.com for pricing information.

Print-only subscriptions: Institutional price is US $970, $1,065 international.

Back print issues: A limited number of print issues are for sale. Single copies are US $80, $90 international (air delivery). Shipping and handling fees will apply; prepay only. To order, write apha.subscriptions@apha.org.

Reprints: For prices and ordering information on 50 or more reprints, check the Reprints section at www.ajph.org. To order smaller quantities of reprints (rush delivery), use the "Purchase Article" link on the article site itself.

Electronic access: Online articles more than 10 years old are available free for personal use at www.ajph.org. Recent articles are available through pay-per-view: single PDF article for $24, single issue access for 24 hours for $33, or entire site access for 24 hours for $38.

Postal information: Periodicals postage paid at Washington, DC, and additional mailing offices. Postmaster: Send address changes to American Journal of Public Health, 800 I St NW, Washington, DC 20001-3710.

Address changes: Send to AJPH, Membership Department (members) or AJPH Subscriptions (subscribers), APHA, 800 I St NW, Washington, DC 20001-3710. Or write to membership.mail@apha.org (members) or apha.subscriptions@apha.org (subscribers).

Indexes: Publications that index or abstract articles from *AJPH* include the following: Ageline, Assia (Applied Social Science Index and Abstracts), Biological Abstracts, Chemical Abstracts, CINAHL, Criminal Justice Abstracts, EMBASE, EMCare, Environmental Abstracts, e-psyche, ERIC, ETOH (Alcohol and Alcohol Problems Science Database), Excerpta Medica, Food Science and Technology, General Science Index, Grateful Med, Hospital Literature Index, Human Resources Abstracts, International Pharmaceutical Abstracts (IPA), Medline, Physical Education Index, Pollution Abstracts, Psychological Abstracts, PsychINFO, Safety Science Abstracts, Sage Family Studies Abstracts, Sage Human Resources Abstracts, Science Citation Index, SCOPUS, SIIC Data Bases, Social Work Research and Abstracts, and Statistical Reference Index (SRI)/LexisNexis.

AJPH

A PUBLICATION OF THE
AMERICAN PUBLIC HEALTH ASSOCIATION

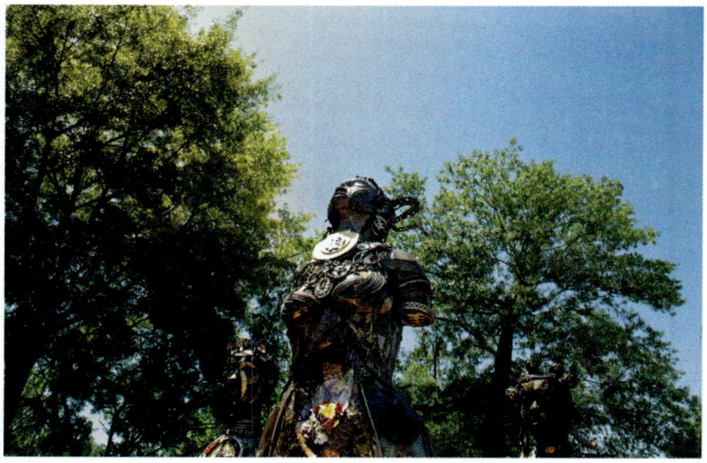

COVER: The Mothers of Gynecology Monument Park is located in Montgomery, Alabama. The erection of the "Mothers of Gynecology" monument honors the sacrifice of Anarcha, Lucy, and Betsey, the enslaved experimental subjects of the so-called "father of gynecology," J. Marion Sims. Created by artist Michelle Browder, the monument stands not far from where Sims's dastardly experiments were conducted. Drawing on a comprehensive reexamination of Sims's career, and archival documents that reveal the lives and fates of Anarcha, Lucy, and Betsey, the "Mothers of Gynecology" acts as a first step toward teaching and reimagining the true story of the nation, facing the injustice of the past, and honoring the courage of overlooked heroes.

Cover concept and selection by Aleisha Kropf. Photo by Andi Rice for *The Washington Post* via Getty Images. Printed with permission.

APHA
AMERICAN PUBLIC HEALTH ASSOCIATION
For science. For action. For health.

Promoting public health research, policy, practice, and education is the *AJPH* mission. As we widen our scope to embrace global issues, we also sharpen our focus to support the needs of public health practitioners. We invite contributions of original unpublished research, opinion and commentary, and letters to the editor.

The *Journal* is printed on acid-free recycled paper.

AJPH May 2026, Vol. 116, No. 5

OPEN ACCESS ONLINE ONLY PODCAST DATA SUPPLEMENT AVAILABLE

EDITOR'S CHOICE

567 Looking Back, Turning Away: The Double Legacy of *An American Health Dilemma*
A. Morabia and G. C. Benjamin

OPINIONS, PRACTICE, & EDUCATION

EDITORIALS FROM THE ACADEMICS

569 From Grit to Greatness: Cultivating a Rural Public Health Pipeline From Scratch
S. Tedders and N. A. Marshall

VACCINE ACCESS

572 Navigating State Politics to Protect Vaccine Policy
L. T. Reinders and R. Hassaballa

575 *AJPH* as a Trusted Source for Child and Adolescent Vaccination Recommendations
R. Kim-Farley, B. O. Ojikutu, and D. T. Lau

EDITORIALS

582 A Radical Reimagining of the Mission of Public Health
G. Markowitz

584 Mortality Risk After Moving From Homelessness Into Supported Housing: A Cautionary Note and a Call to Action
S. W. Hwang

587 Gaps in Surveillance and Data Infrastructure for Postpartum Diabetes Screening in the United States After Gestational Diabetes Mellitus
K. Suvada, R. Chakkalakal, and L. C. M. Johnson

591 The 2025 Drug Overdose Spike That Wasn't: Neither Politics nor Data Errors Explain the Anomaly
L. A. Post, D. Ciccarone, A. L. Lundberg, M. Mason, S. Sharma, G. J. Unick, and N. Dasgupta

594 The Vital Statistics Rapid Release Program Responds
F. B. Ahmad, R. N. Anderson, J. A. Cisewski, L. M. Rossen, and P. D. Sutton

596 The Public Health Potential of Social Media Litigation
H. L. Kent, C. Vidal, and D. G. Aaron

601 Our "Cannabis" Vocabulary Is Eroding Public Health Safeguards
M. E. Rossheim

604 On the 20th Anniversary of the National Board of Public Health Examiners: It Is Long Past Time We Became a Profession
D. J. Petersen, A. Foster, J. W. Corvin, and P. K. Halverson

607 Fifty Years of PL 93-638: Learning From Our Past, Planning for the Future of American Indian Health Governance
T. Parker, L. Teunis, N. Cooeyate, and A. Kelley

610 From "Informant" to "Influencer": Reframing Research Language to Build Trust in Marginalized Communities
A. I. Aguila Gonzalez, B. Faseru, V. Collie-Akers, and E. Ablah

NOTES FROM THE FIELD

615 Addressing Hygiene Poverty and Restoring Dignity: A Community Partnership Through Laundry Love
E. Ablah, N. Long, K. Hollins, C. Miller, C. Owings, K. Weaver, J. Love, C. C. Martinez, T. K. Darby, T. M. Neira, A. Scott, C. M. Pacheco, and S. Finocchario-Kessler

619 A Strategic Alliance as an Implementation Strategy to Achieve Ending the HIV Epidemic Goals Among Latino Men Who Have Sex With Men: Florida and Puerto Rico, 2023
A. Harkness, N. Reyes, C-H. Shrader, M. Tidd, N. Altenberg, G. C. Sánchez, A. C. Gerena, S. Doblecki-Lewis, J. Jaramillo, R. Ledain, S. M. Malavé Rivera, O. Martinez, G. Prado, C. E. Rodríguez-Díaz, R. Saber, S. A. Safren, E. I. Santiago Rodriguez, R. S. Malavé, and E. W. Schrimshaw

AN AMERICAN HEALTH DILEMMA 25 YEARS LATER

625 An American Health Dilemma 25 Years Later
T. M. Brown

628 Black Struggles for Medical Education and Postgraduate Training
K. M. Ludmerer

632 "A Wide Field Is Open Before Her, and Many of Her Sisters": Discovering Early African American Women Physicians
V. N. Gamble

635 Of Miracles, Medicine, and the "Moor's" Leg: What Are We to Do With Race?
R. A. Hogarth

639 Childbearing and Reproductive Health Under Slavery
D. C. Owens

RESEARCH & ANALYSIS

AN AMERICAN HEALTH DILEMMA 25 YEARS LATER

643 Hospitals and the History of Structural Racism in the United States
L. Adolphson and B. Hoffman

649 Enslaved Health and Healing in *An American Health Dilemma*: A Retrospective Review
S. M. Fett

OPEN-THEMED RESEARCH

657 Designed for Disparity: The Structural Origins of Migrant Farmworker Health Inequities in Maryland, 1900–1950
E. Ferrer, T. Sangaramoorthy, and D. Payne-Sturges

665 Changes in All-Cause, Overdose, and Suicide Mortality Risk in the First 2 Years of Supported Housing, United States, 2017–2021
J. Tsai, T. Peltzman, and H. A. Beydoun

674 Reasons for Choosing Telehealth Abortion Based on Food Insecurity Status: United States, 2021–2022
C. E. Williams, A. Becker, L. R. Koenig, L. Peters, and U. D. Upadhyay

683 Societal Costs of Total Abortion Bans in 14 US States After *Dobbs*
I. S. Platt, J. E. Starling, E. Pendl-Robinson, S. Chavez, D. Vohra, and K. Zivin

692 Health Care Use and Health Care–Amenable Mortality Among US Adults With and Without a Bachelor's Degree, 1996–2023
A. Gaffney, S. Woolhandler, S. L. Dickman, E. Schrier, D. McCormick, and D. U. Himmelstein

702 Economic Hardship; Coronavirus Aid, Relief, and Economic Security (CARES) Act Payments; and Self-Rated Health: A Longitudinal Analysis From the Health and Retirement Study, United States, 2020–2022
S. L. Swift, B. P. Horn, B. N. Harding, M. Shendo, T. C. Collins, and A. Zeki Al Hazzouri

711 Psychosocial Risk and Resilience as Moderators of the Association Between Neighborhood Disadvantage and Incident Cardiovascular Disease Across Ethnoracial Groups: Multi-Ethnic Study of Atherosclerosis, United States, 2000–2019
H. Pleasants, J. R. Pike, P. Palta, A. G. Bertoni, T. M. Hughes, Q. Xiao, J. A. Hirsch, and G. S. Bey

722 Population-Level Violence as a Whole
M. D. Esposti, D. K. Humphreys, and J. Murray

732 Projected Increase in HIV Incidence in 11 States if Ryan White Ends: A Simulation Study
M. Schnure, R. Forster, J. L. Jones, C. R. Lesko, D. S. Batey, I. Butler, D. Ward, K. Musgrove, K. N. Althoff, M. K. Jain, K. A. Gebo, D. W. Dowdy, M. Shah, P. Kasaie, and A. T. Fojo

Looking Back, Turning Away: The Double Legacy of *An American Health Dilemma*

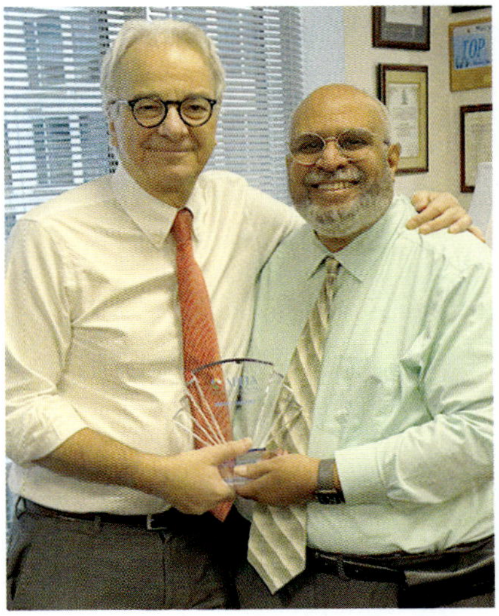

Alfredo Morabia, MD, PhD
Professor, Queens College CUNY and Columbia University
Former Editor-in-Chief, *AJPH* (2015–2025)
Georges C. Benjamin, MD
Chief Executive Officer, American Public Health Association

In 1944, Swedish economist Gunnar Myrdal published the two-volume classic *An American Dilemma: The Negro Problem and Modern Democracy*. When, about 60 years later, physicians W. Michael Byrd and Lynda A. Clayton published two volumes about the medical history of African Americans in the United States, they titled their work *An American Health Dilemma*, deliberately echoing Myrdal's books. Byrd and Clayton, not themselves professional historians, did not offer a comprehensive sociohistorical analysis of race, medicine, and health care in the United States, but they laid the foundations for the documentation of how racism and racially structured medical institutions shaped health outcomes from the colonial period through the end of the 20th century. In this issue of *AJPH*, seven contributions add new blocks on these foundations by revisiting the core insights of the volumes.

Historian Theodore M. Brown, who took the initiative of and supervised the preparation of this issue (bit.ly/40d92Ox), provides a synopsis of these contributions (p. 625). In our reading of this fascinating dossier, some points stand out. Sharla M. Fett's essay (p. 649), focusing on Byrd and Clayton's first volume, argues that both the mental and psychological long-term impact of slavery and the richness of the health subsystem built by slaves have been underestimated until recently. In their essay focusing on the second volume, LeNie Adolfson and Beatrix Hoffman (p. 643) show that historical research has confirmed the role of hospitals as enduring sites of medical racism, institutionalizing segregation, disinvestment, and stigmatization. In their editorials, Deirdre Cooper Owens (p. 639), Rana Asali Hogarth (p. 635), and Kenneth Ludmerer (p. 628) emphasize the continued power of ideas about innate racial difference in clinical practice and professional institutions. Vanessa Northington Gamble (p. 632) contributes to the leveling of a gendered gap in that historiography, highlighting the lives of Rebecca Crumpler and Rebecca Cole, two African American women physicians.

Taken together, these pieces powerfully reaffirm the importance of *An American Health Dilemma*. At the same time, they remain largely centered on medicine—that is, physicians, hospitals, and clinical ideologies—leaving relatively little sustained engagement with population-level public health systems, prevention, or governance. In 2003 the Institute of Medicine reviewed the state of health inequities, finding that disparities in health persisted and that inequities in health care contributed to these disparities (bit.ly/4atFH7r). That work accelerated research in health disparities.

However, a second study, conducted in 2024 by the National Academies of Medicine (formerly the Institute of Medicine), revealed that although progress has been made in our understanding of health disparities, health inequities persist and little has changed with respect to addressing the root causes that have been clarified over the past 20 years (https://bit.ly/46HGEaX). This second report described a series of steps that, if implemented, would address the systematic issues preventing achievement of optimal health for everyone.

This year, the United States is celebrating its 250th year as a nation. However, many of the structural barriers to achieving health equity and optimal health for all have tragically not been addressed. Moreover, the policies of the current administration implemented since early 2025 to demonize diversity, equity, and inclusion initiatives as being discriminatory further undermine efforts to address health inequities. The drastic reductions in research funding related to minority health have resulted in markedly fewer competitive grants (nyti.ms/4kEvgmi), signaling a retreat from the commitments that the book helped to legitimize.

Rejecting diversity and inclusion calls for homogeneity reached by exclusion; rejecting equity worsens the already-existing inequities. These policy decisions have already begun to have a negative impact on the health of underrepresented populations and demonstrate in real time why the very domains illuminated by *An American Health Dilemma* face huge political obstacles.

Revisiting Byrd and Clayton's work 25 years later reinforces the persistence of racism in America as a power-driven and hateful social construct that has a negative impact on the health of everyone. It also demonstrates that persistent policies that support structural racism remain at the core of health equities. Since the first slaves were brought to the English colonies in 1619, the health of the African American population has been an important issue of historical and medical significance. The Freedmen's Bureau, created in 1865, was an early attempt to address these health inequities, and through the years many efforts have been made to document the impact of the vestiges of racism that persist up to today.

Numerous studies, reports, and policy papers have promoted clinical as well as policy solutions to address the root causes that allow these inequities to persist. Few have been successful. The election in 2008 of the first African American president, Barack Obama (bit.ly/461dvYb), was a symbolic perspective that attitudes were changing and that issues around health and social justice inequities were being addressed. The aspiration for change has not translated into action yet. Since January 2025, the country has entered an accelerated phase of obscurantism, one that discounts historical knowledge, undermines scientific inquiry, legitimizes racist ideologies, and threatens profound and lasting consequences for the public's health broadly and the health of racial minorities specifically. Reconciling this dilemma is the central challenge of our day. Deconstructing the systems that foster discrimination and promote inequities is a prerequisite to achieving optimal health for all. AJPH

DOI: https://doi.org/10.2105/AJPH.2026.308493

ORCID iDs:
Alfredo Morabia https://orcid.org/0000-0002-1902-0285

Georges C. Benjamin https://orcid.org/0000-0003-3453-1654

From Grit to Greatness: Cultivating a Rural Public Health Pipeline From Scratch

Stuart Tedders, PhD, and Nandi A. Marshall, DrPH, MPH

ABOUT THE AUTHORS

Stuart Tedders is the dean of the Jiann-Ping Hsu College of Public Health (JPHCOPH) at Georgia Southern University, Statesboro. Nandi A. Marshall is the associate dean for academic affairs of JPHCOPH. She is also the president of the American Public Health Association.

See also Editorials from the Academics, https://bit.ly/3NEdvrc.

The Jiann-Ping Hsu College of Public Health (JPHCOPH) at Georgia Southern University was founded on January 1, 2006, through a generous endowment by Karl E. Peace, MS, PhD, in honor of his late wife, Jiann-Ping Hsu, MA, PhD. Since its inception, the college has achieved initial accreditation from the Council on Education for Public Health in 2011 and two successful reaffirmations. Our mission, vision, and shared values serve as an enduring celebration of Hsu's life, characterized by her "zeal for excellence, consideration of others, intelligence and scholarship, honesty, kindness, and humility."[1] Located in rural Georgia, JPHCOPH works to strengthen the health of rural and underserved communities by reducing disparities through excellence in teaching, research, community engagement, and professional service.

AN AUDACIOUS BEGINNING

Beyond geography, JPHCOPH is shaped by the public health realities of the rural Southeast. Unlike many units formed through reallocation of existing departments, we were built from the ground up by a founding dean, five tenure-track faculty members, three staff members, and 40 graduate students. This was an exceptionally bold undertaking in a region marked by persistent health inequities, limited health care access, chronic disease burden, and underresourced public health infrastructure. In a state often divided between Atlanta and "everyone else," JPHCOPH faced skeptics who doubted a college of public health could be sustained in rural Southeast Georgia. Fortunately, this perspective only strengthened our resolve to bridge widening health gaps.

This "scrappy" beginning required us to live our mission authentically by recruiting faculty willing to invest in a vision rooted in service to rural and underserved communities. These experiences shaped our identity as a college grounded in the understanding that meaningful public health impact, especially in a rural context, requires sustained commitment and resolve.

NAVIGATING THE MODERN ENROLLMENT CRISIS

Today, our academic portfolio is designed specifically for rural and underserved communities. Yet, as we have matured, the challenges have shifted. Enrollment hurdles are acute in the rural Southeast, where rising tuition costs and skepticism about the value of a degree dominate the conversation. Furthermore, demographic shifts and economic uncertainty often push rural youths to enter the workforce immediately to meet family needs.

While significant, these hurdles are the straightforward part of the challenge. The deeper issue is what we call the "visibility crisis." Unlike high-profile clinical roles like nursing or medicine, residents are far less familiar with population-based public health work and systems-level problem-solving. The larger impact of public health is often realized over time and across entire communities, rather than in individual clinical encounters. In rural communities facing urgent economic pressures, long-term solutions are often bypassed for careers deemed more immediate, desirable, or lucrative. Thus, we must work intentionally to make public health visible and attainable. Communicating our passion for making a difference in the community is the JPHCOPH superpower; through this, we not only educate students but also help build the public health workforce essential to the resilience of rural and underserved communities in Georgia.

WORKFORCE PIPELINE STRATEGIES: REACHING THE NEXT GENERATION

To increase visibility, JPHCOPH utilizes a multitiered strategy focused on early exposure and accessibility, introducing public health as a viable career option well before university age. Our goal is to cultivate a mindset of equity and community resilience that persists

AJPH May 2026, Vol. 116, No. 5

regardless of a student's eventual field of study.

This commitment began in 2009 with the launch of Public Health Young Adults Day. For more than 17 years, this initiative has brought high-school students from rural and underserved communities to campus for an interactive half-day of simulations and workshops. For many, this event represents their first exposure to public health beyond traditional clinical roles.

However, interest alone is insufficient if geographic and financial isolation remain as "leaks" in the rural health pipeline. We addressed these hurdles in 2021 by partnering with our dual enrollment office to expand access to our Introduction to Community/Public Health course. This acts as a decisive bridge, allowing students in underserved communities to earn college credit while still in high school and easing the economic pressures that often deter rural families from pursuing higher education. We have also provided access to high-school students in our surrounding areas through the Public and Community Health Pathway partnership with the Bulloch County School System. The curriculum introduces foundational concepts such as epidemiology, prevention, and health equity through practical, community-based applications. A central component of the course is a modified photovoice activity developed by our faculty, in which students document public health issues in their own neighborhoods and connect them to relevant course content. By examining challenges such as access to food, transportation, housing, or safe recreational spaces, students begin to see public health not as an abstract concept but as a powerful tool for improving the well-being of their own rural communities.

To sustain this momentum, we have also worked to establish a Rising Scholars Public Health Institute and integrate global public health into the university-wide core curriculum. Ultimately, we aim to provide a foundational public health perspective for all who engage in our programming, to view their work through an equity and community resilience lens, regardless of their field of study.

A MOVEMENT BUILT TO LAST

We began as a bold experiment in 2006, built on the legacy of Jiann-Ping Hsu. From the beginning, our purpose was clear: to build a home for public health in rural Southeast Georgia, prepare future generations to serve the communities that too often stand at the margins of health systems and policy, and to change lives. Today, JPHCOPH is an impactful college committed to developing a public health workforce grounded in place, purpose, and persistence.

By engaging students across Georgia Southern's campuses and reaching into rural high schools, we are doing more than recruiting students. We are cultivating a pipeline of future public health leaders who understand rural life because they have lived it and because they love it. These students are uniquely positioned to return to their communities as practitioners, researchers, and advocates who can address chronic disease, access to care, environmental risk, and health inequities with cultural humility and local insight. In this way, our work is not simply academic; it is generational.

Our evolution from a small group into a comprehensive college mirrors the resilience we seek to instill in our graduates. We remain steadfast in our commitment to rural and underserved communities, preparing professionals who are ready to stand in the gap where public health infrastructure is thin and need is greatest. As the demands on the public health workforce continue to grow, particularly in rural America, we recognize that no single institution can meet this challenge alone.

Looking ahead to the next decade of JPHCOPH, our vision includes deeper collaboration with rural school districts, local health departments, community organizations, and peer institutions across the country that share a commitment to rural health. By strengthening partnerships with other colleges and schools of public health serving rural regions, we can amplify best practices, expand training pathways, and collectively build a workforce prepared to meet the evolving needs of rural communities nationwide. The work of public health is ongoing, and so is our responsibility to rural Georgia, to future generations, and to the broader effort to ensure health equity wherever people live. AJPH

CORRESPONDENCE

Correspondence should be sent to Dr Nandi A. Marshall, PO Box 8015, Statesboro, GA 30460-8015 (e-mail: nmarshall@georgiasouthern.edu). Reprints can be ordered at https://www.ajph.org by clicking the "Reprints" link.

PUBLICATION INFORMATION

Full Citation: Tedders S, Marshall NA. From grit to greatness: cultivating a rural public health pipeline from scratch. *Am J Public Health*. 2026;116(5): 569–571.

Acceptance Date: February 10, 2026.

DOI: https://doi.org/10.2105/AJPH.2026.308481

ORCID iDs:

Stuart Tedders https://orcid.org/0000-0002-6010-5272

Nandi A. Marshall https://orcid.org/0000-0002-2247-8422

CONTRIBUTORS

Both authors contributed significantly to the conceptualization, drafting, revisions, and final review of the document.

ACKNOWLEDGMENTS

We would like to thank the JPHCOPH faculty, staff, and students, as well as our external partners and stakeholders, for their commitment to the field, our mission, and the growth of our college. We would also like to thank the administration of Georgia Southern University for supporting our efforts.

CONFLICTS OF INTEREST

The authors do not have any potential or actual conflicts of interest to disclose.

REFERENCE

1. Jiann-Ping Hsu College of Public Health. About. 2024. Available at: https://www.georgiasouthern.edu/colleges/public-health/about. Accessed February 9, 2026.

Navigating State Politics to Protect Vaccine Policy

Lina Tucker Reinders, MPH, and Ruaa Hassaballa, PhD(c), MPH

ABOUT THE AUTHORS

Lina Tucker Reinders is with Iowa Public Health Association, Des Moines. Ruaa Hassaballa is with the Kansas Public Health Association, Leawood.

See also *AJPH*'s Vaccine Access Collection, https://bit.ly/4l98J12.

Federal vaccine and broader public health policies are changing rapidly and unpredictably. Public health leaders are understandably concerned about the loss of progress against diseases that have been nearly eliminated from the United States.[1] Preventing further erosion of vaccine confidence and access will require sustained investment in state and local public health infrastructure, protection of public health authority at the community level, and cross-state collaborations such as the Governors Public Health Alliance.[2] Through the Alliance, 15 governors are taking action to support the science of public health in a self-described 100% nonpartisan effort. Notably, all current Alliance members are Democrats, and all but North Carolina and Guam have Democrat-led legislatures. Consequently, their efforts may be perceived as partisan, thus limiting their impact in states aligned with the federal administration. Although the Alliance represents an important effort to uphold evidence-based public health, multistate systems coordination alone is insufficient to protect vaccine access in states with more conservative ideologies.

We admire the goals of the Alliance and look forward to the impact of its work. At the same time, we know that the political, legal, and social contexts shaping public health in conservative (red) states differ in important ways. Whereas the governors committed to the Alliance are leading administrative efforts to protect public health at the systems level, conservative-led states are advancing restrictive local public health and vaccine-related legislation, often with similar bills in multiple states. Even as we continue to assess how federal changes will affect state vaccine policy, we aim to share the perspective of red-state advocates in hopes that our experiences will benefit the efforts of our colleagues who may be encountering public health policy challenges for the first time.

The public health workforce and vaccine advocates across the country are in a precarious state of uncertainty as we work to promote vaccines. Previously, the Centers for Disease Control and Prevention (CDC) and its Advisory Committee on Immunization Practices (ACIP) provided the gold standard for scientific review and vaccine recommendations. Public health teams have long used this institutional guidance to defend against attempts to weaken vaccine policy and other public health measures. Increasingly, however, advocates can no longer rely on federal guidance as a stable reference point in immunization advocacy. When recommendations from professional medical societies, such as the American Academy of Pediatrics, differ from CDC guidance, even when grounded in rigorous evidence, the lack of alignment can be confusing to the public and may be leveraged by antivaccine advocates to undermine trust in public health science, data, and policy.

The questioning of science and misrepresentation of data are not new to advocates in conservative states. Rather, it represents an amplification of the environments in which public health has been working since 2020. Political tensions during the COVID-19 pandemic started with mask mandates and school closures, and grew with the rollout of vaccines, in particular, vaccine mandates. In the years prior to 2020, Iowa saw an average of two bills per legislative session that would have limited vaccine access.[3] The number peaked at 20 in 2022, all sponsored by Republicans and advanced along party lines.

The public health workforce and advocates in conservative-led states depend on strong local partnerships to protect vaccine access and rebuild trust in public health. Local public health authority varies widely, shaping how immunization policy is implemented at the community level. In this context, partnerships may include state and local public health departments, nonprofit organizations, and private-sector allies who, within their respective roles, fill critical gaps in service delivery, data sharing, messaging, and advocacy.

Regional and cross-state networking is particularly important for state policy work. Returning to the previous example, since 2020, Iowa Public Health Association has lobbied on more than 200 bills that would have affected health outcomes in Iowa.[4] Although

AJPH May 2026, Vol. 116, No. 5

some bills aligned with public health practice, the majority were related to vaccines and public health authority. Public health advocates and lobbyists defeated proposed legislation that would have prohibited mRNA vaccines, removed vaccine manufacturers' liability protection, required active and recorded parental consent for every childhood vaccination, and eliminated quarantine authority. The few Iowa bills that passed include limits on vaccine mandates, disclosure of exemptions to school-based vaccine requirements, and the prohibition of mask mandates in schools. Similar legislation was proposed in states in the Midwest and across the country.[5–7]

Multistate networks such as MINK (MO, IA, NE, KS), the Healthy States Collaborative, and the National Network of Immunization Coalitions allow advocates to share policy insights, tactics, and common messaging. Despite the few setbacks, the overwhelming success at stopping bills that would adversely affect health outcomes illustrates how coordinated, cross-state cooperation can blunt the policy impact of well-resourced opposition, even in politically conservative environments.[8]

At the same time, colleagues in state and local governments work diligently to promote vaccines and vaccine access programs (e.g., Vaccines for Children), collect immunization data, and monitor disease through traditional surveillance methods. The extent of their work, however, is limited by the positions and allegiances of the state administration or, at times, by state statutes, such as those that tie school required vaccines to ACIP recommendations.[9] Local public health departments often have greater latitude in how, when, and where they promote vaccination, depending on the direction of their local boards of health. Recently, however, candidates for offices from school boards and local elections to state houses have been seeking the favor of national organizations opposed to vaccine requirements.[10] This tactic is being used in many states, red and blue, to varying degrees of success. The concern is that vaccine policy debates will move from evidence-based public health forums to local governance bodies that may lack technical expertise and compromise vaccine access.

The antivaccine movement represents a minority of opinions regarding vaccines, yet it is organized and well-funded across all states.[8,11] Their ability to recruit parents and advance legislation should not be underestimated. This is precisely why it is critical that communication and partnerships between vaccine advocates, policymakers, and public health leaders remain open across blue and red states. Preventing further erosion of vaccine access and preserving the infrastructure from which to rebuild will require more than isolated state advocacy or coordination among like-minded leaders. Today's political polarization makes the task seem insurmountable. However, we are already seeing how the state and local advocacy in red states complements the systems-level work of the Alliance and other blue states. Together, these efforts strengthen our collective ability to protect and advocate for evidence-based policy decisions. Meeting this moment requires learning from strategies developed in the most constrained policy environments and recommitting to the principle that public health must remain evidence-based, coordinated, community-rooted, and resilient amid political volatility. AJPH

CORRESPONDENCE

Correspondence should be sent to Lina Tucker Reinders, Iowa Public Health Association, 501 SW 7th St, Suite G, Des Moines, IA 50309 (e-mail: Lina@IowaPHA.org). Reprints can be ordered at https://www.ajph.org by clicking the "Reprints" link.

PUBLICATION INFORMATION

Full Citation: Reinders LT, Hassaballa R. Navigating state politics to protect vaccine policy. *Am J Public Health*. 2026;116(5):572–574.

Acceptance Date: February 4, 2026

DOI: https://doi.org/10.2105/AJPH.2026.308485

ORCID iD:

Lina Tucker Reinders https://orcid.org/0009-0005-1100-1556

CONTRIBUTORS

Both authors contributed equally to the work.

ACKNOWLEDGMENTS

We thank the boards of directors and members of the Iowa and Kansas Public Health Associations, and Elizabeth Faber of Iowa Immunizes Coalition.

CONFLICTS OF INTEREST

The authors have no conflicts of interest to disclose.

REFERENCES

1. American Academy of Pediatrics. Statement from leading medical, health and patient advocacy groups on CDC vaccine meeting. 2020. Available at: https://www.aap.org/en/news-room/news-releases/aap/2025/statement-from-leading-medical-health-and-patient-advocacy-groups-on-cdc-vaccine-meeting. Accessed January 21, 2026.
2. Governors Public Health Alliance. December 2025. Available at: https://www.govsforhealth.org. Accessed January 21, 2026.
3. Iowa Legislature. BillBook. Available at: www.legis.iowa.gov. Accessed January 21, 2026.
4. Iowa Legislative Services Agency. Iowa Legislature—lobbyist declarations. Iowa.gov. 2025. Available at: https://www.legis.iowa.gov/lobbyist/reports/declarations. Accessed January 21, 2026.
5. Governor Kim Reynolds. HF 902. Iowa.gov. October 29, 2021. Available at: https://www.legis.iowa.gov/legislation/BillBook?ga=89&ba=HF902. Accessed January 21, 2026.
6. Governor Kim Reynolds. HF 299. Iowa.gov. May 27, 2025. Available at: https://www.legis.iowa.gov/legislation/BillBook?ba=HF%20299&ga=91. Accessed January 21, 2026.

7. Governor Kim Reynolds. HF 847. Iowa.gov. 2025. Available at: https://www.legis.iowa.gov/legislation/BillBook?ba=HF%20847&ga=89. Accessed January 21, 2026.
8. Piper J. Anti-vaxxers are now a modern political force. Politico. September 24, 2023. Available at: https://www.politico.com/news/2023/09/24/anti-vaxxers-political-power-00116527. Accessed January 21, 2026.
9. Association of State and Territorial Health Officials. Impact of the ACIP recommendations on state law. June 23, 2025. Available at: https://www.astho.org/topic/resource/impact-of-acip-recommendations-on-state-law. Accessed January 21, 2026.
10. Moms for Liberty. These candidates and elected officials stand with parents. May 23, 2025. Available at: https://www.momsforliberty.org/pledged-candidates-elected-officials. Accessed January 21, 2026.
11. Nadeem R. How do Americans view childhood vaccines, vaccine research and policy? Pew Research Center. November 18, 2025. Available at: https://www.pewresearch.org/science/2025/11/18/how-do-americans-view-childhood-vaccines-vaccine-research-and-policy/?utm_source=chatgpt.com. Accessed January 21, 2026.

AJPH as a Trusted Source for Child and Adolescent Vaccination Recommendations

Robert Kim-Farley, MD, MPH, Bisola O. Ojikutu, MD, MPH, and Denys T. Lau, PhD

ABOUT THE AUTHORS

Robert Kim-Farley is an associate editor of AJPH *and is with the Departments of Epidemiology and Community Health Sciences, Fielding School of Public Health, University of California, Los Angeles. Bisola O. Ojikutu is an associate editor of* AJPH*; commissioner of public health, Boston, MA; and on the faculty of MassGeneral Brigham, Boston, MA. Denys T. Lau is the editor-in-chief of* AJPH *and is with the Johns Hopkins University, Baltimore, MD; the George Washington University, Washington, DC; and the University of Illinois at Chicago.*

Vaccination is a means to safeguarding millions from vaccine-preventable diseases, and it is estimated that, since 1974, vaccination has averted 154 million deaths worldwide.[1] It remains among the most cost-effective public health interventions in history and is reducing the burden on health care systems worldwide. Yet, starting in 2025, the Centers for Disease Control and Prevention (CDC)—long regarded as the nation's most trusted source of vaccine guidance—has become increasingly politicized on this issue, threatening the transparency and trust on which health professionals and the public alike depend.

In this context, *AJPH* is uniquely positioned, starting with children and adolescents, to serve as a scientifically rigorous and accessible venue for disseminating recommended vaccination schedules.

EROSION OF TRUST IN TRADITIONAL AUTHORITY

Historically, the CDC and its Advisory Committee on Immunization Practices (ACIP) have served as the gold standard for vaccination recommendations in the United States.[2] Their guidance has informed public health policy, shaped clinical practice, and reassured the public of the safety and efficacy of vaccines. However, the recent politicization of ACIP membership, including the appointment of individuals who have publicly expressed vaccine-skeptical views, and interference from leadership in the Department of Health and Human Services holding similar sentiments, have prompted widespread concern within the scientific and medical communities.[3] The American College of Physicians (ACP) expressed alarm at the actions that the current administration has taken to "cast doubt on vaccines, restrict access to vaccines, and contribute to confusion and misinformation about vaccines."[4] The realization that vaccination schedules are now subject to political manipulation rather than scientific rigor undermines confidence in routine preventive care and, in doing so, jeopardizes population health.

AJPH'S ROLE AS A TRUSTED PUBLIC HEALTH INSTITUTION

In this climate of uncertainty, *AJPH* stands out for its unwavering commitment to scientific excellence. Since its first publication in 1911, the *Journal* has been a trusted source of peer-reviewed public health research, policy analysis, and expert commentary.

A recent agreement between *AJPH* and the American Academy of Pediatrics (AAP) permitted the *Journal* to republish the AAP's new, 2026 recommended immunization schedule for children in this issue (Figure 1). This republishing marks the first time in the 115-year history of *AJPH* to do so. It serves as both a first step and pivotal moment in cementing *AJPH*'s role in the dissemination of trusted vaccine guidance to the hundreds of thousands of domestic public health professionals through institutional and online access to the *Journal*. This partnership not only enhances the visibility and accessibility of evidence-based recommendations but also signals a broader commitment of both organizations to scientific integrity and public health advocacy.

THE ENDURING CREDIBILITY OF THE AAP

Since its founding in the 1930s, the AAP has been a leading authority in developing and publishing vaccine recommendations for infants, children, and adolescents in the United States. The AAP's first formal guidance for pediatricians on vaccine use appeared in the mid-1930s; by 1938, the organization had published its first comprehensive immunization recommendations in an eight-page pamphlet that would ultimately become the renowned

AJPH May 2026, Vol. 116, No. 5

"Red Book."[5] The AAP also provides an annual vaccination policy statement in their journal, *Pediatrics*, and maintains a public-facing, simplified schedule on their website HealthyChildren.org.

The AAP's commitment to evidence-based guidance has made its vaccine recommendations a trusted resource for pediatricians and families alike, and the organization has played a pivotal role in shaping national immunization policy, often collaborating with federal agencies while maintaining its independent, science-driven voice.

In January 2026, the AAP, for the first time, published a "Recommended Child and Adolescent Immunization Schedule for Ages 18 Years or Younger" in the United States[6] that differed from those published by the CDC. The AAP recommendations also cover specific medical indications such as pregnancy, immunocompromised individuals, and those with heart disease and diabetes. These recommendations have been endorsed by multiple, prestigious medical and health organizations, including the American College of Obstetricians & Gynecologists (ACOG), the National Medical Association, and the American Academy of Family Physicians (AAFP).

REPUBLICATION AND STRATEGIC PARTNERSHIPS

Given the erosion of the CDC's role as a trusted, single source of vaccine recommendations, the republication of vaccine recommendations from trusted professional bodies in *AJPH* offers key advantages.

By republishing immunization schedules for children and adolescents (and with the goal of adding schedules for adults 19 years of age and older) in a single, annually updated publication, *AJPH* can help eliminate confusion and ensure that public health professionals and health care providers, along with the public, have access to the latest, science-based guidance.

Partnership with the AAP helps ensure that vaccine recommendations are grounded in the best available evidence, reflecting the consensus of experts who are dedicated to advancing public health. *AJPH* can foster a unified front in support of immunization and counteract divisive narratives.

Publishing new vaccine recommendations as they are officially issued by partner organizations, in addition to an annual updated publication of recommended vaccination schedules, would allow *AJPH* to remain agile and responsive to emerging threats, such as novel pathogens or changes in vaccine technology.

In an era of misinformation and skepticism, the endorsement of *AJPH* by leading professional societies to republish their vaccination recommendations reinforces the *Journal*'s reputation as a trustworthy source dedicated to helping rebuild public confidence in vaccination as well as other public health interventions.

AJPH AS A TRUSTED SOURCE FOR VACCINE RECOMMENDATIONS

The republication of the AAP's vaccination schedule in *AJPH* represents more than a procedural change; it constitutes a statement of principle. It reaffirms the *Journal*'s commitment to scientific rigor, transparency, and the protection of public health. It also acknowledges the urgent need for the public health community to come together in defense of evidence-based practice.

It should also be noted that the AAFP publishes an "Adults 19 and Older Immunization Schedule,"[7] and the ACOG no longer endorses the CDC's most recent recommendations, dated May 29, 2025, when it removed the COVID-19 vaccine recommendation for pregnant and lactating individuals.[8]

The fragmentation of vaccine guidance not only confuses clinicians and patients but also provides fertile ground for misinformation and vaccine hesitancy. By supporting *AJPH*'s new role as one of the repositories for vaccine recommendations, the public health community can reclaim the narrative, ensuring that decisions are driven by data rather than ideology.

Moreover, this *AJPH* role is not intended to supplant the CDC or ACIP indefinitely. This role would not confer regulatory authority or substitute for public agencies. However, the stakes are too high to allow political interference to compromise the health of our nation.

LOOKING AHEAD

This partnership between the AAP and *AJPH* (which includes *AJPH*'s republishing of AAP immunization schedules with timely updates as new recommendations emerge) will allow public health departments, policymakers, and health care providers across the country to openly access immunization recommendation through *AJPH*'s website. Community leaders, parents, and patients will also be able to turn to the *Journal* for clear, accessible vaccine schedule recommendations, empowering them to make informed decisions about their health and their children's health. AJPH

Recommended Child and Adolescent Immunization Schedule for Ages 18 Years or Younger

United States 2026

American Academy of Pediatrics
DEDICATED TO THE HEALTH OF ALL CHILDREN®

Vaccines and Other Immunizing Agents in the Child and Adolescent Immunization Schedule*

Monoclonal antibody	Abbreviation(s)	Trade name(s)
Respiratory syncytial virus monoclonal antibody	RSV-mAb	Beyfortus Enflonsia
Vaccine	**Abbreviation(s)**	**Trade name(s)**
COVID-19 vaccine	1vCOV-mRNA	Comirnaty mNexspike Spikevax
	1vCOV-aPS	Nuvaxovid
Dengue vaccine	DEN4CYD	Dengvaxia
Diphtheria, tetanus, and acellular pertussis vaccine	DTaP	Daptacel Infanrix
Haemophilus influenzae type b vaccine	Hib (PRP-T)	ActHIB Hiberix
	Hib (PRP-OMP)	PedvaxHIB
Hepatitis A vaccine	HepA	Havrix Vaqta
Hepatitis B vaccine	HepB	Engerix-B Recombivax HB
Human papillomavirus vaccine	HPV	Gardasil 9
Influenza vaccine (inactivated: egg-based)	IIV3	Multiple
Influenza vaccine (inactivated: cell-culture)	ccIIV3	Flucelvax
Influenza vaccine (recombinant)	RIV3	Flublok
Influenza vaccine (live, attenuated)	LAIV3	FluMist
Measles, mumps, and rubella vaccine	MMR	M-M-R II Priorix
Meningococcal serogroups A, C, W, Y vaccine	MenACWY-CRM	Menveo
	MenACWY-TT	MenQuadfi
Meningococcal serogroup B vaccine	MenB-4C	Bexsero
	MenB-FHbp	Trumenba
Meningococcal serogroup A, B, C, W, Y vaccine	MenACWY-TT/MenB-FHbp	Penbraya
	MenACWY-CRM/MenB-4C	Penmenvy
Mpox vaccine	Mpox	Jynneos
Pneumococcal conjugate vaccine	PCV15	Vaxneuvance
	PCV20	Prevnar 20
Pneumococcal polysaccharide vaccine	PPSV23	Pneumovax 23
Poliovirus vaccine (inactivated)	IPV	Ipol
Respiratory syncytial virus vaccine	RSV	Abrysvo
Rotavirus vaccine	RV1	Rotarix
	RV5	RotaTeq
Tetanus, diphtheria, and acellular pertussis vaccine	Tdap	Adacel Boostrix
Tetanus and diphtheria vaccine	Td	Tenivac Tdvax
Varicella vaccine	VAR	Varivax
Combination vaccines (use combination vaccines instead of separate injections when appropriate)		
DTaP, hepatitis B, and inactivated poliovirus vaccine	DTaP-HepB-IPV	Pediarix
DTaP, inactivated poliovirus, and *Haemophilus influenzae* type b vaccine	DTaP-IPV/Hib	Pentacel
DTaP and inactivated poliovirus vaccine	DTaP-IPV	Kinrix Quadracel
DTaP, inactivated poliovirus, *Haemophilus influenzae* type b, and hepatitis B vaccine	DTaP-IPV-Hib-HepB	Vaxelis
Measles, mumps, rubella, and varicella vaccine	MMRV	ProQuad

*Administer recommended vaccines if immunization history is incomplete or unknown. Do not restart or add doses to vaccine series for extended intervals between doses. When a vaccine is not administered at the recommended age, administer at a subsequent visit when indicated. The use of trade names is for identification purposes only and does not imply endorsement by the AAP.

Updated February 5, 2026

Endorsed by the American Academy of Family Physicians (AAFP), American College of Nurse-Midwives (ACNM), American College of Obstetricians and Gynecologists (ACOG), American Medical Association (AMA), American Pharmacists Association (APhA), Council of Medical Specialty Societies (CMSS), Infectious Diseases Society of America (IDSA), National Association of Pediatric Nurse Practitioners (NAPNAP), National Medical Association (NMA), Pediatric Infectious Diseases Society (PIDS), Pediatric Pharmacy Association (PPA), and Society for Adolescent Health and Medicine (SAHM). (**Endorsements**)

How to use the child and adolescent immunization schedule

1 Determine recommended vaccine by age (**Table 1**)

2 Determine recommended interval for catch-up vaccination (**Table 2**)

3 Assess need for additional recommended vaccines by medical condition or other indication (**Table 3**)

4 Review vaccine types, frequencies, intervals, and considerations for special situations (**Notes**)

5 Review contraindications and precautions for vaccine types (**Appendix**)

6 Review new or updated American Academy of Pediatrics (AAP) guidance (**Addendum**)

Report

- Suspected cases of reportable vaccine-preventable diseases or outbreaks to your state or local health department
- Clinically significant adverse events to the Vaccine Adverse Event Reporting System (VAERS) at www.vaers.hhs.gov (Accessed December 2, 2025) or 800-822-7967
- For RSV-mAb products, clinically significant adverse events to MedWatch Adverse Event Report Program at www.accessdata.fda.gov/scripts/medwatch/index.cfm (Accessed December 2, 2025). If co-administered with other products, then report to VAERS.

Questions or comments

Submit a question or comment to www.aap.org/en/forms/immunization-schedule-questions.

Helpful information

- **Best practices for immunization (including contraindications and precautions):** www.aap.org/immunization and www.immunize.org
- ***Red Book: 2024–2027 Report of the Committee on Infectious Diseases* (33rd Edition):** www.aapRedBook.org
- **Vaccine information statements:** www.immunize.org/vaccines/vis/about-vis
- **Shared decision making:** https://www.aap.org/en/practice-management/providing-patient-and-family-centered-care/shared-decision-making

For the most up-to-date version, visit AAP.org/ImmunizationSchedule

FIGURE 1— American Academy of Pediatrics Recommended Child and Adolescent Immunization Schedule 2026

Note. See full immunization recommendations in the Appendix, available as a supplement to the online version of this article at https://www.ajph.org.
Source. Reproduced with permission from the American Academy of Pediatrics, Recommended Child and Adolescent Immunization Schedule 2026, AAP.org/Immunization Schedule, Updated January 26, 2026. Accessed February 5, 2026.

Table 1 Recommended Child and Adolescent Immunization Schedule for Ages 18 Years or Younger, United States, 2026

American Academy of Pediatrics
DEDICATED TO THE HEALTH OF ALL CHILDREN®

These recommendations must be read with the Notes that follow. For those who fall behind or start late, provide catch-up vaccination at the earliest opportunity as indicated by the outlined purple bars. To determine minimum intervals between doses, see the catch-up schedule (Table 2).

Vaccine and other immunizing agents	Birth	1 mos	2 mos	4 mos	6 mos	8 mos	9 mos	12 mos	15 mos	18 mos	19–23 mos	2–3 yrs	4–6 yrs	7–10 yrs	11–12 yrs	13–15 yrs	16 yrs	17–18 yrs
Respiratory syncytial virus (RSV-mAb [nirsevimab, clesrovimab])	1 dose during RSV season depending on maternal RSV vaccination status (See Notes)					1 dose nirsevimab during RSV season (See Notes)												
Hepatitis B (HepB)	1st dose	2nd dose			3rd dose													
Rotavirus (RV): RV1 (2-dose series), RV5 (3-dose series)			1st dose	2nd dose	See Notes													
Diphtheria, tetanus, and acellular pertussis (DTaP <7 yrs)			1st dose	2nd dose	3rd dose				4th dose				5th dose					
Haemophilus influenzae type b (Hib)			1st dose	2nd dose	See Notes			3rd or 4th dose (See Notes)										
Pneumococcal conjugate (PCV15, PCV20)			1st dose	2nd dose	3rd dose			4th dose										
Inactivated poliovirus (IPV)			1st dose	2nd dose	3rd dose								4th dose					See Notes
COVID-19 (1vCOV-mRNA, 1vCOV-aPS)					1 or more doses of 2025-2026 vaccine (See Notes)							1 or more doses of 2025-2026 vaccine (See Notes) 1 or more doses of 2025-2026 vaccine (See Notes)						
Influenza					1 or 2 doses annually (See Notes)									1 dose annually (See Notes)				
Measles, mumps, and rubella (MMR)					See Notes			1st dose					2nd dose					
Varicella (VAR)								1st dose					2nd dose					
Hepatitis A (HepA)					See Notes			2-dose series (See Notes)										
Tetanus, diphtheria, and acellular pertussis (Tdap ≥7 yrs)															1 dose			
Human papillomavirus (HPV)														2-dose series		See Notes		
Meningococcal (MenACWY-CRM ≥2 mos, MenACWY-TT ≥2years)			See Notes												1st dose		2nd dose	
Meningococcal B (MenB-4C, MenB-FHbp)														See Notes				
Respiratory syncytial virus vaccine (RSV [Abrysvo])															Seasonal administration during pregnancy if not previously vaccinated			
Dengue (DEN4CYD: 9–16 yrs)														Seropositive in areas with endemic dengue (See Notes)				
Mpox																		

Range of recommended ages for all children
Range of recommended ages for catch-up vaccination
Range of recommended ages for certain high-risk groups or populations
Recommended vaccination for those who desire protection
Recommended vaccination based on shared clinical decision-making

FIGURE 1— Continued

Table 2 Recommended Catch-up Immunization Schedule for Children and Adolescents Who Start Late or Who Are More than 1 Month Behind, United States, 2026

American Academy of Pediatrics
DEDICATED TO THE HEALTH OF ALL CHILDREN®

The table below provides catch-up schedules and minimum intervals between doses for children whose vaccinations have been delayed. A vaccine series does not need to be restarted, regardless of the time that has elapsed between doses. Use the section appropriate for the child's age. **Always use this table in conjunction with Table 1 and the Notes that follow.**

Vaccine	Minimum Age for Dose 1	Minimum Interval Between Doses			
		Dose 1 to Dose 2	Dose 2 to Dose 3	Dose 3 to Dose 4	Dose 4 to Dose 5
Children age 4 months through 6 years					
Hepatitis B	Birth	**4 weeks**	**8 weeks *and* at least 16 weeks after first dose:** minimum age for the final dose is 24 weeks		
Rotavirus	6 weeks: Maximum age for first dose is 14 weeks, 6 days.	**4 weeks**	**4 weeks:** maximum age for final dose is 8 months, 0 days		
Diphtheria, tetanus, and acellular pertussis	6 weeks	**4 weeks**	**4 weeks**	**6 months**	**6 months:** A fifth dose is not necessary if the fourth dose was administered at age 4 years or older ***and*** at least 6 months after dose 3
Haemophilus influenzae type b	6 weeks	**No further doses needed** if first dose was administered at age 15 months or older **4 weeks** if first dose was administered before the 1st birthday **8 weeks (as final dose)** if first dose was administered at age 12 through 14 months	**No further doses needed** if previous dose was administered at age 15 months or older **4 weeks** if current age is younger than 12 months and first dose was administered at younger than age 7 months ***and*** at least 1 previous dose was PRP-T (ActHib, Pentacel, Hiberix), Vaxelis, or unknown **8 weeks and age 12 through 59 months (as final dose)** if current age is younger than 12 months ***and*** first dose was administered at age 7 through 11 months; **OR** if current age is 12 through 59 months ***and*** first dose was administered before the 1st birthday ***and*** second dose was administered at younger than 15 months; **OR** if both doses were PedvaxHIB and were administered before the 1st birthday	**8 weeks (as final dose):** This dose only necessary for children age 12 through 59 months who received 3 doses before the 1st birthday	
Pneumococcal conjugate	6 weeks	**No further doses needed** for healthy children if first dose was administered at age 24 months or older **4 weeks** if first dose was administered before the 1st birthday **8 weeks (as final dose for healthy children)** if first dose was administered at the 1st birthday or after	**No further doses needed** for healthy children if previous dose was administered at age 24 months or older **4 weeks:**if current age is younger than 12 months ***and*** previous dose was administered at <7 months old **8 weeks (as final dose for healthy children)** if previous dose was administered between 7–11 months (wait until at least 12 months old); **OR** if current age is 12 months or older ***and*** at least 1 dose was administered before age 12 months	**8 weeks (as final dose):** This dose is only necessary for children age 12 through 59 months regardless of risk, or age 60 through 71 months with any risk, who received 3 doses before age 12 months	
Inactivated poliovirus	6 weeks	**4 weeks**	**4 weeks** if current age is <4 years **6 months (as final dose)** if current age is 4 years or older	**6 months (minimum age 4 years for final dose)**	
Measles, mumps, and rubella	12 months	**4 weeks**			
Varicella	12 months	**3 months**			
Hepatitis A	12 months	**6 months**			
Meningococcal ACWY	2 months MenACWY-CRM 2 years MenACWY-TT	**8 weeks**	See Notes	See Notes	
Children and adolescents age 7 through 18 years					
Meningococcal ACWY	Not applicable (N/A)	**8 weeks**			
Tetanus, diphtheria; tetanus, diphtheria, and acellular pertussis	7 years	**4 weeks**	**4 weeks:** if first dose of DTaP/DT was administered before the 1st birthday **6 months (as final dose):** if first dose of DTaP/DT or Tdap/Td was administered at or after the 1st birthday	**6 months:** if first dose of DTaP/DT was administered before the 1st birthday	
Human papillomavirus	9 years	**Routine dosing intervals are recommended**			
Hepatitis A	N/A	**6 months**			
Hepatitis B	N/A	**4 weeks**	**8 weeks *and* at least 16 weeks after first dose**		
Inactivated poliovirus	N/A	**4 weeks**	**6 months:** A fourth dose is not necessary if the third dose was administered at age 4 years or older ***and*** at least 6 months after the previous dose	A fourth dose of IPV is indicated if all previous doses were administered at <4 years **OR** if the third dose was administered <6 months after the second dose	
Measles, mumps, and rubella	N/A	**4 weeks**			
Varicella	N/A	**3 months** if younger than age 13 years **4 weeks** if age 13 years or older			
Dengue	9 years	**6 months**	6 months		

FIGURE 1— Continued

Table 3 Recommended Child and Adolescent Immunization Schedule by Medical Indication, United States, 2026

American Academy of Pediatrics

DEDICATED TO THE HEALTH OF ALL CHILDREN®

Always use this table in conjunction with Table 1 and the Notes that follow. Medical conditions are often not mutually exclusive. If multiple conditions are present, refer to guidance in all relevant columns. See Notes for medical conditions not listed.

Vaccine and other immunizing agents	Pregnancy	Immunocompromised (excluding HIV infection)[a]	HIV infection CD4 percentage and count[a]: <15% or <200/mm³	HIV infection CD4 percentage and count[a]: ≥15% and ≥200/mm³	CSF leak or cochlear implant	Asplenia or persistent complement component deficiencies	Heart disease or chronic lung disease (CLD)	Kidney failure, End-stage renal disease or on dialysis	Chronic liver disease	Diabetes
RSV-mAb (nirsevimab, clesrovimab)		[blue] 1 dose clesrovimab or nirsevimab during 1st RSV season depending on maternal RSV vaccination status (See Notes); [light] 1 dose nirsevimab 2nd RSV season (See Notes)	[blue]; [light]	[blue]; [light]	[blue]	[blue]	[blue]; [light] 1 dose nirsevimab 2nd RSV season for CLD (See Notes)	[blue]	[blue]	[blue]
Hepatitis B	[blue]	[blue]	[blue]	[blue]	[blue]	[blue]	[blue]	[blue]	[blue]	[blue]
Rotavirus		[hatched]; [dark red] SCID[b]	[hatched]	[hatched]	[blue]	[blue]	[blue]	[blue]	[blue]	[blue]
DTaP/Tdap	DTaP: not applicable; [light] Tdap: 1 dose each pregnancy	[blue]	[blue]	[blue]	[blue]	[blue]	[blue]	[blue]	[blue]	[blue]
Hib		[blue]; [light] HCT[c]: 3 doses	[blue] See Notes	[blue] See Notes	[blue]	[blue] See Notes	[blue]	[blue]	[blue]	[blue]
Pneumococcal		[light]	[light]	[light]	[light]	[light]	[light]	[light]	[light]	[light]
IPV	[hatched]	[blue]	[blue]	[blue]	[blue]	[blue]	[blue]	[blue]	[blue]	[blue]
COVID-19	[blue] *	[light] See Notes	[light] See Notes	[blue]	[blue]	[blue]	[blue]	[blue]	[blue]	[blue]
Influenza inactivated, recombinant	[blue]	[blue] Solid organ transplant: 18 yrs (See Notes)	[blue]	[blue]	[blue]	[blue]	[blue]	[blue]	[blue]	[blue]
LAIV3	[dark red]	[dark red]	[dark red]	[dark red]	[dark red]	[dark red]	[hatched]; [dark red] Asthma, wheezing: 2–4 years[d]	[hatched]	[hatched]	[hatched]
MMR	[dark red] **	[dark red]	[dark red]	[blue]	[blue]	[blue]	[blue]	[blue]	[blue]	[blue]
VAR	[dark red] **	[dark red]	[dark red]	[blue]	[blue]	[blue]	[blue]	[blue]	[blue]	[blue]
Hepatitis A	[blue]	[blue]	[blue]	[blue]	[blue]	[blue]	[blue]	[blue]	[blue]	[blue]
HPV	[dark red] **	[light] 3-dose series (See Notes)	[light] 3-dose series (See Notes)	[light] 3-dose series (See Notes)	[blue]	[blue]	[blue]	[blue]	[blue]	[blue]
MenACWY	[blue]	[blue]	[light]	[light]	[blue]	[light]	[blue]	[blue]	[blue]	[blue]
MenB	[hatched]					[light]				
RSV (Abrysvo)	[blue] Seasonal administration (See Notes)									
Dengue	[hatched]	[dark red]	[dark red]	[hatched]	[yellow]	[yellow]	[yellow]	[yellow]	[yellow]	[yellow]
Mpox	[yellow] See Notes	[yellow]	[yellow]	[yellow]	[yellow]	[yellow]	[yellow]	[yellow]	[yellow]	[yellow]

*For more information, refer to https://www.acog.org/clinical/clinical-guidance/practice-advisory/articles/2020/12/covid-19-vaccination-considerations-for-obstetric-gynecologic-care

- [blue] Recommended for all age-eligible children who lack documentation of a complete immunization series
- [yellow] Not recommended for all children, but recommended for some children based on increased risk for severe outcomes from disease
- [light] Recommended for all age-eligible children, and additional doses may be necessary based on medical condition or other indications. See Notes.
- [hatched] Precaution: Might be indicated if benefit of protection outweighs risk of adverse reaction
- [dark red] Contraindicated or not recommended. **Vaccinate after pregnancy, if indicated

a. For additional information regarding immunization in immunocompromised children, see https://publications.aap.org/redbook/book/755/chapter/14074446/Immunization-and-Other-Considerations-in
b. Severe combined immunodeficiency
c. Hematopoietic cell transplantation
d. LAIV3 contraindicated for children 2–4 years of age with asthma or wheezing during the preceding 12 months

FIGURE 1— Continued

CORRESPONDENCE

Correspondence should be sent to Robert J. Kim-Farley, MD, MPH, UCLA Department of Epidemiology, Room 71-279A CHS, 650 Charles E. Young Drive South, Los Angeles, CA 90095 (email: robert@kimfarley.org). Reprints can be ordered at https://www.ajph.org by clicking the "Reprints" link.

PUBLICATION INFORMATION

Full Citation: Kim-Farley R, Ojikutu BO, Lau DT. *AJPH* as a trusted source for child and adolescent vaccination recommendations. *Am J Public Health*. 2026;116(5):575–581.

Acceptance Date: February 10, 2026

DOI: https://doi.org/10.2105/AJPH.2026.308490

ORCID iD:

Robert Kim-Farley https://orcid.org/0000-0003-3022-6548

CONTRIBUTORS

R. J. Kim-Farley drafted the manuscript. B. O. Ojikutu and D. T. Lau provided revisions.

ACKNOWLEDGMENTS

We thank the American Academy of Pediatrics for agreeing to let *AJPH* publish their 2026 immunization schedule recommendations ("Recommended Child and Adolescent Immunization Schedule for Ages 18 Years or Younger") and help disseminate this important information to the public health community.

CONFLICTS OF INTEREST

The authors declare no conflicts of interest.

REFERENCES

1. Shattock AJ, Johnson HC, Sim SY, et al. Contribution of vaccination to improved survival and health: modelling 50 years of the Expanded Programme on Immunization. *Lancet*. 2024;403(10441):2307–2316. https://doi.org/10.1016/S0140-6736(24)00850-X
2. Centers for Disease Control and Prevention. Advisory Committee on Immunization Practices (ACIP). Available at: https://www.cdc.gov/acip/index.html. Accessed January 31, 2026.
3. Pollard A, Plotkin S. A risk to child health: confusion and concern over changes to US vaccine policy. *Lancet*. 2026;407(10528):553–556. https://doi.org/10.1016/S0140-6736(26)00090-5
4. American College of Physicians. Adult immunization. ACP immunization-related efforts. Available at: https://www.acponline.org/clinical-information/clinical-resources-products/adult-immunization/acp-immunization-related-efforts. Accessed January 31, 2026.
5. Arthur E. AAP has been leading voice on childhood vaccine recommendations since 1930s. AAPNews. July 30, 2025. Available at: https://publications.aap.org/aapnews/news/32762/AAP-has-been-leading-voice-on-childhood-vaccine?autologincheck=redirected. Accessed January 31, 2026.
6. American Academy of Pediatrics. Recommended child and adolescent immunization schedule for ages 18 years or younger. Available at: https://www.aap.org/en/patient-care/immunizations. Accessed January 31, 2026.
7. American Academy of Family Physicians. Adults 19 and older immunization schedule. Available at: https://www.aafp.org/family-physician/patient-care/prevention-wellness/immunizations-vaccines/immunization-schedules/adult-immunization-schedule.html. Accessed January 31, 2026.
8. American College of Obstetricians & Gynecologists. Immunization, infectious disease, and public health preparedness program. Available at: https://www.acog.org/programs/immunization-infectious-disease-public-health. Accessed January 31, 2026.

A Radical Reimagining of the Mission of Public Health

Gerald Markowitz, PhD

ABOUT THE AUTHOR

Gerald Markowitz is with John Jay College and the Graduate Center, CUNY, New York, NY.

See also Ferrer et al., p. 657.

What should be the role of public health in a society that is riven with class conflict, racism, sexism, and other forms of inequality? This has been an essential question since the mid-19th century, when the Sanitarians (19th-century reformers who sought health reforms to combat rampant infectious diseases caused by urbanization) were confronted with massive epidemics and squalid conditions in a number of cities. Unlike the field of medicine in general, public health has understood its charge to be the prevention of disease and ill health for groups of people, rather than the treatment of individual patients. At this moment, when the resources for public health are being restricted, how can this mission still be implemented?

This is the essential question raised by the article in this issue by Ferrer et al., "Designed for Disparity: The Structural Origins of Migrant Farmworker Health Inequities in Maryland, 1900–1950" (p. 657). Over the course of most of the 20th and 21st centuries, there have been major improvements in the health and welfare of Americans in general, and the field of public health has become professionalized. "Designed for Disparity" critiques the "professional" approach because, the authors argue, it came to reenforce structural racism, income inequality, and discrimination against migrant workers. The article demonstrates that the conditions that farm workers faced arose from the structure of the political–economic system, rather than being "independent social determinants of health," which has been the predominant thrust of public health interventions in recent decades. Grounded in the experiences of migrant laborers in Maryland in the first half of the 20th century, the authors show that from the early decades of the 20th century, there was a great disparity between the status of agricultural workers who were White versus those who were African American: some 59% of White agricultural workers had farmer status, whereas African American farmers made up only 21% of overall African American agricultural workers. The abortive interventions by state actors on behalf of the migrant farm workers stand in stark contrast to the actions that migrant farm workers took on their own behalf in the 1960s in California. The United Farm Workers (UFW) organized mostly Mexican and Filipino agricultural workers, especially around issues of unsanitary housing and working conditions. But it soon became clear that the spraying of the pesticide parathion in the fields was making the agricultural workers very ill.[1(pp164,166–167)] One UFW pamphlet declared that "motivated by profit [growers] continued to subject our people to systemic poisoning."[2(p124)] As a result of the farm workers organizing, the UFW was able to sign contracts with 150 grape growers covering 30 000 grape harvesters that gave the workers the right to refuse dangerous work and to decide when it was safe for them to reenter the vineyards after they were sprayed with pesticides.

This broader conception of an activist public health can be traced back to the late 19th century. The dramatic transformation of the American economy in the decades following the Civil War presented new challenges to the Sanitarians and others concerned with protecting the health of residents of the burgeoning cities and industries. By the late 19th and early 20th centuries, the United States experienced revolutionary social and economic changes that transformed the country from a fourth-rate industrial power in the mid-19th century to the most advanced corporate capitalist economy in the world by the first two decades of the 20th century. But these developments had profoundly disparate impacts on different parts of the US population. As one observer noted in 1907, "To unprecedented prosperity . . . there is a seamy side of which little is said."[3(p791)] That seamy side included horrendous housing conditions where landlords could jam residents—mostly immigrants from Eastern and Southern Europe and African Americans fleeing segregation and lynching—into airless, filthy, disease-laden tenements. It included factory owners forcing unskilled laborers to accept an average daily wage in 1870 of $1.66, today's equivalent of $36.86, or $3.70 an hour for a 10-hour day, the standard at the time. It was recognized that such living and working conditions had a profound impact on the health of working people, immigrant and native born alike, in the United States. In 1904, *The Outlook* magazine wrote, "It is becoming as perilous to live in the United States as to participate in actual warfare. . . . The people of the United States may face the situation and understand how cheap human life has become under American conditions."[4(p359)]

How did those who sought to ameliorate health-harming conditions respond to looming social and economic challenges? Before the professionalization of public health, practitioners sought to achieve structural change through radical interventions that brought together public health officials, government bureaucrats, labor leaders, business representatives, reformers, and radical activists in a broad coalition that sought to change the conditions that produced inequalities in death and disease. During the Progressive Era (1890–1914), this coalition was successful in developing a multiclass and multi-interest constituency that brought demands for a more systematic, more integrated approach to ameliorating the excesses of industrial capitalism. But even this important movement had its limitations. Although there were important reforms in housing, sanitation, working conditions, hours of work, and much else, what had not changed were the disparities in housing, work, and environment between the rich and the poor; the working immigrant and the native-born White; African Americans and Whites; Native Americans, Mexican Americans, and Anglos; industrial workers and their managers; and landowners and sharecroppers.

The fundamental issue that Ferrer et al. raise is that although there has been continuous improvement (until the COVID-19 pandemic) in health for all people in the United States over the course of the 20th and 21st centuries, disparities based on race, ethnicity, nature of work, and income remain. And we, as a society, have not seen fit to address the fact that wealth, access to health care, and even life span are not equitable. The narrative that much of the population believes—of ever-more substantial improvement in the health and welfare of Americans in general—needs to be modified to acknowledge that since the Colonial Era, millions of years of life have been lost through the early death of African Americans, Native Americans, the poor, and working-class Whites. We have not yet addressed the fact that American "prosperity" (i.e., the standard of living of middle- and upper-class Americans) is maintained in our society at the expense of the poor and people of color. The brief history presented here suggests that, even in an era of diminished resources, public health can join with labor, undocumented migrants, the unemployed and underemployed, political activists, and other movements for social change to address the inequalities of health that continue to plague American society and to broaden the conception of public health. The model of a broad-based coalition that was achieved at the turn of the 20th century can be the inspiration for public health practitioners and advocates today. This does not necessarily mean increasing budgets for public health departments, but instead addressing inequalities more broadly to ensure good housing for all, raising the minimum wage, and ensuring good quality food at reasonable prices for all, fast and free public transportation, and racial and environmental justice. This will, of course, require a radical reimagining of labor, mobility, and human value, and indeed of public health itself. AJPH

CORRESPONDENCE

Correspondence should be sent to Gerald Markowitz, Department of Interdisciplinary Studies, John Jay College, 524 West 59th St, New York, NY 10019 (e-mail: gmarkowitz@jjay.cuny.edu). Reprints can be ordered at https://www.ajph.org by clicking the "Reprints" link.

PUBLICATION INFORMATION

Full Citation: Markowitz G. A radical reimagining of the mission of public health. *Am J Public Health*. 2026;116(5):582–583.

Acceptance Date: January 21, 2026.

DOI: https://doi.org/10.2105/AJPH.2026.308438

ORCID iD:

Gerald Markowitz https://orcid.org/0000-0002-9021-5536

CONFLICTS OF INTEREST

The author has no conflicts of interest to declare.

REFERENCES

1. Nash L. *Inescapable Ecologies: A History of Environment, Disease and Knowledge.* Berkeley, CA: University of California Press; 2007.
2. Montrie C. *Making a Living: Work and Environment in the United States.* Chapel Hill, NC: University of North Carolina Press; 2008.
3. Reeve AB. The death roll of industry. *Charities and the Commons.* 1907;17:791–794.
4. Slaughter by accident [editorial]. *The Outlook.* October 8, 1904.

Mortality Risk After Moving From Homelessness Into Supported Housing: A Cautionary Note and a Call to Action

Stephen W. Hwang, MD, MPH

ABOUT THE AUTHOR

Stephen W. Hwang is with the MAP Centre for Urban Health Solutions, St. Michael's Hospital, and the Division of General Internal Medicine, Department of Medicine, University of Toronto, Toronto, Ontario.

AJPH May 2026, Vol. 116, No. 5

See also Tsai et al., p. 665.

People experiencing homelessness have a significantly higher risk of death than people who are housed.[1] The factors that account for this excess mortality are manifold and include severe poverty and material deprivation, barriers to accessing health care, inadequately treated mental health conditions and substance use disorders, and the adverse physical and social environments associated with homelessness itself.[2] Reducing the risk of death in this population is an important public health objective, and it would seem reasonable to assume that moving people out of homelessness and into housing should make a substantial contribution toward achieving this goal. After all, permanent housing clearly provides a basic modicum of personal security, protection from the elements, and a stable foundation that can enable access to health care and, potentially, long-term improvements in health status.

In this issue of *AJPH*, Tsai et al. (p. 665) report the findings of a large retrospective cohort study of homeless veterans that examined whether moving into supporting housing was associated with changes in all-cause mortality, overdose mortality, and suicide mortality over a two-year follow-up period. The study capitalizes on the fact that the Department of Housing and Urban Development–Veterans Affairs Supportive Housing (HUD-VASH) program, established in 2008, has been highly successful in helping homeless veterans obtain permanent housing through a combination of rental assistance, case management, and clinical services. The investigators used linked administrative databases to create a cohort of veterans experiencing homelessness who had an initial encounter with the VA system in 2017 through 2019. Deaths in the cohort were identified up to the end of 2021. Veterans who were housed through the HUD-VASH program from 2017 through 2019 were compared with a propensity score–matched cohort of homeless veterans who did not receive HUD-VASH services. Each of the two cohorts comprised 60 888 veterans, making this the largest study of its kind to be conducted to date.

HUD-VASH and other programs that have been proven to be effective in moving people out of chronic homelessness and into stable housing typically use a combination of rent subsidies and intensive supports. Individuals can be housed in scattered-site apartment units with supports from a mobile intensive case management or Assertive Community Treatment (ACT) team (a model known as Housing First), or they can be placed in congregate housing buildings with a support team situated on-site (a model known as permanent supportive housing).[3] Somewhat surprisingly, however, previous studies of housing interventions for homeless individuals have yielded disappointing results regarding their ability to reduce all-cause mortality, despite their effectiveness in ending homelessness. A randomized clinical trial of permanent supportive housing for 423 chronically homeless persons in California found comparably high mortality rates in the treatment and control groups.[4] A randomized trial of a housing and support intervention for 703 homeless adults in France demonstrated no effect on two-year all-cause mortality.[5] Finally, a secondary analysis of data from 2108 participants in a randomized clinical trial of a Housing First intervention in Canada found no statistically significant difference in mortality rates in the intervention group compared with the treatment-as-usual group.[6]

Tsai et al.'s observational study adds three key findings to our understanding of mortality in supported housing programs. First, six months after participants moved into housing, all-cause mortality risk was significantly lower in the HUD-VASH cohort than in the homeless cohort (hazard ratio = 0.88), but at 24 months after moving into housing, all-cause mortality risk was significantly *higher* in the HUD-VASH cohort (hazard ratio = 1.05). Over a two-year observation period, 5.6% of the individuals in the HUD-VASH cohort died. Second, overdose mortality risk was significantly and consistently higher among the HUD-VASH cohort compared with the homeless cohort, with hazard ratios ranging from 2.29 to 1.79 over the observation period. In the HUD-VASH cohort, 13.9% of all deaths were due to overdose. Third, suicide mortality risk was not significantly different between the HUD-VASH and homeless cohorts.

As with any observational study that uses propensity score matching, there is a possibility that unmeasured differences in the baseline characteristics of the two cohorts may have contributed to these findings. In particular, if individuals with high-risk characteristics (e.g., intensity of substance use) that were not accounted for in the propensity score matching were more likely to be selected to receive HUD-VASH services, this could in part account for higher mortality in the cohort that received housing.

This well-designed study provides important insights into the heightened overdose mortality risk associated with the transition period when people move from homelessness into supported housing. This finding serves as a cautionary note and a reminder that a major life change, even one that is widely regarded as positive, can also create unintended risks. For example, leaving home to attend college is associated with a period of increased risk of substance use, including the harmful use of alcohol and opioids.[7] Few would argue, however, that we should therefore stop sending young people to college or expel them from college if they engage in any substance use. Likewise, it would be misguided, or perhaps even ill-intentioned, to use this study's findings to attack or to denigrate the value of Housing First and permanent supportive housing programs.

Instead, the findings of this study should be viewed as an urgent call to action. Although moving people from homelessness into housing yields undeniable benefits for both individuals and society, it also appears to increase the risk of fatal overdose among people who use drugs. As Tsai et al. suggest, this heightened overdose risk is most likely due to a stark change in the physical and social context in which people's drug use is occurring—from a shelter or street corner where bystanders are likely to intervene in the event of overdose, to the privacy of a solitary apartment behind a locked door. Further research is needed to determine if it is possible to identify individuals at highest risk of death by overdose after a move into housing. Most urgently, innovative interventions to reduce the risk of fatal overdose in supportive housing settings must be developed, implemented, and rigorously evaluated. These interventions should include treatment options for individuals who want to reduce or abstain from substance use, and harm reduction options for those who are likely to continue their use. One example of this vital work is a cluster-randomized controlled trial of a multifaceted overdose prevention initiative that is being conducted in permanent supportive housing buildings in New York City.[8] As always, the involvement and expertise of people with lived experience will be essential to the success of these efforts.

This study strongly suggests that the appealing formulation "housing is health" is perhaps overly simplistic. Housing is indeed a fundamental social determinant of health, and safe, decent, affordable housing is critical for population health. However, housing by itself is not sufficient to make a person healthy, let alone reduce their risk of dying. This study by Tsai et al. is an important reminder that the moment a person moves from homelessness into permanent housing is not a capstone achievement, but rather the first step on a long journey toward better health—a journey that we must support with focused attention and the investment of necessary resources. AJPH

CORRESPONDENCE

Correspondence should be sent to Dr. Stephen W. Hwang, St. Michael's Hospital, MAP Centre for Urban Health Solutions, 30 Bond St, Toronto, Ontario M5B 1W8, Canada (e-mail: stephen.hwang@unityhealth.to). Reprints can be ordered at https://www.ajph.org by clicking the "Reprints" link.

PUBLICATION INFORMATION

Full Citation: Hwang SW. Mortality risk after moving from homelessness into supported housing: a cautionary note and a call to action. *Am J Public Health*. 2026;116(5):584–586.

Acceptance Date: January 19, 2026

DOI: https://doi.org/10.2105/AJPH.2026.308426

ORCID iD:
Stephen W. Hwang https://orcid.org/0000-0002-1276-1101

ACKNOWLEDGMENTS

S. W. Hwang is supported by funding from the Canada Research Chairs Program.

CONFLICTS OF INTEREST

The author has no conflicts of interest to disclose.

REFERENCES

1. Aldridge RW, Story A, Hwang SW, et al. Morbidity and mortality in homeless individuals, prisoners, sex workers, and individuals with substance use disorders in high-income countries: a systematic review and meta-analysis. *Lancet*. 2018;391(10117):241–250. https://doi.org/10.1016/S0140-6736(17)31869-X
2. Liu M, Hwang SW. Health care for homeless people. *Nat Rev Dis Primers*. 2021;7(1):5. https://doi.org/10.1038/s41572-020-00241-2

3. National Academies of Sciences, Engineering, and Medicine. *Permanent Supportive Housing: Evaluating the Evidence for Improving Health Outcomes Among People Experiencing Chronic Homelessness.* Washington, DC: National Academies Press; 2018.

4. Raven MC, Niedzwiecki MJ, Kushel M. A randomized trial of permanent supportive housing for chronically homeless persons with high use of publicly funded services. *Health Serv Res.* 2020;55(suppl 2):797–806. https://doi.org/10.1111/1475-6773.13553

5. Tinland A, Loubiere S, Cantiello M, et al. Mortality in homeless people enrolled in the French Housing First randomized controlled trial: a secondary outcome analysis of predictors and causes of death. *BMC Public Health.* 2021;21(1):1294. https://doi.org/10.1186/s12889-021-11310-w

6. Lachaud J, Nisenbaum R, Mejia-Lancheros C, et al. Housing and support intervention and mortality among homeless adults with mental illnesses: a secondary analysis of a randomized clinical trial. *JAMA Netw Open.* 2025;8(7):e2524302. https://doi.org/10.1001/jamanetworkopen.2025.24302

7. Welsh JW, Shentu Y, Sarvey DB. Substance use among college students. *Focus (Am Psychiatr Publ).* 2019;17(2):117–127. https://doi.org/10.1176/appi.focus.20180037

8. Doran KM, Torsiglieri A, Blaufarb S, et al. The POP (Permanent Supportive Housing Overdose Prevention) Study: protocol for a hybrid type 3 stepped-wedge cluster randomized controlled trial. *Implement Sci.* 2023;18(1):21. https://doi.org/10.1186/s13012-023-01278-z

Gaps in Surveillance and Data Infrastructure for Postpartum Diabetes Screening in the United States After Gestational Diabetes Mellitus

Kara Suvada, MPH, Rosette Chakkalakal, MD, MHS, and Leslie C. M. Johnson, MPH, PhD

ABOUT THE AUTHORS

Kara Suvada is with the Department of Epidemiology, Emory University, and the Emory Global Diabetes Research Center, Atlanta, GA. Rosette Chakkalakal is with the Department of Medicine, Division of Internal Medicine, Emory University School of Medicine, and the Emory Global Diabetes Research Center, Atlanta, GA. Leslie C. M. Johnson is with the Department of Family and Preventive Medicine, Emory University School of Medicine, and the Emory Global Diabetes Research Center, Atlanta, GA.

Postpartum diabetes screening after a diagnosis of gestational diabetes mellitus (GDM) is an important yet underexamined component of maternal health in the United States. Although rates of GDM have risen over the past several decades, driven in part by increasing maternal age and body mass index,[1] current clinical data reporting systems are not structured to effectively support public health research on postpartum health care use and long-term outcomes.[2]

In the United States, much of our knowledge about postpartum diabetes screening comes from individual practices, particularly specialty referral centers, and health systems with integrated research teams.[3,4] These data demonstrate that although rates of postpartum diabetes screening among women with a history of GDM have shown gradual improvement, screening uptake remains suboptimal and disparate in terms of race and income, with only about half of eligible women being tested in most settings.[5,6] Notably, despite the majority of women attending follow-up visits with obstetric or primary care providers within the first year after delivery, fewer than 30% undergo recommended postpartum diabetes screening.[7]

Moreover, there is a reliance on information from prospective data collection methods, which are resource intensive, and retrospective reviews of medical records in care settings for surveillance of postpartum diabetes screening.[5] Care fragmentation further impedes surveillance because prenatal care, delivery, postpartum care, and primary care often occur across different health systems, limiting continuity and consistent monitoring.

Routine surveillance of GDM and postpartum diabetes screening is essential for assessing the true burden of GDM, identifying undiagnosed prepregnancy type 2 diabetes, and identifying those at elevated risk for future diabetes, which can be accurately understood only once pregnancy-related glycemia changes resolve after delivery. Strengthening routine postpartum screening is therefore critical to addressing diabetes as a key, yet preventable, contributor to maternal morbidity and mortality in the United States. Here we aim to raise awareness about the lack of routine, generalizable data sources on GDM and postpartum diabetes screening in the United States and to characterize currently available data sources, how they have been or could be used for research, their limitations, and our recommendations for each data set.

DATA CONSIDERATIONS AND ISSUES

We identified nine data sources that include variables related to GDM, postpartum diabetes screening, or both (Box 1 and Table A, available as a supplement to the online version of this article at https://ajph.org).[8] Among these sources, birth certificate information from the National Vital Statistics System provides key nationally representative data on GDM prevalence. However, although these data capture GDM diagnosis at delivery, they do not include use of postpartum care such as diabetes screening. Additional sources such as the Centers for Disease Control and Prevention's Pregnancy Risk Assessment Monitoring System (PRAMS) must be used to assess follow-up care. PRAMS collects self-reported data on maternal experiences before, during, and shortly after pregnancy, including

AJPH May 2026, Vol. 116, No. 5

BOX 1— Current Sources of Gestational Diabetes Data: Description and Limitations

Data Source	Brief Description of Data Set	Limitations
Pregnancy Risk Assessment Monitoring System (PRAMS)	• PRAMS measures health problems and health changes among mothers and their infants before, during, and shortly after pregnancy.	• Self-reported GDM and postpartum testing for diabetes are subject to recall and social desirability bias. • There is evidence that major discrepancies exist between self-reported GDM and birth certificate–ascertained GDM (e.g., Vuncannon et al.[8]), which leads to misclassification and underscreening. • PRAMS samples are relatively small, and the number of women with complete postpartum screening data is even smaller. • If the sample size is too small, data are not released, limiting generalizability further. • Follow-up is only four to six weeks after birth.
National Vital Statistics System (NVSS): CDC WONDER, birth data	• CDC WONDER (birth data) is administered by the NVSS, a federal compilation of vital record data. • This data source is the result of cooperation between the National Center for Health Statistics and the states to provide access to statistical information from birth certificates.	• Postpartum screening for diabetes cannot be assessed with these data alone but can be linked with PRAMS for short-term follow-up outcomes.
National Health and Nutrition Examination Survey (NHANES)	• NHANES measures the health and nutrition of adults and children in the United States. • The survey is nationally representative.	• Question RHQ162 was removed from NHANES during the most recent survey iteration (2021–2023). • Questions RHQ162 and DIQ180 are self-reported, resulting in misclassification and recall bias. • Because of its long duration, three-year postpartum diabetes screening may not truly assess postpartum outcomes. • Cross-sectional data limit assessments of temporality.
National Ambulatory Medical Care Survey (NAMCS)	• The NAMCS collects data on patients and providers in office-based health settings and health centers. • The survey is nationally representative.	• There is not a specific field in the patient record card for recording GDM, only type 1 and type 2 diabetes. • Data are cross sectional, limiting assessments of temporal associations between GDM and follow-up care and screening.
Healthcare Cost & Utilization Project Nationwide Readmissions Database (HCUP NRD)	• The HCUP NRD tracks hospital readmissions by state. • The database is nationally representative.	• The HCUP NRD tracks only readmissions to hospitals, meaning that it does not include office or clinic visits.
Behavioral Risk Factor Surveillance Survey (BRFSS)	• The BRFSS is a telephone survey that collects state-level data on US residents regarding their health-related risk behaviors, chronic health conditions, and use of preventive services. • The survey is nationally representative.	• Cross-sectional data limit assessments of temporality. • There is no question about postpartum diabetes screening.
Electronic health records (EHRs) from hospitals (with health information exchange enhancements)	• EHRs include data from various hospitals, hospital systems, and medical offices or clinics.	• The data may not be nationally representative. • Data sources are not intended for surveillance of conditions (e.g., GDM) or adherence to care guidelines.
Data from health insurance systems, including Medicaid	• Data on claims are collected from large health insurers or employers.	• Accessing data can be challenging (owing to privacy concerns or proprietary reasons). • Data may be under a paywall and prohibitively expensive to examine.
Data from individual practices, specialty referral centers, or integrated care delivery systems	• Data are collected from single or standalone clinics, hospitals, centers, or delivery systems.	• The data are not nationally representative and likely not representative of the local population. • Data sources are not intended for surveillance of conditions (e.g., GDM) or adherence to care guidelines. • Sample sizes are typically small, making it difficult to draw conclusions or offer recommendations.

Note. GDM = gestational diabetes mellitus. Current uses of the data sets for GDM and postpartum diabetes research, along with recommendations, are provided in Table A (available as a supplement to the online version of this article at https://ajph.org).

GDM and, in some years, postpartum screening. However, self-reported measures are prone to recall and social desirability biases. One Georgia-based study reported 65% discordance between self-reported and birth certificate–ascertained GDM.[8]

PRAMS also does not consistently include postpartum screening questions; some waves of data contain these questions and some do not. In addition, PRAMS involves a relatively small sample size, limiting subgroup analyses and generalizability. These limitations underscore the need for linking vital records with other data sources to better track postpartum care and guide interventions.

Other data sources include the National Health and Nutrition Examination Survey (NHANES), the National Ambulatory Medical Care Survey (NAMCS), the Healthcare Cost & Utilization Project Nationwide Readmissions Database (HCUP NRD), the Behavioral Risk Factor Surveillance System (BRFSS), electronic health records (EHRs) from hospitals or health systems, and data from individual clinical practices.

Many of these data sets capture only GDM information and lack information on postpartum screening (e.g., NAMCS, HCUP NRD, BRFSS). National data sets that include GDM or screening information rely on self-reports and are cross sectional, limiting temporal analyses (e.g., NHANES, NAMCS, HCUP NRD, BRFSS). Notably, the GDM question was removed from the most recent NHANES cycle ("During pregnancy, [were you] told you had diabetes?").

EHRs offer valuable, longitudinal data but are often difficult to access because of restrictive data use agreements or high costs, particularly for researchers unaffiliated with participating institutions. Medicaid data and data on payer claims are increasingly being used for public health surveillance generally and could be used as longitudinal data sources, but they may pose the same issues as EHR data. Finally, data from individual clinical practices can provide insight but are limited in scope and generalizability. Record linkage remains a key challenge, especially during transitions between prenatal and postpartum care. Changes in insurance coverage—such as Medicaid churn—may cause women to receive care from different systems, hindering longitudinal follow-up.

RECOMMENDATIONS AND CONCLUSIONS

We offer implementation recommendations in Table A for the data sources described here to improve their utility for GDM monitoring and for postpartum screening surveillance. Although adding or revising questions in national data sets is resource intensive, doing so is essential for robust public health analyses of postpartum health. If direct questions about postpartum screening cannot be added, variables regarding the timing of recent pregnancies (e.g., "When was your last pregnancy?" "How many weeks or months ago were you last pregnant?") could help define cohorts of individuals with GDM or other pregnancy-related conditions. Structuring data to enable linkage with future health care use and bolstering existing health information exchange networks would help identify care gaps and emerging trends.

Future directions should include incorporating postpartum health questions into national data sets and establishing mother–baby linkages within EHRs or surveys, as mothers often engage more consistently with pediatric care than with postpartum providers. Integration of continuous glucose monitoring data through remote platforms also offers promise for enhanced postpartum glycemic surveillance.[9] Together, these improvements would strengthen our capacity to monitor postpartum health and address persistent contributors to maternal morbidity and mortality in the United States. AJPH

CORRESPONDENCE

Correspondence should be sent to Kara Suvada, MPH, Emory University, 1518 Clifton Rd, Atlanta, GA 30329 (e-mail: ksuvada@emory.edu). Reprints can be ordered at https://www.ajph.org by clicking the "Reprints" link.

PUBLICATION INFORMATION

Full Citation: Suvada K, Chakkalakal R, Johnson LCM. Gaps in surveillance and data infrastructure for postpartum diabetes screening in the United States after gestational diabetes mellitus. *Am J Public Health*. 2026;116(5):587–590.

Acceptance Date: December 14, 2025

DOI: https://doi.org/10.2105/AJPH.2025.308408

ORCID iDs:

Kara Suvada https://orcid.org/0000-0003-2785-835X

Leslie C. M. Johnson https://orcid.org/0000-0003-4574-847X

CONTRIBUTORS

K. Suvada contributed to the design and drafting of the editorial and to interpretation of data sources. R. Chakkalakal contributed to interpretation of data sources, provided clinical insight to the work, and revised the editorial for important intellectual and clinical content. L. C. M. Johnson conceived the idea for the work, contributed to the drafting of the editorial, and served as the senior author.

CONFLICTS OF INTEREST

The authors have no conflicts of interest to disclose.

REFERENCES

1. Zhou T, Du S, Sun D, et al. Prevalence and trends in gestational diabetes mellitus among women in the United States, 2006–2017: a population-based study. *Front Endocrinol (Lausanne)*. 2022;13:868094. https://doi.org/10.3389/fendo.2022.868094
2. Vounzoulaki E, Khunti K, Abner SC, Tan BK, Davies MJ, Gillies CL. Progression to type 2 diabetes in women with a known history of gestational diabetes: systematic review and meta-analysis. *BMJ*. 2020;369:m1361. https://doi.org/10.1136/bmj.m1361

3. Ortiz FM, Jimenez EY, Boursaw B, Huttlinger K. Postpartum care for women with gestational diabetes. *MCN Am J Matern Child Nurs.* 2016;41(2):116–122. https://doi.org/10.1097/NMC.0000000000000215

4. Herrick CJ, Keller MR, Trolard AM, Cooper BP, Olsen MA, Colditz GA. Postpartum diabetes screening among low income women with gestational diabetes in Missouri 2010–2015. *BMC Public Health.* 2019;19(1):148. https://doi.org/10.1186/s12889-019-6475-0

5. Tovar A, Chasan-Taber L, Eggleston E, Oken E. Postpartum screening for diabetes among women with a history of gestational diabetes mellitus. *Prev Chronic Dis.* 2011;8(6):A124.

6. Dietz PM, Vesco KK, Callaghan WM, et al. Postpartum screening for diabetes after a gestational diabetes mellitus–affected pregnancy. *Obstet Gynecol.* 2008;112(4):868–874. https://doi.org/10.1097/AOG.0b013e318184db63

7. Eggleston EM, LeCates RF, Zhang F, Wharam JF, Ross-Degnan D, Oken E. Variation in postpartum glycemic screening in women with a history of gestational diabetes mellitus. *Obstet Gynecol.* 2016;128(1):159–167. https://doi.org/10.1097/AOG.0000000000001467

8. Vuncannon DM, Chandrasekaran S, Luong J, Stevenson IC, Johnson LCM. 1235-P: gestational diabetes mellitus in Georgia, United States—agreement between maternal self-report and birth certificate documentation. *Diabetes.* 2024;73(suppl 1):1235-P. https://doi.org/10.2337/db24-1235-P

9. Painter SL, Lu W, Schneider J, James R, Shah B. Drivers of weight loss in a CDC-recognized digital diabetes prevention program. *BMJ Open Diabetes Res Care.* 2020;8(1):e001132. https://doi.org/10.1136/bmjdrc-2019-001132

The 2025 Drug Overdose Spike That Wasn't: Neither Politics nor Data Errors Explain the Anomaly

Lori Ann Post, PhD, Daniel Ciccarone, MD, MPH, Alexander Lars Lundberg, PhD, Maryann Mason, PhD, Shivangi Sharma, MS, George Jay Unick, PhD, and Nabarun Dasgupta, PhD

ABOUT THE AUTHORS

Lori Ann Post, Alexander Lars Lundberg, Maryann Mason, and Shivangi Sharma are with the Department of Emergency Medicine, Northwestern Feinberg School of Medicine, Chicago, IL. Daniel Ciccarone is with Family and Community Medicine, University of California, San Francisco. George Jay Unick is with the School of Social Work, University of Maryland at Baltimore. Nabarun Dasgupta is with the Gillings School of Global Public Health, University of North Carolina at Chapel Hill.

See also Ahmad et al., p. 594.

Starting in August 2023, drug overdose deaths (DODs) entered the longest decline in more than 40 years.[1,2] The "great deceleration" brought cautious optimism to public health leaders and academics alike. That optimism was shaken in June 2025 when the National Center for Health Statistics (NCHS) National Vital Statistics System (NVSS) released provisional estimates for January 2025 suggesting that overdose deaths had spiked, abruptly reversing the national downward trend.[3] According to an NPR segment that aired on June 18, 2025 ("U.S. Drug Overdose Deaths Rise Again After Hopeful Decline"), public health officials and academics reacted with concern.[4]

Because of the inertia of large national numbers, a national rise in January 2025 after many months of decline was implausible. Amid declining overdose deaths, the NVSS algorithm used to account for incomplete autopsies and national projections was revised. The first revision contradicted evidence of continuing declines and coincided with sudden restrictions in other federal data sources, amplifying suspicion. Some interpreted the anomaly as a potential sign of political interference.[5]

HOW OVERDOSE DEATHS ARE TRACKED

Overdose deaths are classified in the NVSS by either underlying cause of death (UCD) or multiple causes of death. Because toxicology and death investigation reports often become available months after the date of death, provisional data are incomplete. To address this issue, the NCHS developed predicted provisional counts—referred to here as UCD Predict—which are created from a predictive model based on UCD and multiple cause of death inputs that provides estimates of 12-month moving sums of overdose deaths. Regression-based adjustments are applied to provisional UCD data to approximate final totals.[3] Historically, these predicted values have tracked well with observed data once reporting delays are resolved.

Provisional estimates began to break down when fentanyl, a powerful synthetic opioid, reshaped the overdose epidemic. It has driven DODs, accounting for 92% of all opioid deaths and 70% of all DODs at peak (August 2023).[1] Fentanyl began displacing heroin around 2013 in the Midwest, Northeast, and South but not markedly in the West until approximately 2019.[1,6,7] This nonlinear, noncontiguous, regionally staggered diffusion of fentanyl destabilized statistical models trained on slower-moving historical patterns. As a result, models trained on the explosive growth of 2022 performed poorly when applied to 2023, when DODs declined.

We examined national death data (observed and predicted) from the NVSS (January 2015–March 2025). Our analysis drew on four related NVSS provisional data series: UCD counts and three versions of UCD Predict that were downloaded at three different intervals and were subject to different algorithms, all of which ostensibly adjusted for delayed reporting and underreporting but involved different baselines, starting with 2015.

NVSS observed UCD counts represent the official record of DODs once reporting is complete. To complement these data, we reviewed 12-month moving sums from UCD Predict. During our study period, three versions of UCD Predict were available: the original series, accessed in July 2024; a revision released in February 2025; and a second revision released in July 2025.

First, we plotted three versions of UCD Predict to assess trend concordance and identify time periods of divergence (Figure 1). This approach allowed visual comparisons of how revisions to UCD Predict altered the apparent trajectory of overdose deaths. Second, we quantified the difference between predicted and observed; using UCD Observed and UCD Predict, we subtracted observed national counts from predicted counts at each monthly time point (Figure 1). This calculation yielded a deviation series for each of the three versions of UCD Predict, highlighting the degree to which DODs from each model were overestimated or underestimated; the aim was to assess whether the apparent January 2025 spike in UCD Predict represented a genuine reversal in DODs, a data or coding error, or a statistical artifact of predictive modeling.

SHIFTING PREDICTIONS AND THE ILLUSION OF SPIKES

We use "spike" to denote a change that is both (1) directionally inconsistent with the previous trend and (2) large relative to the typical month-to-month change in the 12-month moving sum, which already smooths random month-to-month variation. Figure 1 compares three iterations of the UCD Predict series. The original green line tracks observed NVSS UCD counts closely. In winter 2025, the NCHS retroactively revised the series back to 2015 (blue) using data from 2022–2023, when deaths were still rising in large states. This first revision overestimated data from January and February 2024, creating the illusion of a spike and a reversal of the 17-month deceleration.

The anomaly was unlikely to be political manipulation: neither the Biden administration in 2024 nor the Trump administration in 2025 had an apparent reason to inflate mortality. Instead, the anomaly was a model artifact. A second revision released in August 2025 (red) corrected the discrepancy, clarifying that the January 2025 "spike" was an artifact. Although the three iterations of UCD Predict may seem minor against the backdrop of more than 114 000 DODs (12-month moving sum) in August 2023, comparing them with the observed counts reveals substantial deviations.

In January 2015, there were 47 523 observed DODs. The original UCD Predict estimated 48 126, a deviation of 603 (green). The first revision estimated 48 856, a deviation of 1333 (blue), and the second and most recent revision estimated 48 060, a deviation of 537 (red).

By January 2024 and January 2025, the numbers of observed deaths were 105 521 and 78 883, respectively, whereas the first revision (blue) estimated 110 909 and 82 138 (overestimating by 5388 and 3255, respectively). The first revision even underestimated December 2024 deaths by 137, an implausible negative deviation.

Because of these inconsistencies, the NCHS revised the model again. The original UCD Predict consistently underpredicted deaths during inflection points of

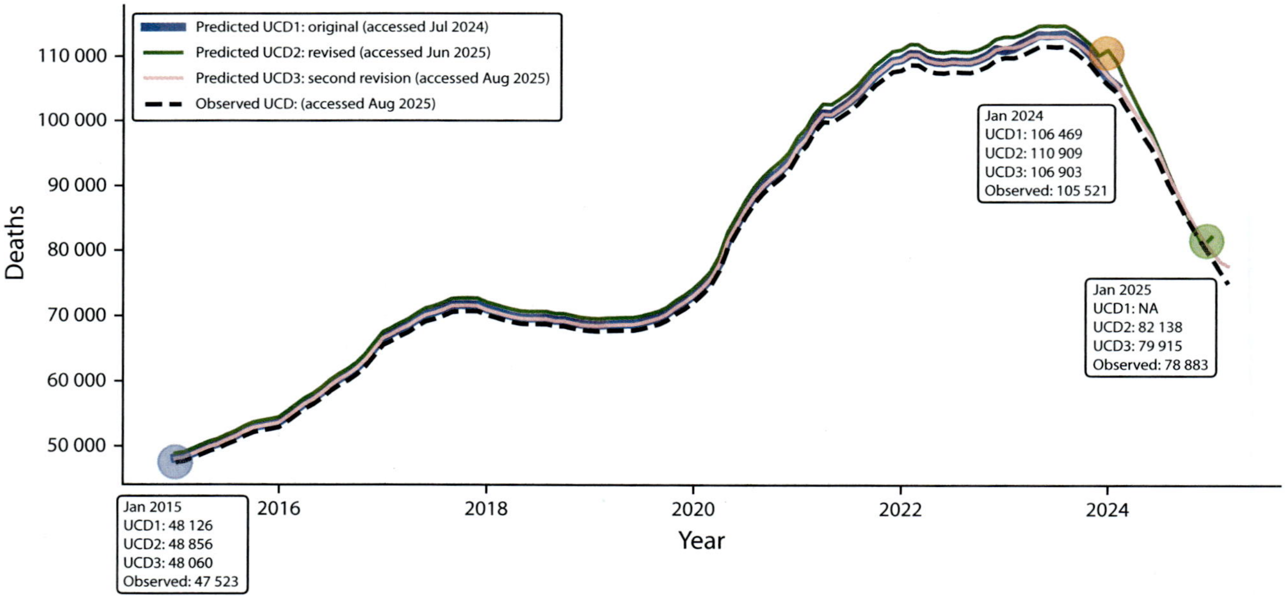

FIGURE 1— Twelve-Month Moving Sum of Drug Overdose Deaths: United States, UCD Predict, 2024–2025

Note. NA = not applicable; UCD = underlying cause of death.

acceleration, plateau, and deceleration around 2023–2024. The first revision (blue) overshot in early 2024 and early 2025 while undershooting in fall 2024. This volatility misled commentators, with some suggesting a national resurgence. Drug epidemiologists, however, recognized the discordance and pressed for clarification.

The second revision (red line) improved the fit by retroactively adjusting counts back to 2015, reducing both overpredictions and underpredictions. This episode illustrates how predictive models trained on years of exponential growth can generate spurious spikes when applied to a decelerating epidemic.

This sequence of revisions highlights two lessons. First, predictive surveillance is highly vulnerable when epidemics shift phases. Models based on past data may be misleading during transitions, creating false inflection points. Second, transparency is critical: methodological changes that affect provisional estimates should be announced in advance, accompanied by a concise change log describing what changed, when, and why, reiterated with each affected release. It is of note that confidence in the NVSS remains essential because death certificate data underpin overdose surveillance and response.

Importantly, these data releases were not a political conspiracy. Instead, they reflected the challenge of modeling an epidemic with sudden outbreaks, regional diffusion, supply changes, and seasonality. The artifact briefly suggested a resurgence but was resolved with updated models. NCHS epidemiologists confirmed that the anomaly resulted from applying growth-era algorithms to a period of decline. Their transparency clarified the discrepancy.

WHY USE UCD PREDICT IF IT IS SUBJECT TO ERROR?

UCD Predict provides the timeliest national data available, data that are central to monitoring overdose deaths. All surveillance systems are imperfect proxies subject to time lags, misreporting, underreporting, coding variations, and incomplete case ascertainment. Yet even with these challenges, UCD Predict remains the best near-real-time mortality source.

Importantly, UCD Predict has generally performed well. For the past decade, provisional predicted values have closely tracked observed counts and aligned with other surveillance systems, underscoring the model's reliability and utility. The recent anomalies do not negate this performance but instead highlight the importance of recognizing the limits of predictive modeling during volatile phases. To reduce confusion, we recommend that the NCHS announce planned methodological changes in advance. Even so, the overdose crisis remains dynamic: national rates are declining, but the pace is slowing.[2] AJPH

CORRESPONDENCE

Correspondence should be sent to Lori Ann Post, PhD, Northwestern University Feinberg School of Medicine, 420 E Superior St, Chicago, IL 60646 (e-mail: lori.post@northwestern.edu). Reprints can be ordered at https://www.ajph.org by clicking the "Reprints" link.

PUBLICATION INFORMATION

Full Citation: Post LA, Ciccarone D, Lundberg AL, et al. The 2025 drug overdose spike that wasn't: neither politics nor data errors explain the anomaly. *Am J Public Health*. 2026;116(5):591–593.

Acceptance Date: December 1, 2025

DOI: https://doi.org/10.2105/AJPH.2025.308412

ORCID iDs:

Lori Ann Post https://orcid.org/0000-0002-6261-3254

Daniel Ciccarone https://orcid.org/0000-0002-2355-5477

Alexander Lars Lundberg https://orcid.org/0000-0002-9743-8441

Maryann Mason https://orcid.org/0000-0001-6524-1532

Shivangi Sharma https://orcid.org/0009-0003-5951-281X

George Jay Unick https://orcid.org/0000-0001-6939-3162

Nabarun Dasgupta https://orcid.org/0000-0002-4098-605X

CONTRIBUTORS

L. A. Post was responsible for conception, design of the work, and final approval of the work. D. Ciccarone, A. L. Lundberg, M. Mason, G. J. Unick, and N. Dasgupta reviewed the work, data analyses, and interpretation of the analyses and made edits to the initial and final versions of the article. S. Sharma was responsible for data acquisition and initial figures.

ACKNOWLEDGMENTS

This study was funded in part by the National Institutes of Health (grant NIH/NIDA 1R21DA058583-01).

CONFLICTS OF INTEREST

The authors have no conflicts of interest to declare.

REFERENCES

1. Post LA, Ciccarone D, Unick GJ, et al. Decline in US drug overdose deaths by region, substance, and demographics. *JAMA Netw Open*. 2025;8(6):e2514997. https://doi.org/10.1001/jamanetworkopen.2025.14997
2. Centers for Disease Control and Prevention. National Vital Statistics System. Available at: https://www.cdc.gov/nchs/nvss/index.htm. Accessed December 20, 2025.
3. Ahmad FB, C J, Rossen LM, Sutton P. Provisional drug overdose death counts. Available at: https://www.cdc.gov/nchs/nvss/vsrr/drug-overdose-data.htm. Accessed December 20, 2025.
4. NPR. U.S. drug overdose deaths rise again after hopeful decline. Available at: https://www.npr.org/2025/06/18/nx-s1-5436711/overdose-drugs-cdc. Accessed December 20, 2025.
5. Dasgupta N, Sibley A, Miller C. The math ain't mathing. Available at: https://www.opioiddata.org/this-ad-didnt-age-well. Accessed December 20, 2025.
6. Shover CL, Falasinnu TO, Dwyer CL, et al. Steep increases in fentanyl-related mortality west of the Mississippi River: recent evidence from county and state surveillance. *Drug Alcohol Depend*. 2020;216:108314. https://doi.org/10.1016/j.drugalcdep.2020.108314
7. Wilson N, Kariisa M, Seth P, Smith H, IV, Davis NL. Drug and opioid-involved overdose deaths—United States, 2017–2018. *MMWR Morb Mortal Wkly Rep*. 2020;69(11):290–297. http://dx.doi.org/10.15585/mmwr.mm6911a4

The Vital Statistics Rapid Release Program Responds

Farida B. Ahmad, MPH, Robert N. Anderson, PhD, Jodi A. Cisewski, MPH, Lauren M. Rossen, PhD, and Paul D. Sutton, PhD

ABOUT THE AUTHORS

The authors are with the National Center for Health Statistics, Centers for Disease Control and Prevention, Hyattsville, MD.

See also Post et al., p. 591.

We appreciate the editorial by Post et al. (p. 584) discussing provisional drug overdose data from the National Vital Statistics System, highlighting the utility and timeliness of this information for monitoring national trends in drug overdose mortality. The editorial describes several important issues related to provisional drug overdose mortality data, including the presence of reporting lags that contribute to incomplete data in recent time periods and the need to regularly reassess and update the algorithms used to adjust provisional death counts for underreporting. These issues are critical for data users to understand, and the National Center for Health Statistics (NCHS) provides several resources such as Technical Notes pages and reports with detailed information about the data and corresponding limitations.[1,2] Recognizing that many data users may not use these resources, here we provide additional clarification on how provisional drug overdose mortality data are produced and updated.

The National Vital Statistics System collects and disseminates vital statistics data for the United States and its territories, releasing provisional death data in summary reports and data files to provide the public with near-real-time trends in mortality through the Vital Statistics Rapid Release Program.[3] The Provisional Drug Overdose Death Counts dashboard has provided the public with early estimates of drug overdose deaths since August 2017, representing the earliest and most complete estimates of drug overdose death counts in the United States for public health surveillance and monitoring of emerging trends.

Drug overdose deaths can require additional investigation before death certificate data are completed (e.g., autopsy, toxicology, and death scene investigation). Because of such delays, drug overdose death data may not be complete for more than six months and the cause of death is temporarily listed as "pending investigation," resulting in underestimates relative to final counts. The Provisional Drug Overdose Death Counts dashboard provides both reported death counts and predicted death counts identified through underlying cause of death codes, the latter of which are adjusted for reporting lags to provide a more complete picture of recent drug overdose mortality trends. The methods used to generate these predicted counts are described in detail in a report published in 2018.[2]

Briefly, historical provisional data files are compared with final data to determine how complete provisional data are at given lags (e.g., four months and six months). Adjustment factors are generated by modeling completeness as a function of the percentage of records with manner of death "pending investigation" and the month and year. It is important to note that these adjustments are always based on the estimated reporting lags from past data years, because current reporting lags cannot be estimated until data are finalized sometime in the future. This is a critical limitation, as reporting lags vary over time, by cause of death, and by other factors.

Since the inception of these estimates, NCHS has continuously monitored, reevaluated, and updated the adjustment factors used to generate predicted counts to reflect the most recent estimates of reporting lags. The adjustment factors have been regularly updated with each new final data year with the exception of 2020 to 2022; during the COVID-19 pandemic, there were disruptions in timeliness associated with the pandemic. Updates resumed with the 2023 data year, and it was that update that created the aberration noted by Post et al. for the January 2024 and January 2025 predicted counts. The reason for this aberration was that the relationship between completeness and the percentage of records in which manner of death was "pending investigation" was weaker for the 2023 data year than in previous years; similarly, completeness was lower in January 2023 than it had been in earlier years.

When the 2023-based adjustment factors were applied to the more recent provisional data for 2024 to 2025, the predicted 12-month ending counts for January of each year were overadjusted

AJPH May 2026, Vol. 116, No. 5

(i.e., they were too high). (It should be noted that although the predicted 12-month ending count was overestimated, a continued decrease in counts from the previous 12-month period was reported.) Given these aberrations in the trend lines, further evaluations were done to confirm that this issue was an artifact of 2023 reporting lags, and NCHS revised the adjustment factors on the basis of available provisional 2024 data to correct the anomaly.

With each improvement or update, NCHS has summarized and explained the changes in the Technical Notes included below the key charts and tables of the dashboard. Users are also typically alerted to changes with a banner placed at the top of the dashboard summarizing the changes and directing the user to read the Technical Notes for additional information. Because of the rapid periodicity of provisional drug overdose estimate releases, advance notice of changes is not always feasible; as noted, however, information on changes in methodology is provided at the time of release.

NCHS continues to make improvements to the timeliness and availability of provisional data, ensuring that the data are accurate and reliable and that the methods and limitations are well documented in Technical Notes and reports. These data remain a critical resource for tracking recent drug overdose mortality trends across the United States. AJPH

CORRESPONDENCE

Correspondence should be sent to Farida B. Ahmad, MPH, 3311 Toledo Rd, Hyattsville, MD 20782 (e-mail: fbahmad@cdc.gov). Reprints can be ordered at https://www.ajph.org by clicking the "Reprints" link.

PUBLICATION INFORMATION

Full Citation: Ahmad FB, Anderson RN, Cisewski JA, Rossen LM, Sutton PD. The Vital Statistics Rapid Release Program responds. *Am J Public Health*. 2026;116(5):594–595.

Acceptance Date: February 5, 2026

DOI: https://doi.org/10.2105/AJPH.2026.308478

ORCID iDs:

Farida B. Ahmad https://orcid.org/0000-0002-1064-5131

Robert N. Anderson https://orcid.org/0000-0002-2944-6028

Jodi A. Cisewski https://orcid.org/0000-0002-7841-6079

Lauren M. Rossen https://orcid.org/0000-0003-3823-1982

Paul D. Sutton https://orcid.org/0000-0002-7398-2709

CONTRIBUTORS

All of the authors contributed to the writing, editing, and reviewing of the article.

ACKNOWLEDGMENTS

The National Center for Health Statistics acknowledges the efforts of vital statistics jurisdictions to improve the timeliness and quality of drug overdose death data.

Note. The findings and conclusions in this article are those of the authors and do not necessarily represent the official position of the Centers for Disease Control and Prevention.

CONFLICTS OF INTEREST

The authors report no conflicts of interest.

REFERENCES

1. Ahmad FB, Cisewski JA, Rossen LM, Sutton P. Provisional drug overdose death counts. Available at: https://www.cdc.gov/nchs/nvss/vsrr/drug-overdose-data.htm. Accessed January 26, 2026.
2. Rossen LM, Ahmad FB, Spencer MR, Warner M, Sutton P. Methods to adjust provisional counts of drug overdose deaths for underreporting. Available at: https://www.cdc.gov/nchs/data/vsrr/report006.pdf. Accessed January 26, 2026.
3. National Center for Health Statistics. Vital Statistics Rapid Release. Available at: https://www.cdc.gov/nchs/nvss/vsrr.htm. Accessed January 26, 2026.

The Public Health Potential of Social Media Litigation

Hayden L. Kent, Carol Vidal, MD, PhD, MPH, and Daniel G. Aaron, MD, JD

ABOUT THE AUTHORS

Hayden L. Kent and Daniel G. Aaron are with the S.J. Quinney College of Law, University of Utah, Salt Lake City. Carol Vidal is with the Johns Hopkins University School of Medicine, Baltimore, MD.

AJPH May 2026, Vol. 116, No. 5

After 16-year-old Mason Edens died from a self-inflicted gunshot wound, his mother discovered that he had watched at least 15 TikTok videos promoting suicide, five of which promoted the lethal method he used. In March 2024, she sued TikTok and ByteDance, the owner of TikTok, commenting that "[t]hey're not going to self-regulate until there's true accountability."[1] The Edens family represents just one in a growing chorus that believes social media companies are contributing to a growing youth mental health crisis. Amid high rates of teen social media use (averaging 4.8 hours per day) and recognition of social media's mental health risks, the surgeon general issued a major public health advisory in 2023 in which he called for warning labels on social media platforms, and numerous plaintiffs have sued social media companies for compensation and accountability. Here we discuss the role of courts in addressing social media's harms, incentivizing safer platform designs, increasing transparency, and filling regulatory gaps.

SOCIAL MEDIA'S PUBLIC HEALTH IMPLICATIONS

Among US adolescents, 53% report feeling at least somewhat "addicted" to digital media,[2] a phenomenon that has raised concerns about health and safety risks. Some researchers have linked social media use to rising rates of youth depression and suicide-related behaviors,[3] noting that the quality rather than sheer duration of digital screen time has the most impact on adolescent mental health.[3] Although more research is needed to understand causal mechanisms, strong evidence indicates that social media use negatively affects sleep and is associated with myriad behavioral health problems.[4] Harms may fall disproportionately on minority and younger age groups,[5] those with underlying mental health issues, and compulsive users.

A confluence of factors lead to these risk associations, including the time spent on the platforms, the algorithm's content output, the interactions it prioritizes, the disruptive impact on essential activities, and the unique vulnerabilities of adolescent brain development.[5] Features, including "likes," infinite scroll, and curated content, are optimized to retain user attention and generate advertising revenue. Platforms generally downplay risks despite concerns about how these features may exploit the adolescent brain's sensitivity to reward and social feedback.[6]

However, quality engagement on social media can benefit mental health by increasing access to support among marginalized individuals (e.g., LGBTQ+ [lesbian, gay, bisexual, transgender, or queer] or disability communities), decreasing mental health stigma, and lowering barriers to educational resources, although the information presented may not necessarily be accurate. Social media may also provide tools for mental health care delivery and intervention.

THE GROWING LITIGATION LANDSCAPE

In 2021 a whistleblower leaked the "Facebook Files," a portfolio of documents that included an internal study showing that 13.5% of UK adolescent girls said Instagram worsened their suicidal thoughts.[7] On November 18, 2021, a bipartisan coalition of 10 state attorneys general began investigating whether Meta—and later ByteDance—violated consumer protection laws and harmed public health by targeting young users.[8]

State investigations have culminated in a wave of lawsuits against social media companies in both federal and state courts. Plaintiffs, making claims largely for negligence, product liability, and violations of consumer protection law, accuse the platforms of designing features to foster compulsive use, thereby significantly contributing to the population-level mental health decline in this age group.

Thirty states have sued in state courts (Box 1), yet most of the litigation is centralized in federal multidistrict litigation (MDL) in northern California. The still-growing Social Media Adolescent Addiction MDL, involving 35 states, four tribal nations, and hundreds of personal injury

BOX 1— National Scope of Lawsuits Against Social Media Companies

State/Court	Company (Companies) Sued	Case Name	Date Filed
California/US District Court for the District of Northern California	Meta, Alphabet/Google, Snap, ByteDance/TikTok	*In re: Social Media Adolescent Addiction/ Personal Injury Products Liability Litigation*	Consolidated October 6, 2022
California/Superior Court for the State of California for the County of Los Angeles	Meta, Alphabet/Google, Snap, ByteDance/TikTok	*Social Media Cases JCCP*	Consolidated September 15, 2022
Indiana/Superior Court of Allen County	TikTok	*State of Indiana v TikTok Inc. et al.*	October 7, 2022
Arkansas/Cleburne County Circuit Court	TikTok	*State of Arkansas ex rel. Tim Griffin, Attorney General v TikTok Inc., et al*	March 28, 2023
Arkansas/Polk County Circuit Court	Meta	*State of Arkansas v Meta Platforms, Inc.*	March 28, 2023
Utah/Third Judicial District Court, Salt Lake County	TikTok	*Utah Division of Consumer Protection v TikTok, Inc.*	October 10, 2023
Vermont/Chittenden Superior Court	Meta	*State of Vermont v Meta Platforms, Inc.*	October 10, 2023
District of Columbia/Superior Court of the District of Columbia Civil Division	Meta	*District of Columbia v Meta*	October 24, 2023
Massachusetts/Suffolk County Superior Court	Meta	*Commonwealth of Massachusetts v Meta Platforms, Inc. and Instagram, LLC*	October 24, 2023
Mississippi/Chancery Court for the First Judicial District of Hinds County	Meta	*State of Mississippi ex rel. Lynn Fitch, Attorney General v Meta Platforms et al.*	October 24, 2023
New Hampshire/Merrimack County Superior Court	Meta	*State of New Hampshire v Meta Platforms, Inc. et al.*	October 24, 2023
Oklahoma/District Court of Osage County	Meta	*State of Oklahoma, ex rel., Gentner Drummond, Attorney General of Oklahoma v Meta et al.*	October 24, 2023
Tennessee/Chancery Court of Davidson County Tennessee for the Twentieth Judicial District at Nashville	Meta	*State of Tennessee, ex rel., Jonathan Skrmetti, Attorney General and Reporter v Meta Inc.*	October 24, 2023
Iowa/District Court for Polk County	TikTok	*State of Iowa ex rel. Brenna Bird v TikTok, Inc. et al.*	January 17, 2024
Nevada/Clark County District Court	TikTok	*State of Nevada v TikTok Inc., et al.*	January 30, 2024
Kansas/Shawnee County District Court	TikTok	*State of Kansas ex rel. Kris W. Kobach, Attorney General v TikTok, Inc. et al.*	March 6, 2024
Nebraska/Lancaster County District Court	TikTok	*State of Nebraska ex rel. Michael T. Hilgers, Attorney General v TikTok Inc., et al.*	May 22, 2024
Utah/Third Judicial District Court, Salt Lake County	TikTok	*Utah Division of Consumer Protection v TikTok, Inc.*	June 3, 2024
Nevada/Clark County District Court	Meta	*State of Nevada v Meta Platforms, Inc.*	June 30, 2024
Nevada/Clark County District Court	Snap Inc.	*State of Nevada v Snap Inc.*	June 30, 2024
New Mexico/First Judicial District Court, County of Santa Fe	Snap Inc.	*State of New Mexico ex rel. Raúl Torrez, Attorney General v Snap Inc.*	September 5, 2024
Arkansas/Phillips County Circuit Court	Alphabet	*State of Arkansas ex rel. Tim Griffin, Attorney General v Alphabet Inc.*	September 30, 2024
Texas/District Court of Galveston County	TikTok	*State of Texas v TikTok et al.*	October 3, 2024
California/Santa Clara County Superior Court	TikTok	*People of the State of California v TikTok, Inc. et al.*	October 8, 2024
Illinois/Circuit Court of Cook County	TikTok	*The People of the State of Illinois v TikTok Inc., et al.*	October 8, 2024
Louisiana/21st Judicial District Court, Parish of Livingston	TikTok	*State of Louisiana v TikTok Inc. et al.*	October 8, 2024
Massachusetts/Suffolk County Superior Court	TikTok	*Commonwealth of Massachusetts v TikTok, Inc. et al.*	October 8, 2024
Mississippi/Chancery Court for the First Judicial District of Hinds County	TikTok	*State of Mississippi ex rel. Lynn Fitch, Attorney General v TikTok, Inc.*	October 8, 2024
North Carolina/Superior Court Wake County	TikTok	*State of North Carolina ex rel. Joshua H. Stein, Attorney General v TikTok Inc.*	October 8, 2024

Continued

BOX 1— Continued

State/Court	Company (Companies) Sued	Case Name	Date Filed
New Jersey/Superior Court of New Jersey Chancery Division, Essex County	TikTok	*Matthew J. Platkin, Attorney General of the State of New Jersey, and Cari Fais, Acting Director of the New Jersey Division of Consumer Affairs v TikTok Inc. et al.*	October 8, 2024
New York/New York County Superior Court	TikTok	*People of the State of New York v TikTok, Inc. et al.*	October 8, 2024
South Carolina/Richland County Court of Common Pleas	TikTok	*State of South Carolina ex rel. Alan Wilson, Attorney General v TikTok, Inc. et al.*	October 8, 2024
Vermont/Washington Superior Court	TikTok	*State of Vermont v TikTok Inc.*	October 8, 2024
Washington/Superior Court for the State of Washington, King County	TikTok	*State of Washington v TikTok Inc et al.*	October 8, 2024
Kentucky/Scott County Circuit Court	TikTok	*Commonwealth of Kentucky, ex rel. Russell Coleman, Attorney General v TikTok Inc., et al.*	October 9, 2024
Oregon/Multnomah County Circuit Court	TikTok	*State of Oregon ex rel. Ellen F. Rosenblum, Attorney General v TikTok, Inc. et al.*	October 9, 2024
District of Columbia/Superior Court of the District of Columbia Civil Division	TikTok	*District of Columbia v TikTok Inc.*	October 10, 2024
Montana/District Court of Lewis and Clark County	TikTok	*State of Montana et al. v TikTok Inc. et al.*	October 24, 2024
New Hampshire/Merrimack County Superior Court	TikTok	*State of New Hampshire v TikTok, Inc.*	October 25, 2024
Texas/District Court of Galveston County	TikTok	*State of Texas v TikTok et al.*	January 9, 2025
Virginia/Richmond County Circuit Court	TikTok	*State of Virginia v TikTok, Inc. et al.*	January 17, 2025
New Jersey/Superior Court of New Jersey Chancery Division, Essex County	Discord	*Matthew J. Platkin, Attorney General of the State of New Jersey, and Cari Fais, Acting Director of the New Jersey Division of Consumer Affairs v Discord Inc.*	April 17, 2025
Alabama/Montgomery County Circuit Court	TikTok	*State of Alabama, ex rel. Steve Marshall, Attorney General v TikTok et al.*	April 29, 2025
Nevada/Clark County District Court	Alphabet	*State of Nevada v Alphabet, Inc.*	June 16, 2025
Utah/Third Judicial District Court, Salt Lake County	Snap Inc.	*Utah Division of Consumer Protection v Snap Inc.*	June 30, 2025
Minnesota/County of Hennepin	TikTok	*State of Minnesota, by its Attorney General, Keith Ellison v TikTok Inc.*	August 19, 2025
Nevada/Clark County District Court	MediaLab.AI (holding company of Kik)	*State of Nevada v Medialab AI, Inc.*	August 19, 2025
Florida/Circuit Court of the First Judicial District in and for Santa Rosa County	Snap. Inc.	*Office of the Attorney General et al v Snap Inc.*	October 22, 2025

plaintiffs and local governmental entities, has consolidated federal claims against Meta, Alphabet (parent company of Google and YouTube), Snap Inc., and ByteDance.

MDL proceedings combine similar cases to save time and cost and are a frequent fixture in public health litigation. MDL cases have been established in litigation over asbestos, opioid prescription drugs, and Monsanto's pesticide Roundup, among others. In theory, MDLs manage pretrial affairs before cases return to their original court for trial. In practice, cases can become trapped in an MDL with thousands of other cases, and the pressure to settle becomes significant.[9] Eight plaintiffs in the social media MDL are scheduled for trial in 2026, and the outcomes will likely influence the direction of the remaining cases. Most claims have survived the platforms' early efforts to defeat them, suggesting that this litigation holds significant potential to address existing public health harms.

PUBLIC HEALTH'S POSSIBLE GAINS

In the absence of comprehensive regulation, litigation may offer a critical mechanism to drive corporate accountability and reform. Acquired funds can be directed toward digital media literacy education, mental health initiatives, nonprofit advocacy, and research efforts to better understand social media's impacts. Litigation also creates financial pressure that can shift business incentives away from maximizing engagement at any cost, potentially inspiring proactive changes that limit problematic platform features.

Likewise, lawsuits can force transparency and public accountability. Document requests could expose internal platform operations and knowledge of harm. However, MDL proceedings are sometimes secretive, a dynamic noted in the prescription opioid MDL,[10] and defendants may condition monetary recovery on confidentiality. To maximize public health impact, settlement provisions must enable disclosure, and plaintiffs should scrutinize any requests to seal important documents. Already, state cases have spurred the release of internal documents highlighting ByteDance's knowledge of the app's addictiveness.[11]

Litigation remains an imperfect vehicle for achieving systemic reform. Legal action is costly and slow. Tensions may arise between the goal of public health and the motivations of plaintiffs and their counsel, such as incentives to accept settlement offers that are tied to confidentiality requirements or that provide insufficient accountability.[9] Plaintiffs also face the burden of showing causation, that social media caused them harm. Plaintiffs may point to peer-reviewed evidence of social media's mental health harms and companies' internal documents that reach similar findings, but plaintiffs who use multiple social media platforms or engage in other activities that represent potential causes of harm may face a taller causation burden. Another barrier is Section 230 of the Communications Decency Act, which shields platforms from liability for user content. But recent lawsuits argue that harms stem from addictive design features and not solely user content. Courts have shown a growing receptivity to plaintiffs' public health claims,[12] signaling a possible rejection of broad immunity under Section 230.

Despite the litigation, social media platforms remain popular and can provide community, education, and bonding over shared hardships. To maximize public health value, litigation should not wholly dismantle social media but incentivize structural platform redesigns that align with public health objectives while minimizing known harms, such as by restricting use of minor users' data, removing personalized recommendation features, hiding "like" counts, and strengthening content moderation efforts.[13]

Ultimately, litigation is likely to play a supporting role, furnishing resources and information to mount bottom-up pressure and building toward comprehensive regulation needed to fully address social media's health harms.

PUBLIC HEALTH COMMUNITY GUIDANCE

With litigation ongoing, public health practitioners need not sit idle. They can support the development of digital literacy and responsible social media use initiatives. Delivery methods can range from school health curricula to public health campaigns. Public health scholars can shape the narrative by quantifying the burden that social media–related harms place on schools and health systems and by further researching causal relationships, evidence-based remedies, and links between social media use and other public health concerns, such as cyberbullying and exposure to risky behaviors or extremist content.[5] Finally, public health researchers can advocate for clear industry guardrails, improved design standards, and greater government oversight.

Litigation against social media companies is an imperfect solution and is unlikely to remedy nonhealth harms, including the platforms' wider effects on the environment and democratic governance. Still, it could serve as a catalyst for developing a national approach to addressing social media's health impacts on vulnerable populations such as youths. And it could provide a model for addressing emerging technology-related harms such as those arising from artificial intelligence–powered chatbots. AJPH

CORRESPONDENCE

Correspondence should be sent to Hayden L. Kent, 383 South University St, Salt Lake City, UT 84112 (e-mail: hayden.kent@law.utah.edu). Reprints can be ordered at https://www.ajph.org by clicking the "Reprints" link.

PUBLICATION INFORMATION

Full Citation: Kent HL, Vidal C, Aaron DG. The public health potential of social media litigation. *Am J Public Health*. 2026;116(5):596–600.

Acceptance Date: December 19, 2025

DOI: https://doi.org/10.2105/AJPH.2025.308413

ORCID iDs:

Hayden L. Kent https://orcid.org/0009-0003-3379-2251

Carol Vidal https://orcid.org/0000-0001-5104-2284

Daniel G. Aaron https://orcid.org/0000-0003-4490-7504

CONTRIBUTORS

H. L. Kent conceptualized the project and wrote and revised the original draft. C. Vidal wrote portions of the article and edited the full article. D. G. Aaron conceptualized the project, supervised the process, and edited the full article.

CONFLICTS OF INTEREST

Daniel G. Aaron receives funding from Arnold Ventures. The authors report no other conflicts of interest.

REFERENCES

1. Goggin B. Did TikTok videos inspire a teen's suicide? His mom says she found graphic evidence. Available at: https://www.nbcnews.com/tech/social-media/tiktok-suicide-videos-lawsuit-social-media-self-harm-rcna146680. Accessed July 22, 2025.
2. Bickham D, Hunt E, Bediou B, Rich M. Adolescent media use: attitudes, effects, and online experiences. Available at: https://digitalwellnesslab.org/pulse-surveys/adolescent-media-use-attitudes-effects-and-online-experiences. Accessed November 16, 2025.
3. Mantey DS, Yockey RA, Springer AE. Digital screen time and suicidality during high school: how important is cyberbullying? A mediation analysis using the Youth Risk Behavioral Surveillance Survey, 2011–2019. *Prev Med.* 2023;166:107330. https://doi.org/10.1016/j.ypmed.2022.107330
4. Li TMH, Chan NY, Li CT, et al. The associations of electronic media use with sleep and circadian problems, social, emotional and behavioral difficulties in adolescents. *Front Psychiatry.* 2022;13:892583. https://doi.org/10.3389/fpsyt.2022.892583
5. American Psychological Association. American Psychological Association health advisory on social media use in adolescence. Available at: https://www.apa.org/topics/social-media-internet/health-advisory-adolescent-social-media-use. Accessed November 16, 2025.
6. Vidal C, Sussman C. Problematic social media use or social media addiction in pediatric populations. *Pediatr Clin North Am.* 2025;72(2):291–304. https://doi.org/10.1016/j.pcl.2024.08.005
7. Romo V. Whistleblower's testimony has resurfaced Facebook's Instagram problem. Available at: https://www.npr.org/2021/10/05/1043194385/whistleblowers-testimony-facebook-instagram. Accessed August 1, 2025.
8. Duffy C. State attorneys general launch investigation into Meta-owned Instagram's impact on kids. Available at: https://www.cnn.com/2021/11/18/tech/meta-instagram-kids-attorneys-general-investigation. Accessed July 24, 2025.
9. Aaron DG. Public health in the opioid litigation. Available at: https://loyola-chicago-law-journal.scholasticahq.com/article/77237-public-health-in-the-opioid-litigation. Accessed December 18, 2025.
10. Oliva JD. Opioid multidistrict litigation secrecy. Available at: https://papers.ssrn.com/abstract=3411746. Accessed July 19, 2025.
11. Hunton. Massachusetts AG unveils internal TikTok documents in lawsuit alleging child addiction strategies. Available at: https://www.hunton.com/privacy-and-information-security-law/massachusetts-ag-unveils-internal-tiktok-documents-in-lawsuit-alleging-child-addiction-strategies. Accessed July 19, 2025.
12. Bergman M. Assaulting the citadel of Section 230 immunity: products liability, social media, and the youth mental health crisis. *Lewis Clark Law Rev.* 2023;26(4):1159.
13. American Psychological Association. Potential risks of content, features, and functions: the science of how social media affects youth. Available at: https://www.apa.org/topics/social-media-internet/youth-social-media-2024. Accessed August 22, 2025.

Our "Cannabis" Vocabulary Is Eroding Public Health Safeguards

Matthew E. Rossheim, PhD, MPH

ABOUT THE AUTHOR

The author is with the Department of Health Administration and Health Policy, Texas College of Osteopathic Medicine, University of North Texas Health Science Center, Fort Worth.

Imagine if cigarette companies had convinced Americans to describe tobacco laws as "recreational nicotine policy" or if bottles of vodka were labeled "nonmedical ethanol." It sounds absurd, because it is. Yet, the same linguistic sleight of hand is happening now to support the rapid commercialization of intoxicating tetrahydrocannabinol (THC) products.

Misleading terms such as "recreational," "medical," "adult use," "cannabis," and "hemp" now dominate policy debates, media reporting, public opinion surveys, and even scientific discourse. Although often framed as neutral descriptors, these words act as powerful framing devices. They normalize use, lower perceived risks, and blur critical distinctions between reducing criminal penalties and expanding retail access. As states debate legislation, the president calls for rescheduling, and intoxicating hemp derivatives proliferate nationwide,[1] the vocabulary we use is shaping the policies we face. Words do not merely describe policy environments; they help construct them.

Using language to shape public opinion is hardly new. Tobacco companies promoted terms such as "environmental tobacco smoke" to make secondhand exposure sound less harmful.[2] E-cigarette marketers popularized the term "vapor" to downplay the risks of aerosolized chemicals. This strategy works: using more accurate terminology increases risk perception, which is strongly associated with supporting tobacco-free policies.[3]

HOW INDUSTRY LANGUAGE MASKS RISK AND EXPANDS MARKETS

A prominent example in THC discourse is the term "recreational" marijuana, which evokes casual, low-risk activities. In stark contrast, today's THC products carry substantial risks including addiction, psychosis, impairment, traffic crashes, injuries, and poisonings.[4] The label recreational was not coined by clinicians or epidemiologists; it emerged from ballot initiatives and industry messaging designed to make commercial THC products sound like low-risk entertainment.

"Medical marijuana" sounds reassuring, but it is a political label, not a medical one. Clinical evidence does not support cannabis as an effective treatment for most conditions that qualify patients for state programs.[5] The only cannabinoid medications approved by the Food and Drug Administration (FDA) are those designed to treat HIV/AIDS-related anorexia, chemotherapy-induced nausea and vomiting, and certain pediatric seizure disorders. In state dispensaries, "medical" products routinely include smoked/vaped flower and high-potency concentrates (often 70%–95% THC), products fundamentally different from FDA-approved medications.

Research supports that state medical programs facilitate use unrelated to qualifying conditions; for example, from 2018 to 2021, Arizona's medical market showed a 120-pound per-day sales spike on average during the week of 4/20.[6] Medical programs also serve as the pathway to commercial markets. Support for legalization is much higher when THC products are described as "medical."[7] This appears related to perceptions that "medical" use is more moral and less addictive, harmful, and impairing.[7] Because "nonmedical" is implicitly defined against "medical," both terms reinforce the misconception that THC products carry inherent therapeutic value.

Many professionals avoid the word marijuana because of its racialized history and have adopted cannabis as a more neutral alternative. However, cannabis evokes the image of a natural plant, contrasting sharply with today's THC market, which increasingly relies on synthesized cannabinoids.[8] The botanical term obscures distinctions between plant material and manufactured intoxicants, potentially lowering risk perceptions.

Overly broad terminology creates confusion that industry actors exploit. Cannabis refers to a plant used to create products in many categories: textiles, cosmetics, nutritious foods, and nonintoxicating cannabidiol (CBD). None of these products are the focus of contemporary THC policy debates.

AJPH May 2026, Vol. 116, No. 5

When states pass "cannabis laws," they are not regulating soap or lotions; they are expanding commercial access to intoxicants. This market expansion raises equity concerns, consistent with patterns observed in alcohol and tobacco markets: the populations most exposed to harms—including youths, lower-income communities, and historically marginalized groups—are often the least resourced to absorb the resulting health and social consequences.[9]

Companies also exploit the word "hemp." By calling their intoxicating THC products hemp, they attempt to evade marijuana laws while framing regulatory efforts as irrational attacks on harmless, nonintoxicating goods. In efforts to reduce associated harms, several states have recently enacted laws to regulate intoxicating hemp products. However, in doing so, many inadvertently created state-legalized THC markets for products that remain federally illicit. Public Law 119–37, enacted on November 12, 2025, further clarifies the federal illegality of these products by redefining hemp to explicitly exclude products containing synthesized cannabinoids or more than 0.3% intoxicating cannabinoids by weight or 0.4 milligrams per container. This policy direction was recommended in the National Academies of Sciences, Engineering, and Medicine 2024 report *Cannabis Policy Impacts Public Health and Health Equity*.[4] The law includes a one-year implementation period and represents an important step toward protecting public health that industry groups are already mobilizing to overturn.

"Adult use" is another industry-driven framing term that conveys a false sense of strong youth protections. The THC industry often cites alcohol and tobacco as models of effective regulation. Yet, alcohol and tobacco remain the substances most commonly used by underage youths.[10] Evidence demonstrates that expanded retail availability increases access for everyone—including youths—regardless of age gating.[11]

Terms such as "cannabis reform" and "liberalization" suggest that expanding access is inherently progressive; critics are cast as prohibitionists, polarizing debates. This rhetoric blurs two distinct policy domains: decriminalization, which advances social justice by reducing penalties for possessing small quantities, and commercialization, which expands retail markets, use, and associated harms. Misleading language collapses them into a false dichotomy—criminalize or commercialize—and public health and equity suffer in both scenarios.[12]

Rescheduling illustrates similar dynamics. Scheduling is intended to reflect abuse potential, pharmacological effects, and demonstrated safety and efficacy. That evidence has not changed in ways that would justify rescheduling. Yet on December 18, 2025, the president issued an executive order directing agencies to expedite rescheduling to Schedule III, framing it as a way to expand research—an emphasis reflected in the order's title.

However, the primary barriers to clinical research are FDA drug approval requirements, which rescheduling does not change. Schedule III substances—such as dronabinol (Marinol)—must be FDA approved, prescribed by a licensed clinician, and dispensed through a pharmacy registered by the Drug Enforcement Administration. Rescheduling will not make today's marijuana markets federally legal or meaningfully expedite research.

The real impetus for rescheduling is tax deductions. Rescheduling makes THC products more profitable to sell and makes them appear more medically legitimate than evidence supports. The disconnection between scientific criteria and commercial motivations underscores how THC policy narratives are increasingly shaped by industry framing rather than scientific evidence.

Language is not merely symbolic; it shapes how the public perceives risk and how policymakers set regulatory priorities. As intoxicating THC products proliferate—and with Public Law 119–37 clarifying the federal illegality of many such products—states should reconsider how their terminology, definitions, and policies align with public health goals.

RECLAIMING PUBLIC HEALTH VOCABULARY

Borrowing from tobacco control, states that prohibit the commercial and medical sale of THC products could be described as having "100% THC-free policies" or "comprehensive THC prevention policies." By contrast, states authorizing commercial THC markets constitute weak prevention environments characterized by widespread retail availability, expansive advertising, and an industry empowered to lobby for increasingly permissive regulations.

Importantly, THC must be defined broadly enough to encompass cannabinoids with similar effects. As companies reengineer products to exploit definitional gaps,[1,8] statutory language and policy discourse must evolve to prevent so-called loopholes from expanding commercial access.

Industry actors have strategically framed expanded intoxicant markets as modern, recreational, medical, and adult only. Public health must reclaim the vocabulary, not to oppose decriminalization but to ensure clarity regarding the implications of commercialization.

We cannot effectively shape policy using terminology that obscures risk, minimizes complexity, and echoes industry messaging. If public health does not define the vocabulary, industry will. And once the language is lost, policy battles become far more difficult to win. AJPH

CORRESPONDENCE

Correspondence should be sent to Matthew E. Rossheim, PhD, MPH, Texas College of Osteopathic Medicine, University of North Texas Health Science Center, 3500 Camp Bowie Blvd, Fort Worth, TX 76107 (e-mail: matthew.rossheim@unthsc.edu). Reprints can be ordered at https://www.ajph.org by clicking the "Reprints" link.

PUBLICATION INFORMATION

Full Citation: Rossheim ME. Our "cannabis" vocabulary is eroding public health safeguards. *Am J Public Health*. 2026;116(5):601–603.

Acceptance Date: December 30, 2025

DOI: https://doi.org/10.2105/AJPH.2025.308415

ORCID iD:
Matthew E. Rossheim https://orcid.org/0000-0003-4388-5251

CONFLICTS OF INTEREST

The author manages an independent consulting firm and receives compensation for presentations and consultations, including expert work in litigation against the alcohol, cannabis, tobacco, and kratom industries. Neither the author nor his consulting firm accepts funding from these industries.

REFERENCES

1. Rossheim ME, LoParco CR, Tillett KK, et al. Intoxicating cannabis products in vape shops: United States, 2023. *Am J Prev Med*. 2024;67(5):776–784. https://doi.org/10.1016/j.amepre.2024.07.001
2. Eubanks SY, Glantz SA. *Bad Acts: The Racketeering Case Against the Tobacco Industry*. American Public Health Association; 2013.
3. Rossheim ME, Zhao X, Soule EK, et al. Aerosol, vapor, or chemicals? College student perceptions of harm from electronic cigarettes and support for a tobacco-free campus policy. *J Am Coll Health*. 2022;70(6):1754–1760. https://doi.org/10.1080/07448481.2020.1819293
4. National Academies of Sciences, Engineering, and Medicine. *Cannabis Policy Impacts Public Health and Health Equity*. National Academies Press; 2024. https://doi.org/10.17226/27766
5. Hsu M, Shah A, Jordan A, Gold MS, Hill KP. Therapeutic use of cannabis and cannabinoids: a review. *JAMA*. 2026;334(4):345–359. https://doi.org/10.1001/jama.2025.19433
6. Meier MH, Meier MA, Anderson SF, et al. The effects of the 4/20 cannabis holiday and adult-use cannabis legalization on medical cannabis sales and medical cannabis patient registration in Arizona. *Int J Drug Policy*. 2023;114:103974. https://doi.org/10.1016/j.drugpo.2023.103974
7. Mikos RA, Kam CD. Has the "M" word been framed? Marijuana, cannabis, and public opinion. *PLoS One*. 2019;14(10):e0224289. https://doi.org/10.1371/journal.pone.0224289
8. Rossheim ME, Tillett KK, Vasilev V, et al. Types and brands of derived psychoactive cannabis products: an online retail assessment, 2023. *Cannabis Cannabinoid Res*. 2024;9(6):1478–1481. https://doi.org/10.1089/can.2023.0266
9. Kephart LL, Rees VW, Giovenco DP, Subramanian SV. The unequal geography of recreational cannabis retailers in the U.S. *Am J Prev Med*. 2025;69(2):107643. https://doi.org/10.1016/j.amepre.2025.107643
10. Substance Abuse and Mental Health Services Administration. Key substance use and mental health indicators in the United States: results from the 2024 National Survey on Drug Use and Health. Available at: https://www.samhsa.gov/data/sites/default/files/reports/rpt56287/2024-nsduh-annual-national-report.pdf. Accessed December 1, 2025.
11. Rossheim ME, Treffers RD, Sparks AC, et al. The evolving alcohol landscape: implications for public health and policy. *J Stud Alcohol Drugs*. 2025;86(3):323–329. https://doi.org/10.15288/jsad.24-00339
12. Jernigan DH, Ramirez RL, Castrucci BC, Patterson CD, Castillo G, eds. *Cannabis: Moving Forward—Protecting Health*. American Public Health Association; 2021. https://doi.org/10.2105/9780875533186

On the 20th Anniversary of the National Board of Public Health Examiners: It Is Long Past Time We Became a Profession

Donna J. Petersen, ScD, MHS, CPH, Allison Foster, MBA, CPH, Jaime W. Corvin, PhD, MSPH, CPH, and Paul K. Halverson, DrPH, CPH

ABOUT THE AUTHORS

Donna J. Petersen and Jaime W. Corvin are with the University of South Florida College of Public Health, Tampa. Allison Foster is with the National Board of Public Health Examiners, Washington, DC. Paul K. Halverson is with the Oregon Health & Science University, Portland State University School of Public Health, Portland, OR.

AJPH May 2026, Vol. 116, No. 5

It has been nearly 25 years since Al Sommer and Mohammed Akhter[1,2] called for public health to become a profession and 20 years since that call was answered with the creation of the National Board of Public Health Examiners.[3–5] Since the first Certified in Public Health (CPH) exam was offered in 2008, more than 14 000 people have earned a CPH, including those with and without public health degrees from all over the world.[6] These numbers are insufficient to raise the status of public health as a critical and credible profession essential to assuring the public's interest in attaining and maintaining good health. Here we issue an urgent call for the field to throw its entire weight behind certification to finally and fully affirm our status as professionals, promote quality in preprofessional and postprofessional education, and honor our responsibility to be accountable to the public we serve.

As a mission-driven enterprise, public health attracts people from many different disciplines who share a set of values and a mutual desire to improve quality of life through improvements in health. Its disciplinary diversity is one of the great strengths of public health. It is also one of its greatest weaknesses, as this diversity perpetuates the idea that public health is not a singular profession and that anyone who chooses to work in it is, by definition, a public health professional.

The Oxford Languages dictionary defines a profession as "a paid occupation, especially one that involves prolonged training *and a formal qualification*" (emphasis added).[7] A profession is a vocation, requiring specialized training and skills based on an established body of knowledge. Professionals adhere to professional standards, belong to professional associations, and follow industry-specific codes of ethics.[8] For all other health professions, board certification is considered the gold standard for credentialing.[9]

Importantly, a profession is also associated with a level of respect, typically tied directly to the recognition granted through certification. In public health, as the only health care profession without a required certification, the absence is glaring. The lack of a unifying credential signifying that individuals have earned professional status weakens the public health profession at a time when the public would be best served by a recognized profession respected for its specific contributions to the public good.

Sommer and Akhter, in calling for the development of certification on behalf of their respective organizations (the Association of Schools of Public Health, now the Association of Schools and Programs of Public Health, and the American Public Health Association [APHA]),[1,2] simply realized that public health as a field received too little attention and its workers too little respect given the enormity of their responsibility and the challenging environments within which they toiled on behalf of an unknowing public. Public health has been called an invisible shield, which has a romantic cache but in practical terms perpetuates a lack of acknowledgment, credibility, and status in the community and among other peer professional groups. In fact, public health is a profession, and it deserves to be recognized, fully and respectfully, for the important work it does.

The effort to create a board focused on public health certification was a collaborative one between APHA and the Association of Schools of Public Health. A joint task force recommended the creation of the National Board of Public Health Examiners; the inaugural board, convened in 2005, enhanced this academic–practice partnership including representatives from the Association of Prevention Teaching and Research, the Association of State and Territorial Health Officers, and the

National Association of City and County Health Officials.

The National Board of Medical Examiners was selected through an open bid process to guide the development of the CPH exam. The stellar reputation of the board and the rigorous development and testing of the exam assured the field that the exam was valid and reliable; it consistently demonstrates psychometric rigor.

When the exam was launched in 2008, there was support but also skepticism from within academia and across the practice field. Some felt that public health was somehow different from other professions; to some who did not believe that public health is a discipline, certification did not make sense. Others thought it highly unlikely that higher wages would be available for certified individuals in resource-constrained governmental agencies or believed that certification was redundant for those with earned degrees in public health. Supporters saw certification as a means to elevate the entire field, consistent with the broad vision for public health itself. Furthermore, certification would create parity with other health professions and assure the public that the workforce was qualified.

Initially, eligibility was limited to alumni and, later, graduate students of schools and programs accredited by the Council on Education for Public Health. In response to requests from people working in the field, eligibility was expanded in 2016, realizing the original vision to professionalize the field by offering certification to the public health workforce regardless of specialty area, work setting, or academic background. Expanding eligibility to the workforce encouraged a reorientation of the exam to reflect the work performed by professionals rather than the curriculum learned by graduates. The National Board of Public Health Examiners 2017 "Job Task Analysis" altered the content but also confirmed considerable overlap between the jobs performed by the workforce and the competencies required by the Council on Education for Public Health.[10]

Schools and programs that require or strongly encourage their students to take the CPH can use data on examinee performance to assess the quality of their curricula and to ensure that their students are well prepared at the time of graduation. Students benefit by graduating with both a degree and certification, confirming their membership in the public health profession. Yet, many schools and programs neither require nor encourage certification. The reluctance of academic public health leaders to support certification has two profound consequences: (1) it renders nearly every governmental public health agency bereft of certified professionals, and (2) it renders invisible the thousands of public health alumni who contribute to the public's health through other governmental agencies, the private sector, and the nonprofit sector.

Earning certification confers on the individual a responsibility to maintain certification through lifelong professional development. This requirement was one of the major reasons a certification system was proposed; it created another element of parity with all other health professionals, enabled lifelong learners to earn credit for their efforts, and created another opportunity for greater synergy between academic public health and the public health workforce.[11] These synergies led the board to expand its membership to include representatives from both the Council on Education for Public Health and the Public Health Accreditation Board; advocates are highlighting where in these two accreditation processes data on certification can be helpful in demonstrating compliance.

More recently, the board has been approached by health department leaders who see value in incorporating the CPH into their professional development programs. More than 20 health departments have engaged with the board to promote certification for their employees. It requires a significant investment and political will to have large numbers of employees attend exam preparation courses and then sit for the exam. But the rewards are equally significant in gaining a workforce with greater morale, a shared language and body of knowledge, a renewed commitment to the values and the ethical practice of public health, and access to a system that promotes lifelong learning.

The goal of professionalizing public health cannot wait for academic leaders to get over their reluctance to embrace certification or for state and local agencies to recognize the value of certification and secure the necessary investment. Immediate action is essential to achieve this objective now. The imperative voiced 20 years ago remains, even though we find ourselves in a very different moment in history.

Indeed, the fact that the qualifications of some members of our workforce are being questioned solely on the basis of their personal characteristics cannot go unanswered. A new generation of leaders must, with all due haste, mobilize and embrace our collective responsibility to ensure the health and sustainability of the public health workforce. It is vital to our long-term interests that we do so. Certification bolsters the workforce, fuels pride, and encourages respect. Academic and practice leaders need to come together to assure the public that a dedicated, externally validated workforce is acting every day to promote their interest in maintaining good health and a high quality of life. By embracing certification, we will become the visible shield needed to protect the health of the public and guide stronger policies and better practice. It is time for us to deliver on this promise. AJPH

CORRESPONDENCE

Correspondence should be sent to Allison Foster, 1405 S Fern St #256, Arlington, VA 22202 (e-mail: afoster@nbphe.org). Reprints can be ordered at https://www.ajph.org by clicking the "Reprints" link.

PUBLICATION INFORMATION

Full Citation: Petersen DJ, Foster A, Corvin JW, Halverson PK. On the 20th anniversary of the National Board of Public Health Examiners: it is long past time we became a profession. *Am J Public Health*. 2026;116(5):604–606.

Acceptance Date: October 15, 2025

DOI: https://doi.org/10.2105/AJPH.2025.308361

ORCID iDs:

Allison Foster https://orcid.org/0000-0002-6468-7783

Jaime W. Corvin https://orcid.org/0009-0002-7936-7755

CONTRIBUTORS

D.J. Petersen generated the first draft. All of the authors contributed to the conceptualization and revisions of the article.

ACKNOWLEDGMENTS

We thank Charles Mahan and Al Sommer for early conversations that inspired this article.

CONFLICTS OF INTEREST

The authors have no conflicts of interest, financial or otherwise, related to the work reported in this article.

REFERENCES

1. Sommer A, Akhter MN. It's time we became a profession. *Am J Public Health*. 2000;90(6):845–846.
2. Akhter MN. Professionalizing the public health workforce: the case for certification. *J Public Health Manag Pract*. 2001;7(4):46–49.
3. Gebbie K, Goldstein BD, Gregorio DI, et al. The National Board of Public Health Examiners: credentialing public health graduates. *Public Health Rep*. 2007;122(4):435–440.
4. Goldstein BD. Credentialing in public health: the time has come. *J Public Health Manag Pract*. 2008;14(1):1–2.
5. Goldstein B. Credentialing of the public health workforce. *Commonwealth*. 2008;14(1):137–162.
6. National Board of Public Health Examiners. CPH eligibility requirements. Available at: https://www.nbphe.org. Accessed March 20, 2025.
7. Oxford Languages. Definition of profession. Available at: https://languages.oup.com/google-dictionary-en. Accessed January 6, 2025.
8. Greenwood E. Attributes of a profession. *Soc Work*. 1957;2(3):45–55. http://www.jstor.org/stable/23707630.
9. Chappell KB, Howard MS, Lundmark V, Ivory C. Credentialing and certification: overview, science, and impact on policy, regulation, and practice. *Int Nurs Rev*. 2021;68(4):551–556. https://doi.org/10.1111/inr.12721.
10. Foster A, King LR, Bender K. Are public health academia, professional certification, and public health practice on the same page? *J Public Health Manag Pract*. 2018;24(suppl 3):S47–S50.
11. Dwelle TL, Halverson PK, Petersen DJ. Not so strange bedfellows: how practice and academic together will ensure the future of the public health workforce. *J Public Health Manag Pract*. 2015;21(suppl 6):S11–S12.

Fifty Years of PL 93-638: Learning From Our Past, Planning for the Future of American Indian Health Governance

Tassy Parker, PhD, RN, Larissa Teunis, DrPH, MPA, Norman Cooeyate, MCRP, and Allyson Kelley, DrPH, MPH

ABOUT THE AUTHORS

Tassy Parker, Larissa Teunis, and Norman Cooeyate are with the Center for Native American Health, Health Sciences Center, University of New Mexico, Albuquerque. Allyson Kelley is with Allyson Kelley & Associates PLLC, Sisters, OR.

As we write this editorial, 50 years have passed since the enactment of PL 93-638—the Indian Self-Determination and Education Assistance Act of 1975—which aimed to transfer control of health care and education from the federal government to Tribal Nations. It remains the most significant piece of legislation supporting Tribal sovereignty in modern US history. However, PL 93-638 falls short of fulfilling its trust and treaty obligations to uphold equitable, accessible, and culturally grounded health care for American Indian/Alaska Native (AI/AN) communities.[1]

FIFTY YEARS, PERSISTENT DISPARITIES

In 2006, Jones's landmark article "The Persistence of American Indian Health Disparities" emphasized that these inequities stem not only from poor access to health care but also from more profound disparities in wealth, power, and structural opportunities—conditions PL 93-638 sought to correct by empowering Tribal leadership.[2]

PL 93-638 was followed by the Indian Health Care Improvement Act (PL 94–437) in 1976, reaffirming the federal government's obligation to elevate the health status of AI/AN people by expanding preventive services and funding for the Indian Health Service (IHS).[3] Over subsequent decades, Title I of PL 93-638 expanded contracting options with the Bureau of Indian Affairs and IHS, and by 2000, Title V allowed Tribes to compact and assume control over health care delivery. As of April 2025, 118 compacts and 145 funding agreements exist between IHS and Tribes or Tribal organizations, reflecting significant progress in self-governance.[4]

PROMISES WITHOUT INFRASTRUCTURE

Despite these advances, the promise of self-determination remains only partially realized. More than half of federally recognized Tribes have negotiated self-governance compacts, yet many lack resources, staffing, and infrastructure to manage their own systems.[1] Contract support costs remain a significant barrier—particularly when IHS fails to reimburse Tribal programs for third-party billing costs because of insufficient congressional funding.

AI/AN people access the IHS health care system through three primary systems: IHS facilities, Tribal health programs, and urban Indian health organizations, collectively known as "I/T/U." Although some AI/ANs have access through state-funded programs or private insurance companies, for AI/ANs living in rural and reservation areas, I/T/U systems are often the only places to access health care. Nearly 20% of AI/ANs are uninsured, making up the largest uninsured population in the United States.[1]

Chronic underfunding, leadership gaps, inadequate facilities, equipment shortages, and persistent staffing deficits have led to serious quality and access issues. IHS is funded at just 50% of need, and the US Government Accountability Office has placed the agency at high risk, citing possible fraud, waste, abuse, and mismanagement.[1] A 2019 Office of Inspector General report found that IHS lacked formal structures, clear policies, and defined roles and lines of authority.[5] This lack of organization has resulted in minimal accountability and has left agency leaders with little confidence in IHS's ability to sustain care.

The IHS strategic plan for 2025 through 2029 aims to transform operations into a unified, centrally managed system, but this approach does not prioritize self-determination or Tribal sovereignty.[6] Instead, it risks recentralizing authority and perpetuating a colonial system that has consistently failed to meet AI/AN health needs. IHS realignment efforts have largely bypassed legally mandated Tribal Consultation,

AJPH May 2026, Vol. 116, No. 5

offering Tribal leaders rushed in-person "listening sessions" instead of meaningful engagement, according to comments made during the Virtual Urban Confer held July 28, 2025. PL 93-638 was designed to empower Tribes, yet in practice, it falls short. Ultimately, little has changed since the 1975 Government Accountability Office report, which identified multiple structural and bureaucratic obstacles.[7]

A NEW MODEL OF HEALTH

The life expectancy of AI/AN people born in 2021 is 65.2 years—10 years less than the general population and the lowest life expectancy of any racial or ethnic group in the United States.[8] This stark disparity highlights the urgent need for additional support, funding, and training to enable Tribes to self-govern their health services and systems. When Tribes design and run their own health systems, services better reflect community needs, incorporate language and culture, and integrate traditional medicine, which helps address historical trauma and the distrust of health care providers.[9–11]

Current IHS practices fail to reflect core AI/AN values, such as relationship, trust, reciprocity, community, and connection to the land. By contrast, models such as the Southcentral Foundation's Nuka System of Care—a customer-owned, relationship-based system developed by an Alaska Native–owned nonprofit health care organization that serves more than 70 000 individuals—demonstrate that health systems aligned with these values can more effectively serve the needs of AI/AN populations.[10] Expanding and adapting models such as these across IHS could guide the transformation toward culturally grounded, community-driven health systems that elevate the health, well-being, and welfare of AI/AN people. Without these structural reforms, expecting Tribes to "fix" an underperforming and misaligned system negates the original treaty and trust obligations of the US government.

Proposed fiscal year 2026 funding cuts to US Department of Health and Human Services (HHS) programs and ongoing efforts to reorganize federal health systems threaten to destabilize AI/AN health services further. These moments of wide-scale change prompt critical questions: Will Tribal voices shape the next 25 years of public health and health care delivery, transitioning federal Indian policy from self-determination to self-governance? Or will the federal government continue to offer promises it cannot or will not keep?

REENVISIONING PL 93-638 IN 2050

PL 93-638 was a landmark in Tribal self-determination, yet its structure and chronic underfunding continue to limit genuine sovereignty, reducing self-governance to delegated federal authority rather than independent control. IHS retains significant control under Titles I and V, limiting true Tribal governance. Tribes must be restored as equal partners in a phased fashion, with IHS redefined as an advocate and negotiator rather than an operator. Historical paternalistic practices must be explicitly identified, dismantled, and replaced with Indigenous-led frameworks for technical assistance and governance to improve health outcomes for AI/AN communities. Current colonial health models—driven by economic, political, and corporate interests—undermine Tribal sovereignty and perpetuate inequities. A decolonized health system must center Indigenous governance, community priorities, and culturally grounded care to achieve lasting health equity.[12] Halfway through the next 50 years, the following systematic and sustained actions can lead to progress toward promoting AI/AN well-being:

- IHS must deconstruct systems that have failed to deliver quality care. New health systems should be built based on Tribal values, practices, and wisdom, with Tribes leading the design and governance.
- IHS must provide tailored training and technical assistance for Tribal leaders and communities based on their level of readiness to design and govern their own health care systems. Even though Tribes are sovereign nations, their contracted and compacted health systems might mimic the federal system, which has produced poor and unreliable outcomes.
- HHS must examine health disparities for AI/AN communities through the lens of structural and social determinants of health, including inadequate education, poverty, cultural barriers, and poor health care services. Addressing the root causes of limited health care access, underfunding, and disparities in quality and treatment are essential to achieving health equity.
- The federal government must promote insurance coverage and parity for AI/AN people, addressing economic, political, and socioeconomic factors that contribute to poor health and premature death.
- HHS leadership must change how IHS is funded and operated in HHS. Funding must honor treaty rights

and the federal promise to elevate AI/AN health to the highest level in the nation.

- The federal government must require administrators to engage in Tribal Consultation as a foundational step in developing and implementing federal policies and programs affecting AI/AN people. Such actions should include those with lived experience and cultural knowledge to help shape funding decisions and define community needs. Federal approaches must shift from paternalistic control to models rooted in reciprocity, community ownership, and cultural sovereignty.

Now is the time to honor treaty rights, trust responsibilities, and Tribal sovereignty through robust implementation of PL 93-638. The success of Tribes reclaiming and reimagining their futures, destinies, and equity in quality care and health as self-determined and self-governed must be celebrated and supported. The next 25 years should be marked by a transition from federal control to true Tribal self-governance, with Tribes leading and designing health systems that reflect their unique cultural values and meet their communities' needs. AJPH

CORRESPONDENCE

Correspondence should be sent to Dr. Tassy Parker, 1001 Medical Arts Blvd NE, Albuquerque, NM 87102 (e-mail: TaParker@salud.unm.edu). Reprints can be ordered at https://www.ajph.org by clicking the "Reprints" link.

PUBLICATION INFORMATION

Full Citation: Parker T, Teunis L, Cooeyate N, Kelley A. Fifty years of PL 93-638: learning from our past, planning for the future of American Indian health governance. *Am J Public Health*. 2026;116(5): 607–609.

Acceptance Date: November 20, 2025.

DOI: https://doi.org/10.2105/AJPH.2025.308374

ORCID iD:

Larissa Teunis https://orcid.org/0000-0001-7144-9073

CONTRIBUTORS

T. Parker conceptualized the editorial and led the overall intellectual direction of the work. L. Teunis drafted the editorial and contributed to conceptual development. N. Cooeyate reviewed the editorial for consistency and provided contextual and cultural guidance. A. Kelley critically reviewed the editorial. All authors contributed to writing and editing and take full responsibility for the integrity of the work presented.

ACKNOWLEDGMENTS

This editorial is dedicated to those we have lost because the system failed them. They left us too soon. A better system could have extended their lives and the well-being of their communities and families.

CONFLICTS OF INTEREST

The authors have no conflicts of interest to disclose.

REFERENCES

1. Racehorse VA. Tribal health self-determination: the role of Tribal health systems in actualizing the highest attainable standard of health for American Indians and Alaska Natives. *Columbia Human Rights Law Review*. In press.
2. Jones DS. The persistence of American Indian health disparities. *Am J Public Health*. 2006;96(12): 2122–2134. https://doi.org/10.2105/ajph.2004.054262
3. Warne D, Frizzell LB. American Indian health policy: historical trends and contemporary issues. *Am J Public Health*. 2014;104(suppl 3):S263–S267. https://doi.org/10.2105/ajph.2013.301682
4. Indian Health Service. Self-governance tribes. Available at: https://www.ihs.gov/selfgovernance/tribes. Accessed December 10, 2025.
5. US Department of Health and Human Services. Organizational challenges to improving quality of care in Indian Health Service hospitals. August 27, 2025. Available at: https://oig.hhs.gov/reports/all/2019/organizational-challenges-to-improving-quality-of-care-in-indian-health-service-hospitals. Accessed November 3, 2025.
6. Indian Health Service. Indian Health Service strategic plan. Fiscal years 2025–2029. 2025. Available at: https://www.ihs.gov/sites/newsroom/themes/responsive2017/display_objects/documents/2024_Letters/Enclosure_DTLL_DUIOLL_100124.pdf. Accessed August 5, 2025.
7. US Government Accountability Office. The Indian Self-Determination Act: many obstacles remain (HRD-78-59). 1978. Available at: https://www.gao.gov/assets/hrd-78-59.pdf. Accessed November 3, 2025.
8. Parker T, Kelley A. American Indian and Alaska Native life expectancy. *JAMA*. 2023;330(21): 2053–2054. https://doi.org/10.1001/jama.2023.22614
9. Roubideaux Y. Perspectives on American Indian health. *Am J Public Health*. 2002;92(9):1401–1403. https://doi.org/10.2105/ajph.92.9.1401
10. Southcentral Foundation. Nuka system of care. 2025. Available at: https://www.southcentralfoundation.com/nuka-system-of-care. Accessed December 10, 2025.
11. Reese SE, Dang A, Liddell JL. "We'd just patch ourselves up": preference for holistic approaches to healthcare and traditional medicine among members of a state-recognized tribe. *J Holist Nurs*. 2024;42(1):34–48. https://doi.org/10.1177/08980101231169867
12. Barcham M. Decolonizing public healthcare systems: designing with Indigenous peoples. *She Ji*. 2022;8(4):454–472. https://doi.org/10.1016/j.sheji.2022.10.004

From "Informant" to "Influencer": Reframing Research Language to Build Trust in Marginalized Communities

Amanda I. Aguila Gonzalez, PhD, MPH, Babalola Faseru, MBChB, MPH, CPH, Vicki Collie-Akers, PhD, and Elizabeth Ablah, PhD, MPH, CPH

ABOUT THE AUTHORS

Amanda I. Aguila Gonzalez and Elizabeth Ablah are with the Department of Population Health, University of Kansas School of Medicine-Wichita. Babalola Faseru and Vicki Collie-Akers are with the Department of Population Health, University of Kansas Medical Center, Kansas City.

AJPH May 2026, Vol. 116, No. 5

To ensure that research findings are relevant, equitable, and reflective of human experiences, it is essential that diverse communities engage in research. Historically, Black/African American and Hispanic/Latinx communities have been underrepresented,[1–3] resulting in knowledge gaps, limited generalizability, and interventions that do not adequately serve all populations.[3] Effective engagement requires culturally sensitive recruitment strategies and inclusive language.

Language is not a neutral tool for communication; it reflects and reinforces cultural understanding and interpersonal and community power dynamics.[4] In community-based research, terminology can facilitate or hinder meaningful engagement, trust, relationship building, information sharing, and the sense of agency that community members experience throughout the process.[5,6] Developing a safe and inclusive environment is essential, and language that is culturally insensitive unnecessarily reinforces barriers to creating this environment. Researchers' use of inclusive framing language can empower community members, fostering a sense of collaboration, understanding, and respect.[5]

INFORMANT INTERVIEWS IN COMMUNITY-BASED RESEARCH

Strong community relationships are essential for social and behavioral health researchers and practitioners (henceforth referred to as "researchers") to effectively address community issues. Community members' perspectives and insights highlight community needs, assets, and priorities that can guide culturally relevant and appropriate solutions. To foster connectivity and trust, community-based methods such as needs assessments, asset mapping, listening sessions, and key informant interviews are foundational.[6]

Key informant interviews, which originated in anthropology and ethnography,[7] are widely used in social, behavioral, and medical research to gain deep insights from knowledgeable individuals, often in a social or cultural context.[5,6,8] Conducted in private, safe settings, these interviews help researchers understand diverse community perspectives on specific topics.

However, the term "key informant" may negatively affect community participation and trust, as it carries deeply negative connotations, especially among Black/African American and Hispanic/Latinx communities. Negative associations regarding the term "informant" are rooted in systemic racism,[9] civil rights abuses, and experiences during the "war on drugs."[10] The term "informant" implicitly evokes feelings of surveillance, betrayal, and exploitation, resulting in mistrust and reluctance to participate in qualitative research.[11,12] Accordingly, it is critical that we as researchers carefully consider the cultural connotations and emotional impact of the term "key informant."

The term "informant" is derived from a word meaning to inform, instruct, or teach.[13] The original intent of the term "key informant" in community-based research was to highlight the esteemed role of the community member. It was intended to acknowledge and honor the unique wisdom, cultural insights, and lived experiences shared by those being interviewed.[8] Previous studies have outlined the ideal qualities of key informants, including being willing to engage, having a key role within a community, being knowledgeable about the issue researchers are studying, and having the ability to share experiences and insights in a unique way.[7,8] Through this lens, community members are recognized for actively shaping the direction of research, its methods and results, and interpretations of the data.

However, using the word "informant" can unintentionally reinforce mistrust among communities of color, especially Black/African American and Hispanic/Latinx populations. This mistrust stems from historical trauma related to systemic racism, harmful law enforcement practices, and negative associations with the term "informant" as a "snitch" or "betrayer" within these communities.[14–16] Within the Black/African American community, the term "informant" may evoke negative associations with law enforcement and the criminal legal system. In one study, individuals who reported negative encounters with the police had higher levels of medical and institutional mistrust than those without such experiences.[14]

Similarly, for the Hispanic/Latinx, the word "informant," often referred to as "*informante de policía*" (i.e., police informant), connotes a sense of surveillance betrayal: that someone is monitoring their community and reporting information to authorities. In Spanish, the term "informant" may be associated with the terms "*chota*," "*soplón*," or "*chivato*," depending on the country of origin. These terms are commonly used to describe police informants, often perceived as traitors in the Hispanic/Latinx community.[17] Promoting research opportunities using "key informant interviews" may provoke fear, such as concerns about community backlash for being labeled an informant or anxiety that information shared could be used by the government to discriminate against or harm individuals. This fear may affect the likelihood of Hispanic/Latinx community members engaging in research.

Furthermore, distrust of medical research, especially in the Black/African American community, stems from historical exploitation and harmful medical practices inflicted upon Black individuals and other racial and ethnic minorities. For example, the Tuskegee Syphilis Study involved Black men who were recruited without being accurately informed about the study's true purpose and denied necessary medical treatment.[18,19] Research conducted with Black/African American adults has indicated that the phrase "medical research" carries negative connotations, often equating participation with being a "guinea pig" subjected to experimentation.[12] Widespread mistrust among members of the Black/African American community toward medical research and governmental institutions has been identified as a significant barrier to their participation in research studies.[12]

In addition, the term "informant" may unintentionally suggest to individuals in some communities that researchers expect community members to share sensitive or valuable information with authorities and outsiders, which can feel exploitative and undermine trust-building efforts. Moreover, this positions researchers as authority figures, fundamentally at odds with community-based research approaches. Particularly within Black/African American and Hispanic/Latinx communities, using this term might cause individuals to become wary of their own or others' involvement in research, reduce overall engagement, and foster distrust toward researchers. Such outcomes would directly oppose the goals of community-based research. This mistrust hinders the development of essential research that accurately reflects community diversity and prevents the creation of culturally appropriate methods and intervention strategies. Therefore, there is a critical need for alternative, inclusive language.

BUILDING A SHARED VOCABULARY: CASE STUDY IN WICHITA, KS

Facts Not Fear Wichita (FNFICT) was a community-based project from 2021 through 2024 in Wichita, Kansas, funded through the City of Wichita by the US Department of Health and Human Services' Office of Minority Health. These funds were designed to advance health literacy and ensure equitable community responses to COVID-19, including Black/African American and Hispanic/Latinx Wichitans. Community members' provision of information regarding their most pressing needs and concerns served as a cornerstone of this project's community-based approach. Although several significant needs were identified, two emerged as primary areas of interest: mental illness and substance use.

Consistent with a participatory approach, FNFICT partners included community champions and faith-based leaders from the Black/African American and Hispanic/Latinx communities, who supported and helped advance project efforts; these partners shaped and influenced research and outreach strategies to ensure that these were culturally responsive and appropriate to the needs of the communities. Researchers developed key informant interview scripts and engaged community members in discussing recruitment strategies. During these conversations, challenges in engaging community members surfaced regarding use of the "key informant" interview terminology.

Participating community partners, who were themselves members of the communities of focus, expressed concerns that promoting interview opportunities using the term "informant"

AJPH May 2026, Vol. 116, No. 5

would be disrespectful and insensitive to the communities' experiences, trust, and association with this term. Additionally, interviews addressing substance use would likely include discussions about illegal substances, further increasing community members' apprehension. Such concerns could significantly undermine the trust that the project team had worked to build. Given that the FNFICT project had previously provided various resources, such as health education resources and mobile vaccination clinics, to these communities, some community members worried that using the term might suggest an expectation to them to reciprocate by serving as "key informants," potentially implying a betrayal of their communities.

PROPOSED VERBIAGE

To build trust and address concerns about discrimination or exploitation, collaborative research language was developed through an inclusive and equitable process. Guided by a community-based research framework, rooted in cultural humility, openness, and collaboration,[5] Black/African American and Hispanic/Latinx community partners were engaged in discussions about terminology to ensure that it reflected their values, perspectives, and lived experiences. The researchers sought to use language that would encourage participation from Black/African American and Hispanic/Latinx communities in qualitative interviews and would strengthen trust.

This process emphasized shared decision-making with community partners, invited feedback and critique, and created space to reflect on how language can either foster inclusion or perpetuate marginalization.[5] Community partners served as equal contributors to the research process. Discussions occurred virtually, facilitated by a researcher who ensured adherence to the community-based research principles and self-identified within one of the populations of focus.

One key concern raised was the use of the term "key informant," which was viewed as carrying negative connotations. Alternatives such as "community member," "participant," and "expert" were considered and deemed acceptable. However, the intent was to preserve the original, revered intention behind the "key informant" concept by adopting a term currently viewed as more culturally appropriate and positively received: "key influencer."

The term "influencer" started becoming popular in the American language during the early 2000s and saw further growth throughout the 2010s with the rise of social media platforms like Facebook, Instagram, TikTok, and X.[20] In that context, an "influencer" refers to someone who generates interest in a product, service, or topic by highlighting it on their social media account, typically to a large audience.[21–23] Social and behavioral scientists, however, use the concept more broadly to describe individuals who have the capacity or authority to shape the behaviors or health-related decisions of others.[20] Key community influencers possess unique insights into the strengths and challenges faced by their communities, and they offer valuable feedback to researchers.[5] These influencers are often trusted community members and leaders whose experiences, expertise, and perspectives can positively affect health behaviors and encourage community support for addressing specific health issues.

For the FNFICT project, the term "key influencer" emerged through multiple meetings with representatives from local community health organizations that advocate for Black/African American and Hispanic/Latinx health. Weekly two-hour virtual meetings were conducted for three months that included four Black/African American and three Hispanic/Latinx individuals, along with representatives of other racial and ethnic groups. Once interview scripts and recruitment materials were drafted, they were presented for feedback on cultural appropriateness and responsiveness. Community partners expressed that recruitment language would not be effective without changes and suggested the adoption of "key influencer."

The team recognized that the term "key influencer" may also imply that an individual holds power in the community that may shape attitudes, norms, and behaviors. By contrast, the original term "informant" refers to someone with insider or specialized knowledge about the community, regardless of their influence over others. To address "influencer" power dynamics, it was important for the group to establish a collaborative definition of this term. The team defined "key influencer" as a leader in one's community or neighborhood who was engaged in community efforts to improve health and well-being, was a trusted source of information among peers, and was willing to share one's experiences and insights. Some community health organization representatives did not identify as influencers in their communities, yet the team emphasized inclusivity and the importance of integrating diverse voices.

Recruitment was led by researchers and community members who were members of the communities they intended to serve and were regarded as trusted individuals within their respective communities, which helped build trust and encourage participation. To avoid perceptions of bias or commercialization, researchers provided a brief description of the interviews, including the types of questions asked and how their input would be used.

Although the acceptability of the term was not measured quantitatively, anecdotal evidence suggested that adopting "key influencer" may reduce stigma, encourage participation, and avoid associations with being a "police informant." This linguistic shift could enable more effective recruitment and foster stronger community trust and engagement.

This approach bolsters the idea that the community's voices need to be included and amplified. By failing to adapt our research terminology and processes to the unique needs of the communities we serve, we are unintentionally creating further gaps between researchers and the community, which may lead to reduced engagement and a lack of trust, potentially exacerbating health disparities. It is critical for future research studies to implement similar community-based research frameworks to ensure that research processes and procedures are culturally responsive and representative of the communities intended to be served.

CONCLUSION

Using more inclusive language creates space for community reflection, underscoring to community members that their voices and experiences are valuable and contribute meaningfully to research. Community perspectives on health issues can help researchers more effectively allocate limited resources to address specific community needs. Additionally, when researchers use culturally sensitive and appropriate language, it fosters trust throughout the research process. The term "influencer" better reflects participants' roles as respected and knowledgeable community leaders whose insights positively shape research outcomes and community benefits.[24] This shift in terminology not only promotes respect and dignity but actively dismantles historical barriers of suspicion and fear associated with research participation.[25] As research efforts continue to advance, it is essential for researchers to adapt language to ensure inclusivity and demonstrate respect. This is particularly important for better understanding and effectively addressing health disparities that affect racial and ethnic communities. AJPH

CORRESPONDENCE

Correspondence should be sent to Amanda I. Aguila Gonzalez, Department of Population Health, University of Kansas School of Medicine-Wichita, 1010 N. Kansas St, Wichita, KS 67214 (e-mail: aaguilagonzalez@kumc.edu). Reprints can be ordered at https://www.ajph.org by clicking the "Reprints" link.

PUBLICATION INFORMATION

Full Citation: Aguila Gonzalez AI, Faseru B, Collie-Akers V, Ablah E. From "informant" to "influencer": reframing research language to build trust in marginalized communities. *Am J Public Health*. 2026; 116(5):610–614.

Acceptance Date: January 19, 2026

DOI: https://doi.org/10.2105/AJPH.2026.308428

ORCID iDs:

Amanda I. Aguila Gonzalez https://orcid.org/0000-0002-2332-5874

Elizabeth Ablah https://orcid.org/0000-0003-4550-2162

CONTRIBUTORS

All authors contributed to the development of the manuscript and reviewed and approved the final version.

ACKNOWLEDGMENTS

This work was supported by grant 1 CPIMP211300-01-00 issued by the Office of the Assistant Secretary for Health of the US Department of Health and Human Services (HHS) as part of a financial assistance award totaling $4 000 000, with 100% funded by the Office of Minority Health/OASH/HHS.

Note. The contents are solely the responsibility of the authors and do not necessarily represent the official views of, nor an endorsement by, the Office of Minority Health/OASH/HHS, or the US Government. For more information, please visit https://minorityhealth.hhs.gov.

CONFLICTS OF INTEREST

The authors have no conflicts of interest to disclose.

HUMAN PARTICIPANT PROTECTION

This study was approved by the institutional review board at the University of Kansas Medical Center (STUDY00160306).

REFERENCES

1. Gwizdala KL, Pugh EA, Carter L, Carmichael OT, Newton RL Jr. Impact of COVID-19 pandemic on research participation among older African Americans. *Alzheimer Dis Assoc Disord.* 2022;36(4): 350–353. https://doi.org/10.1097/WAD.0000000000000512
2. Webber-Ritchey KJ, Lane-Cordova AD. Health disparities and COVID-19 pandemic: increasing clinical research participation among African Americans. *J Health Dispar Res Pract.* 2021;14(2): 1–13.
3. Ceballos RM, Knerr S, Scott MA, et al. Latino beliefs about biomedical research participation: a qualitative study on the US–Mexico border. *J Empir Res Hum Res Ethics.* 2014;9(4):10–21. https://doi.org/10.1177/1556264614544454
4. Saaida M. Language, culture, and power: exploring the dynamics of communication across differences. *Zenodo.* 2023. https://doi.org/10.5281/zenodo.10884324
5. Collins SE, Clifasefi SL, Stanton J, et al. Community-based participatory research (CBPR): towards equitable involvement of community in psychology research. *Am Psychol.* 2018;73(7):884–898. https://doi.org/10.1037/amp0000167
6. Sanders Thompson VL, Ackermann N, Bauer KL, Bowen DJ, Goodman MS. Strategies of community engagement in research: definitions and classifications. *Transl Behav Med.* 2021;11(2): 441–451. https://doi.org/10.1093/tbm/ibaa042
7. Tremblay MA. The Key Informant Technique: a nonethnographic application. *Am Anthropol.* 1957;59(4):688–701. https://doi.org/10.1525/aa.1957.59.4.02a00100
8. Pahwa M, Cavanagh A, Vanstone M. Key informants in applied qualitative health research. *Qual Health Res.* 2023;33(14):1251–1261. https://doi.org/10.1177/10497323231198796
9. Scott-Jones G, CAADC, Kamara MR, PE. The traumatic impact of structural racism on African Americans. *Dela J Public Health.* 2020;6(5):80–82. https://pmc.ncbi.nlm.nih.gov/articles/PMC8352535
10. Hall MF. The "war on drugs": a continuation of the war on the African American family. *Smith Coll Stud Soc Work.* 1997;67(3):609–621. https://doi.org/10.1080/00377319709517509
11. Corbie-Smith G, Thomas SB, Williams MV, Moody-Ayers S. Attitudes and beliefs of African Americans toward participation in medical research. *J Gen Intern Med.* 1999;14(9):537–546. https://doi.org/10.1046/j.1525-1497.1999.07048.x
12. Scharff DP, Mathews KJ, Jackson P, Hoffsuemmer J, Martin E, Edwards D. More than Tuskegee:

understanding mistrust about research participation. *J Health Care Poor Underserved.* 2010;21(3):879–897. https://doi.org/10.1353/hpu.0.0323

13. Oxford English Dictionary. Informer. Available at: https://www.oed.com/dictionary/informer_n?tl=true. Accessed May 13, 2025.
14. Alang S, McAlpine D, McClain M, Hardeman R. Police brutality, medical mistrust and unmet need for medical care. *Prev Med Rep.* 2021;22:101361. https://doi.org/10.1016/j.pmedr.2021.101361
15. Feldman JM, Gruskin S, Coull BA, Krieger N. Killed by police: validity of media-based data and misclassification of death certificates in Massachusetts, 2004–2016. *Am J Public Health.* 2017;107(10):1624–1626. https://doi.org/10.2105/AJPH.2017.303940
16. Neuschatz JS, DeLoach DK, Hillgartner MA, et al. The truth about snitches: an archival analysis of informant testimony. *Psychiatr Psychol Law.* 2021;28(4):508–530. https://doi.org/10.1080/13218719.2020.1805810
17. SpanishDictionary.com. Soplón vs chivato. 2025. Available at: https://www.spanishdict.com/compare/sopl%C3%B3n/chivato. Accessed February 4, 2025.
18. Vonderlehr RA, Clark T, Wenger OC, Heller JR. Untreated syphilis in the male negro: a comparative study of treated and untreated cases. *JAMA.* 1936;17:260–265. https://doi.org/10.1001/jama.1936.02770370020006
19. Center for Disease Control and Prevention. The Untreated Syphilis Study at Tuskegee. Available at: https://www.cdc.gov/tuskegee/about/timeline.html. Accessed January 29, 2025.
20. Powell J, Pring T. The impact of social media influencers on health outcomes: systematic review. *Soc Sci Med.* 2024;340:116472. https://doi.org/10.1016/j.socscimed.2023.116472
21. Engel E, Gell S, Heiss R, Karsay K. Social media influencers and adolescents' health: a scoping review of the research field. *Soc Sci Med.* 2024;340:116387. https://doi.org/10.1016/j.socscimed.2023.116387
22. Freberg K, Graham K, McGaughey K, Freberg LA. Who are the social media influencers? A study of public perceptions of personality. *Public Relat Rev.* 2011;37(1):90–92. https://doi.org/10.1016/j.pubrev.2010.11.001
23. Zou W, Zhang WJ, Tang L. What do social media influencers say about health? A theory-driven content analysis of top ten health influencers' posts on Sina Weibo. *J Health Commun.* 2021;26(1):1–11. https://doi.org/10.1080/10810730.2020.1865486
24. Israel BA, Schulz AJ, Parker EA, Becker AB. Review of community-based research: assessing partnership approaches to improve public health. *Annu Rev Public Health.* 1998;19:173–202. https://doi.org/10.1146/annurev.publhealth.19.1.173
25. Yancey AK, Ortega AN, Kumanyika SK. Effective recruitment and retention of minority research participants. *Annu Rev Public Health.* 2006;27:1–28. https://doi.org/10.1146/annurev.publhealth.27.021405.102113

Addressing Hygiene Poverty and Restoring Dignity: A Community Partnership Through Laundry Love

Elizabeth Ablah, PhD, MPH, CPH, Nadine Long, MPA, Kara Hollins, MPH, Callie Miller, Charell Owings, Kimberly Weaver, Jody Love, MBA, Clarissa Carrillo Martinez, MBA, Tatiana K. Darby, MPH, Ton Miras Neira, BA, Angela Scott, Christina M. Pacheco, JD, MPH, and Sarah Finocchario-Kessler, PhD, MPH

Hygiene poverty is a term describing the inability to afford essential hygiene products such as laundry detergent, toothpaste, menstrual products, or diapers, which profoundly affects dignity. Few community-level strategies have been developed to improve access to hygiene or "dignity" products. This case study from Kansas highlights the process and outcomes of a successful community-driven intervention that originated in one county and was adopted by 10 other Kansas counties. (*Am J Public Health*. 2026;116(5): 615–618. https://doi.org/10.2105/AJPH.2025.308410)

AJPH May 2026, Vol. 116, No. 5

Laundry Love is a national "neighboring movement" that encourages collaboration among residents, organizations, and laundromats to reduce barriers to clean laundry.[1] Through coordination with the national organization, Laundry Love sites receive various resources for chapter startup. Local organizers are encouraged to approach the owner of a laundromat near an underresourced community, describe the intention of the initiative, and work with them to identify a date and time to host a Laundry Love event.

INTERVENTION AND IMPLEMENTATION

The Barton County Local Health Equity Action Team (BCLHEAT) established monthly four-hour Laundry Love events, determining that participants could wash up to five loads at no cost, with no eligibility criteria. Participation was open to all laundromat patrons during events, an intentional choice to promote dignity, avoid stigma, reduce administrative burden, and build rapport and trust with community members. A consistent monthly schedule helped participants plan transportation. A Communities Organizing to Promote Equity (COPE) community health worker (CHW) attended events to build relationships with attendees and offer referrals to local social or health services, as needed.

The BCLHEAT organized and staffed events, promoted events, managed payments, and provided supplemental supports (e.g., establishing bank accounts, food basket distribution). Volunteers welcomed attendees, distributed supplies, and tracked key data (e.g., numbers served, amount spent). Efforts were made to create a welcoming environment; one member sponsored snacks, coloring activities for families with children, and seasonal events (e.g., Santa and Mrs. Claus at a December event).

During a COPE learning collaborative with 19 other Kansas counties,[2] the BCLHEAT shared its model, noting that Laundry Love was relatively easy to establish, supported nationally, and responsive to the pervasive challenge of hygiene poverty. Following this presentation, the BCLHEAT provided technical assistance to interested counties.

PLACE, TIME, AND PERSONS

Barton County (population 25 493) is a nonmetropolitan community[3] in central Kansas with a median income of $56 733.[4] In January 2022, a community coalition was formed through the COPE initiative, an academic–community partnership designed to address the health disparities exacerbated by the COVID-19 pandemic.[5] The BCLHEAT consisted of three stakeholder groups: a CHW hired through COPE, organizational representatives (e.g., nonprofits, service providers, local businesses), and residents who self-identified as having lived experience of inequities (e.g., poverty, racism). The BCLHEAT was one of 20 Kansas coalitions formed through COPE, and each had the discretion to direct their efforts and budget ($50 000 over three years) toward locally identified disparities.

By summer of 2022, after hosting several community events, the BCLHEAT began discussing their next initiative. Members noted growing requests for assistance with laundry because of the high cost of detergent, transportation barriers, and limited access to washing and drying machines. Recognizing this as a pressing community need, the coalition explored solutions, including the national Laundry Love initiative.[1]

PURPOSE

Poverty is a well-documented public health issue in the United States. Individuals experiencing poverty have higher rates of chronic disease, mental illness, and poorer overall health outcomes than those with higher incomes.[6] One critical yet often overlooked aspect of poverty is hygiene. Hygiene poverty is the inability to afford essential products such as laundry detergent, toothpaste, menstrual products, or diapers.[7] Beyond material deprivation, hygiene poverty undermines self-worth and dignity. Families with low incomes are disproportionately affected, often forced to choose between clean clothing and other necessities (e.g., food, shelter). In one national study, 69% of low-income families reported skipping laundry or dishwashing to save money, and 63% reported washing only their children's clothing.[8]

Limited access to hygiene resources is associated with poorer educational, employment, and physical health outcomes.[2,9] Among children, inadequate hygiene contributes to social rejection and bullying in school.[10] Students from low-income households who cannot afford hygiene products are more likely to miss school chronically, which is linked to poor reading skills, lower grades, and higher dropout rates.[11]

EVALUATION AND ADVERSE EFFECTS

Between August 2022 and September 2024, the Barton County Laundry Love effort achieved the following:

- Hosted 27 Laundry Love events, serving 530 families and 1227 individuals with more than 3,000 loads of laundry.
- Secured support from 18 local businesses, civic organizations, churches, and other partners, with seven providing multi-month sponsorships.
- Raised $10 600 in revenue through $400 monthly sponsorships. Expenses totaled $8142 ($7157 in quarters and $985 in supplies such as snacks and a cooler), leaving a balance of $2457. Laundry detergent was donated through the national Laundry Love partnership with Earth Breeze.
- Established cross-sector collaborations that were later leveraged to address other health needs; the United Way established a regional nonprofit network, bringing together more than 40 nonprofits to coordinate and streamline efforts.

The initiative inspired replication across nine other Kansas counties. As of May 30, 2024, COPE Local Health Equity Action Team–initiated Laundry Love statewide programs, not including Barton County, had achieved the following:

- Supported nearly 2500 individual encounters through 94 laundry events, tailored to local needs (e.g., providing quarters for apartment-based laundry units, offering meals, coordinating transportation, distributing laundry baskets).
- Facilitated nearly 180 CHW referrals to local health and social services.

All CHWs hired through COPE were trained to follow up with each client at least three times over a 10-day period to support and ensure referral completion. In the 10 counties included in this analysis, CHWs achieved 95% referral completion (n = 2560). This high proportion suggests strong potential for improving health outcomes. The most commonly accessed services in these counties included food and household items (54%; n = 1440), transportation (7%; n = 191), and housing support (7%; n = 178).

An unanticipated outcome was the program's role in fostering social cohesion. Nonprofit volunteers formed meaningful relationships with residents by engaging in spaces where residents naturally congregate, thereby consistently building trust over time. CHWs facilitated referrals to employment opportunities, crisis services, and other essential resources. Notably, clients referred one another to services, featuring the emergence of peer-to-peer support networks. One BCLHEAT member described the impact:

> We have connected domestic abuse victims to our local crisis center, connected people to jobs, passed on information about resources, talked to clients about their lives, and built trust and connections between the non-profits that volunteer and the people that walk through the door. Clients also have helped each other. Though our volunteers are well-versed, there are some specific issues that we may not be as knowledgeable about. We have had clients referring each other to services based on

specific asks that they have heard us discussing. It is heartwarming to see the connections that have been built. One thing I like to mention when talking about the program is that this is a way for us to go to those in need instead of them having to come to us and ask for help. We are there, consistently, and that goes a long way.

What began as a response to a basic hygiene need has evolved into a monthly community gathering that fosters trust, mutual support, and community pride.

SUSTAINABILITY

Several factors likely contribute to the sustainability of the Laundry Love intervention. First, the ongoing demand for dignity-related products and services reflects the widespread nature of hygiene poverty. Such efforts are imperative when holistically addressing the physical health (e.g., infections, illnesses) and mental health (e.g., stress, anxiety) of low-income individuals and families. Second, institutional infrastructure has been established through the national Laundry Love organization, which provides free laundry detergent and offers guidance for organizing community laundry events. Third, during the early development of the Barton County Laundry Love initiative, the local United Way (represented by a BCLHEAT member) formally adopted Laundry Love as a permanent community program, thereby securing stable funding. Finally, sustainability will be strengthened through the implementation of a rigorous evaluation framework. In this study, we did not collect event-specific data on the number of referrals from CHWs in Barton County, which represents a missed opportunity. A more systematic evaluation could generate data to justify continued investment and support for this initiative in Barton County and in communities across Kansas, the United States, and beyond.

PUBLIC HEALTH SIGNIFICANCE

Few community-level strategies in the United States directly address hygiene poverty or expand access to "dignity" products, such as clean clothing and bedding. Most intervention literature stems from low- and middle-income countries, where water, sanitation, and hygiene (WASH) programs are often implemented during humanitarian crises. This gap underscores the need for sustained, community-based strategies in the United States that extend beyond emergency relief. Laundromats are increasingly recognized as promising avenues for reaching and supporting disenfranchised populations,[12] making them particularly relevant for hygiene-focused initiatives. Against this backdrop, the current case study from Kansas documents the process and outcomes of a community-driven practice to expand laundry access. This initiative contributed to developing local systems for sustainability and inspired replication across nine additional Kansas counties. AJPH

ABOUT THE AUTHORS

Elizabeth Ablah is with the Department of Population Health, University of Kansas School of Medicine, Kansas City. Nadine Long is with Sauerwein-Long Consulting, LLC, Wichita, KS. Kara Hollins is with the Department of Family Medicine and Community Health, University of Kansas Medical Center, Kansas City. Callie Miller is with Housing Opportunities, Inc, Great Bend, KS. Charell Owings is with United Way of Central Kansas, Great Bend, KS. Kimberly Weaver is with We Are Wyandotte, Community Health Council of Wyandotte County, Kansas City, KS. Jody Love is with the Healthy Bourbon County Action Team, Fort Scott, KS. Clarissa Carrillo Martinez is with the Department of Population Health, University of Kansas School of Medicine, Kansas City. Tatiana K. Darby is with Openfields, Kansas City, MO. Ton Miras Neira is with the Department of Family Medicine and Community Health, University of Kansas Medical Center, Kansas City. Angela Scott is with the Department of Family Medicine and Community Health, University of Kansas Medical Center, Kansas City. Christina M. Pacheco is with the Department of Population Health, University of Kansas School of Medicine, Kansas City. Sarah Finocchario-Kessler is with the Department of Population Health, University of Kansas School of Medicine, Kansas City, KS.

CORRESPONDENCE

Correspondence should be sent to Christina M. Pacheco, JD, MPH, 3901 Rainbow Blvd MS 1030, Kansas City, KS 66106 (e-mail: cpacheco@kumc.edu). Reprints can be ordered at https://www.ajph.org by clicking the "Reprints" link.

PUBLICATION INFORMATION

Full Citation: Ablah E, Long N, Hollins K, et al. Addressing hygiene poverty and restoring dignity: a community partnership through Laundry Love. *Am J Public Health*. 2026;116(5):615–618.

Acceptance Date: December 14, 2025

DOI: https://doi.org/10.2105/AJPH.2025.308410

ORCID iDs:

Elizabeth Ablah https://orcid.org/0000-0003-4550-2162

Jody Love https://orcid.org/0009-0007-3932-2030

Ton Miras Neira https://orcid.org/0009-0007-5248-7630

Christina M. Pacheco https://orcid.org/0000-0002-6288-0221

CONTRIBUTORS

E. Ablah, N. Long, C. M. Pacheco, and S. Finocchario-Kessler conceptualized and supervised the parent project. N. Long, K. Knapp, J. Love, C. Carrillo Martinez, and T. K. Darby supervised on-the-ground project implementation across regions of the state. C. Miller and C. Owings conceptualized and led the Barton County initiative, and K. Weaver conceptualized and led the Wyandotte County initiative. T. Miras Neira and A. Scott conceptualized and supervised the community health worker component of the parent project. E. Ablah and N. Long led manuscript development. K. Knapp, T. Miras Neira, and A. Scott contributed to data analysis and interpretation. All authors contributed to critical revision of the manuscript, approved the final version for publication, and agree to be accountable for all aspects of the work.

ACKNOWLEDGMENTS

This work was supported by the Kansas Department of Health and Environment through a Centers for Disease Control and Prevention (CDC) grant (OT21-2103). Author effort was additionally supported by the National Institutes of Health (NIH); Christina M. Pacheco and Sarah Finocchario-Kessler were supported by the National Institute of General Medical Sciences (P20GM139733).

An earlier version of this work was presented at the American Public Health Association Annual Meeting; Minneapolis, MN; October 30, 2024.

We thank the Barton County and Wyandotte County Local Health Equity Action Teams (LHEATs) and their members, Laundry Love volunteers, and community members who trusted us with their time, experiences, and stories, making this work possible. We specifically acknowledge Vicki Richardson, a Barton County LHEAT member, for identifying hygiene poverty as a critical need in Barton County and bringing this intervention forward to the LHEAT for action. We are also grateful to local laundromat partners and community organizations across the state that provided space, supplies, and logistical support to our many LHEATs that undertook this intervention in their respective communities. Additionally, we recognize the broader Communities Organizing to Promote Equity (COPE) network, including LHEAT members, community health workers, administrative staff, partnering organizations, and community residents, for their instrumental roles in the design, implementation, and shared learning that support health equity efforts across Kansas communities.

Note. The contents are solely the responsibility of the authors and do not necessarily represent the official views of the CDC or the NIH.

CONFLICTS OF INTEREST

The authors declare that they have no conflicts of interest.

HUMAN PARTICIPANT PROTECTION

This study was approved by the institutional review board at the University of Kansas Medical Center (IRB# STUDY00148455). Informed consent was obtained from participants.

REFERENCES

1. Laundry Love. Love. Dignity. Detergent. The Laundry Love initiative. Available at: https://laundrylove.org. Accessed February 23, 2025.
2. Greene VW. Personal hygiene and life expectancy improvements since 1850: historic and epidemiologic associations. *Am J Infect Control*. Aug 2001;29(4):203–206. https://doi.org/10.1067/mic.2001.115686
3. US Department of Agriculture, Economic Research Service. *Rural-Urban Continuum Codes*. 2025. Available at: https://www.ers.usda.gov/data-products/rural-urban-continuum-codes. Accessed March 17, 2026.
4. US Census Bureau. QuickFacts. Barton County, Kansas. Population, Census, 2020 & 2010. Available at: https://www.census.gov/quickfacts/fact/table/bartoncountykansas/POP010220. Accessed February 18, 2025.
5. Pacheco CM, Bridges KM, Ellerbeck EF, et al. Communities organizing to promote equity: engaging local communities in public health responses to health inequities exacerbated by COVID-19—protocol paper. *Front Public Health*. 2024;12:1369777. https://doi.org/10.3389/fpubh.2024.1369777
6. Walker ER, Druss BG. Cumulative burden of comorbid mental disorders, substance use disorders, chronic medical conditions, and poverty on health among adults in the USA. *Psychol Health Med*. 2017;22(6):727–735. https://doi.org/10.1080/13548506.2016.1227855
7. Knighton SC. Ideal or real: a call to harness infection prevention education and resources through the lens of equity, inclusion and hygiene poverty. *Am J Infect Control*. 2022;50(10):1077–1078. https://doi.org/10.1016/j.ajic.2022.07.026
8. Feeding America. In short supply: American families struggle to secure everyday essentials. 2011. Available at: https://www.feedingamerica.org/sites/default/files/research/in-short-supply/in-short-supply-executive.pdf. Accessed March 17, 2026.
9. World Health Organization. Sanitation. Updated March 22, 2024. Available at: https://www.who.int/news-room/fact-sheets/detail/sanitation. Accessed March 17, 2026.
10. van der Geest S. Hygiene and sanitation: medical, social and psychological concerns. *CMAJ*. 2015; 187(17):1313–1314. https://doi.org/10.1503/cmaj.150588
11. Utah Education Policy Center. Research brief: chronic absenteeism. 2012. Available at: https://uepc.utah.edu/our-work/posts/2012/july/research-brief-chronic-absenteeism-2012.php. Accessed March 17, 2026.
12. Tsai J, Solis V, Schick V. Medical care needs of laundromat users in San Antonio, Texas: a potentially unique setting for health interventions. *J Community Health*. 2023;48(1):1–9. https://doi.org/10.1007/s10900-022-01137-w

A Strategic Alliance as an Implementation Strategy to Achieve Ending the HIV Epidemic Goals Among Latino Men Who Have Sex With Men: Florida and Puerto Rico, 2023

Audrey Harkness, PhD, Nequiel Reyes, MPH, Cho-Hee Shrader, PhD, Maeleigh Tidd, PhD, Nicole Altenberg, BS, Glorián Carrasquillo Sánchez, MPH, Amanda Cruz Gerena, MS, Susanne Doblecki-Lewis, MD, Jahn Jaramillo, MPH, Ron Ledain, MBA, Souhail M. Malavé Rivera, PhD, Omar Martinez, JD, Guillermo Prado, PhD, Carlos E. Rodríguez-Díaz, PhD, Rana Saber, MS, Steven A. Safren, PhD, Edda I. Santiago Rodriguez, DrPH, Ruth Soto Malavé, MD, and Eric W. Schrimshaw, PhD

Evidence-based interventions for Ending the HIV Epidemic inadequately reach Latino men who have sex with men, particularly in Florida and Puerto Rico, stressing the need for implementation strategies. SOMOS Alianza (San Juan, Orlando, Miami Organizational Strategic Alliance) connects implementers, community members, and researchers pursuing Ending the HIV Epidemic goals among Latino men who have sex with men. We describe SOMOS Alianza, present its post–one-year outcomes, and explore how strategic alliances serve as implementation strategies that reduce HIV disparities. (*Am J Public Health*. 2026;116(5):619–624. https://doi.org/10.2105/AJPH.2025.308390)

AJPH May 2026, Vol. 116, No. 5

SOMOS Alianza (San Juan, Orlando, Miami Organizational Strategic Alliance) is a network of implementers, community members, and researchers. Collaboratively, we work to end the HIV epidemic affecting Latino men who have sex with men (LMSM).[1,2]

INTERVENTION AND IMPLEMENTATION

SOMOS Alianza functions as an implementation strategy promoting the reach of evidence-based interventions such as preexposure prophylaxis, HIV treatment, and mental health treatments to LMSM. Our development of this alliance was guided by "network weaving," which involves building relationships across organizations to support local implementation.[3,4] We chose network weaving based on its conceptual fit with our implementation goals (i.e., unifying implementation networks with shared challenges) and its alignment with our values of centering different forms of expertise and reducing hierarchy.[4]

PLACE, TIME, AND PERSONS

SOMOS Alianza was supported by an Ending the HIV Epidemic grant to build strategic alliances across jurisdictions to reach Ending the HIV Epidemic goals using implementation research. Our focus is on reducing the impact of HIV on LMSM in Miami, Florida; Orlando, Florida; and San Juan, Puerto Rico—regions where LMSM are disproportionately affected.

SOMOS Alianza's inaugural meeting was February 6 to 7, 2023, and included 27 members: 14 individuals involved in implementing HIV services for LMSM, 12 HIV researchers, and 1 LMSM community member. Implementer roles varied across leadership and client-facing positions; implementers came from clinics, health departments, and advocacy groups. Our initial meeting took place in Orlando, during which we developed our vision and discussed barriers to and facilitators of delivering services to LMSM. For the remainder of the year, we held monthly online meetings driven by cocreated priorities. Monthly meetings included member updates and discussions on navigating the sociopolitical climate when conducting HIV implementation research and practice; adapting a referral tool for HIV services designed for LMSM in Miami for use in Puerto Rico and Orlando; and networking to increase collaborations, grant writing, and sharing best practices for engaging LMSM.

SOMOS Alianza concluded the funding period with a meeting in San Juan December 4 to 5, 2023, during which members shared implementation successes and challenges and planned next steps. Although SOMOS Alianza began as a project led by the first author (A. H.), it was collaborative from inception; we invited collaborators from each jurisdiction and role to share expertise and guidance with the network. We spent substantial time decentralizing SOMOS Alianza leadership, with members voting on meeting structures (e.g., length, frequency, topics), cocreating working groups, and selecting working group leaders. Our analysis indicates that this approach effectively increased network connectivity by reducing structural bridges (i.e., critical actors whose removal would disconnect two otherwise separate network clusters).

PURPOSE

We formed SOMOS Alianza for several reasons. Miami, Orlando, and San Juan are highly affected by HIV, particularly among LMSM.[1,2] Yet evidence-based clinical interventions for preventing HIV (e.g., preexposure prophylaxis) have limited reach among LMSM in these regions.[5,6] In addition to similar HIV health and healthcare disparities across these regions, there is significant migration between them, with Orlando and Miami being primary destinations for Puerto Rican migrants to the continental United States[7,8] Given these connections, we determined that a strategic alliance using our collective expertise to build implementation research and practice efforts collaboratively could help us achieve Ending the HIV Epidemic goals among LMSM. Our mission was to develop a regional network to accelerate implementation of evidence-based HIV prevention and treatment interventions through coordinated learning, rather than isolated efforts.

EVALUATION AND ADVERSE EFFECTS

SOMOS Alianza members completed REDCap (research electronic data capture)[9] surveys at baseline, six months, and one year to evaluate the process of SOMOS Alianza and determine whether we met our objective of increasing members' collaborative implementation research and practice efforts for LMSM. Members completed a sociocentric (whole) network inventory on REDCap in which they identified research and implementation activities that they engaged in during the past six months (e.g., paper writing or collaboration, scientific or community presentation, local HIV service implementation, LMSM referral to another organization for HIV service).

For each activity endorsed, members named SOMOS Alianza members involved. They then listed members they knew (i.e., by name or contact) and identified collaborative implementation research or practice activities relevant to LMSM that they engaged in together (e.g., sharing resources, codeveloping ideas, funding, networking). Lastly, we asked members to report their experiences with SOMOS Alianza and any benefits they experienced (outlined in Table 1).

We used the R environment (R Foundation for Statistical Computing, Vienna, Austria) to conduct descriptive statistics of the networks and Cytoscape[10] to visualize them. SOMOS led to a less fragmented, more connected, and stronger collaborative network overall (Figure 1). From baseline to 12 months, members created 204 new relationships. The network diameter, which refers to the "longest shortest path," or the maximum number of people it would take to "get across" the entire network using the shortest possible route (suggesting a more connected network), decreased from six to three, and the network density (i.e., a fraction of the number of connections that exist vs how many could exist) increased by 140% (from 0.208 to 0.499). The clustering coefficient also increased, indicating a stronger network (from 0.542 to 0.623). In-degree centrality, or the number of people who knew each member, is a measure of an individual's influence in a network; this increased by an average of 7.56 members from baseline to 12.96 members at 12-month follow-up. Additional information is found in Figure 1.

Implementation research and practice activities occurring among SOMOS members also increased over time. At baseline, members reported 367 implementation research and practice activities, which increased to 510 at 6 months and 779 at 12 months. Activities that increased the most were (1) learning about implementing HIV services for LMSM from another SOMOS member (+292.9%), (2) sharing resources with another SOMOS member to help with implementing HIV services for LMSM (+191.6%), (3) sharing information about implementing HIV

TABLE 1— SOMOS Alianza Members' Experiences in the Network Over Time: Miami, FL; Orlando, FL; San Juan, PR; 2023

Variable and Member Type (n = 27)	6-Mo Survey, Mean ±SD or No. (%)	12-Mo Survey, Mean ±SD or No. (%)
Evaluation of the SOMOS Alianza process[a]		
SOMOS Alianza builds trust		
Overall	3.62 ±0.85	3.88 ±0.59
Implementation/community members	3.40 ±1.06	3.8 ±0.77
Research members	3.91 ±0.30[b]	4.00 ±0.00[b]
SOMOS Alianza builds knowledge		
Overall	3.62 ±0.85	3.85 ±0.61
Implementation/community members	3.40 ±1.06	3.8 ±0.77
Research members	3.91 ±0.30[b]	3.91 ±0.30[b]
SOMOS Alianza builds collaboration and partnerships		
Overall	3.62 ±0.85	3.85 ±0.61
Implementation/community members	3.33 ±1.05	3.8 ±0.77
Research members	4.00 ±0.00[b]	3.91 ±0.30[b]
SOMOS Alianza increases the reach of HIV prevention and treatment services to Latino men who have sex with men		
Overall	3.69 ±0.84	3.77 ±0.65
Implementation/community members	3.53 ±1.06	3.8 ±0.77
Research members	3.91 ±0.30[b]	3.73 ±0.47[b]
SOMOS Alianza benefits[c]		
Enhanced ability to address an important issue		
Overall	20 (76.9)	25 (96.2)
Implementation/community members	10 (71.4)[b]	14 (93.3)
Research members	10 (83.3)	11 (100.0)[b]
Developed new skills		
Overall	15 (57.7)	21 (80.8)
Implementation/community members	9 (64.3)[b]	11 (73.3)
Research members	6 (50.0)	10 (90.9)[b]
Heightened public profile		
Overall	19 (73.1)	19 (76.0)
Implementation/community members	9 (64.3)[b]	10 (71.4)[b]
Research members	10 (83.3)	9 (81.8)[b]
Increased use of my expertise or services		
Overall	19 (76.0)	22 (88.0)
Implementation/community members	8 (61.2)[d]	11 (78.6)[b]
Research members	11 (91.7)	11 (100.0)[b]
Acquired useful knowledge about services, programs, or people in the community		
Overall	25 (96.2)	25 (96.2)
Implementation/community members	13 (92.9)[b]	14 (93.3)
Research members	12 (100.0)	11 (100.0)[b]
Enhanced ability to affect public policy		
Overall	14 (58.3)	16 (66.7)
Implementation/community members	8 (66.7)[d]	7 (53.8)[e]
Research members	6 (50.0)	9 (81.8)[b]

Continued

TABLE 1— Continued

Variable and Member Type (n = 27)	6-Mo Survey, Mean ±SD or No. (%)	12-Mo Survey, Mean ±SD or No. (%)
Developed valuable relationships		
Overall	26 (100.0)	25 (96.2)
Implementation/community members	14 (100.0)[b]	14 (93.3)
Research members	12 (100.0)	11 (100.0)[b]
Enhanced ability to meet the needs of my community, clients, or participants		
Overall	23 (92.0)	25 (96.2)
Implementation/community members	12 (92.3)[e]	14 (93.3)
Research members	11 (91.7)	11 (100.0)[b]
Enhanced ability to have a greater impact, more than I could have on my own		
Overall	21 (91.3)	22 (91.7)
Implementation/community members	10 (90.9)[f]	11 (84.6)[e]
Research members	11 (91.7)	11 (100.0)[b]
Enhanced ability to contribute to the community		
Overall	23 (92.0)	24 (92.3)
Implementation/community members	12 (92.3)[e]	13 (86.7)
Research members	11 (91.7)	11 (100.0)[b]
Acquired additional financial support, funding, or grants		
Overall	11 (45.8)	13 (54.2)
Implementation/community members	6 (50.0)[e]	5 (38.5)[e]
Research members	5 (41.7)	8 (72.7)[b]

Note. SOMOS Alianza = San Juan, Orlando, Miami Organizational Strategic Alliance.
[a]Response options were from 1 (strongly disagree) to 4 (strongly agree).
[b]Indicates missing value of n = 1.
[c]Response options were yes or no. Percentages reflect proportion of respondents who indicated yes and are from the total number of individuals who answered that question (excluding missing values).
[d]Indicates missing values of n = 3.
[e]Indicates missing values of n = 2.
[f]Indicates missing values of n = 4.

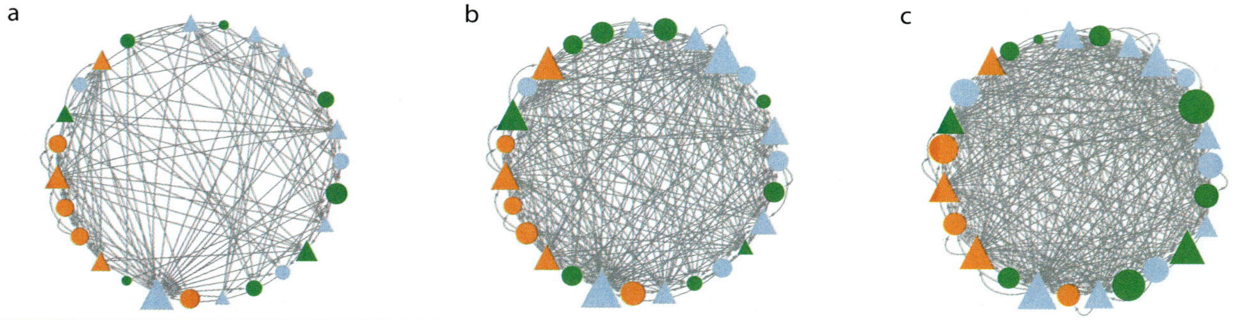

a	b	c
Network density: 0.208	Network density: 0.385	Network density: 0.499
# Connections: 146	# Connections: 270	# Connections: 350
Network diameter: 6	Network diameter: 3	Network diameter: 3
Clustering coefficient: 0.542	Clustering coefficient: 0.575	Clustering coefficient: 0.623

FIGURE 1— Growth in Connectivity in the SOMOS Alianza Network at (a) Baseline, (b) 6 Months, and (c) 12 Months: Miami, FL; Orlando, FL; San Juan, PR; 2023

Note. SOMOS Alianza = San Juan, Orlando, Miami Organizational Strategic Alliance. Study population size was n = 27. Nodes represent members. Blue = Miami; green = Orlando; orange = San Juan. Circle = implementer or community member; triangle = researcher. Larger node = more connections; smaller node = fewer connections.

services for LMSM with another SOMOS member (+176.9%), and (4) sharing resources with another SOMOS member to help them implement HIV services for LMSM (+129.7%). We also observed this overall increase in activities at the dyadic level: at baseline, 93 SOMOS member dyads engaged in at least one implementation research or practice activity together. By contrast, at 6 months and 12 months, there were 177 and 257 members, respectively, who engaged in at least one implementation research and practice activity with another member (Figure A, available as a supplement to the online version of this article at http://www.ajph.org).

Our final network analysis showed that SOMOS members increased their collaborative activities. At baseline, members reported 135 implementation research and practice activities, which increased to 199 at 6 months and 217 at 12 months. Additionally, 70 unique member dyads engaged in at least one collaboration, which increased at 6 months and 12 months, respectively, to 123 and 141 dyadic collaborations, (Figure B, available as a supplement to the online version of this article at http://www.ajph.org). Collaborative activities that increased the most among SOMOS members were program or health services grant submission (+325.0%), implementing programs to support HIV service engagement (+300.0%), scientific conference presentations (+137.0%), nonscientific and community presentations (+100.0%), and research grant submissions (+50.0%).

Consistent with our network analyses, Table 1 indicates that SOMOS fostered trust, knowledge, and collaboration among members. The network also enhanced members' abilities to address critical issues, supported skill development, and increased members' public profile and use of their expertise. Both implementation and community members and research members benefited from their involvement, although research members generally reported higher scores.

SUSTAINABILITY

Sustainability has been a key challenge for SOMOS Alianza. The network was funded through a unique, nonrenewable one-year National Institutes of Health Ending the HIV Epidemic award, supporting essential process-oriented activities (e.g., trust and relationship building, cocreating priorities) to inform community-grounded implementation research.[11,12] Identifying funding for longer-term process work has been difficult.

Subsequent research funding engages all members but is less focused on sustaining these foundational processes. During a funding gap, members voluntarily continued virtual meetings (during the grant-funded period, members received percentage effort, honoraria, or consultation fees and travel funding), highlighting the network's value. Integrating SOMOS Alianza into health departments is a potential path for sustainability but would require resources and might encounter barriers (e.g., outer setting factors,[13] such as coordinating across different departments of health and state and federal priorities). However, potential returns are significant, including sustained collaboration, service coordination, and efficiently scaling implementation strategies across jurisdictions. Continued evaluation of SOMOS Alianza's impact may inform investments and long-term sustainability.

PUBLIC HEALTH SIGNIFICANCE

Our findings suggest that SOMOS is a useful implementation strategy for promoting collaborations among researchers, implementers, and community members to advance implementation research and practice. Although all members reported positive experiences, we observed nonsignificant trends that researchers particularly benefited. This highlights the importance of examining how to ensure that network benefits are equitably beneficial to all; strategies such as rotating or shared implementer and researcher leadership could help to address this challenge. Our findings also indicate that strategic alliances such as SOMOS Alianza could serve as implementation strategies to achieve Ending the HIV Epidemic goals for different populations affected by HIV in various geographic regions or for other health conditions affecting populations experiencing health disparities. In our project, we were unable to examine the impact of SOMOS Alianza on local HIV incidence; however, this is an area that could be further explored in future work. AJPH

ABOUT THE AUTHORS

Audrey Harkness, Maeleigh Tidd, Nicole Altenberg, and Guillermo Prado are with the School of Nursing and Health Studies, University of Miami, Coral Gables, FL. Nequiel Reyes, Jahn Jaramillo, and Susanne Doblecki-Lewis are with the Miller School of Medicine, University of Miami. Cho-Hee Shrader is with the School of Nursing, Rutgers University, New Brunswick, NJ. Glorián Carrasquillo Sánchez, Souhail M. Malavé Rivera, and Edda I. Santiago Rodriguez are with the School of Public Health, University of Puerto Rico, San Juan. Amanda Cruz Gerena, Omar Martinez, and Eric W. Schrimshaw are with the Department of Population Health Sciences, University of Central Florida, Orlando. Ron Ledain is with Care Resource, Miami. Carlos E. Rodríguez-Díaz is with the School of Public Health, Boston University, Boston, MA. Rana Saber is with the Feinberg School of Medicine, Northwestern University, Chicago, IL. Steven A. Safren is with the Department of Psychology, University of Miami. Ruth Soto Malavé is with Puerto Rico CONCRA, San Juan, PR.

CORRESPONDENCE

Correspondence should be sent to Audrey Harkness, PhD, University of Miami School of Nursing and Health Studies, 5030 Brunson Dr, Coral Gables, FL 33146 (e-mail: aharkness@miami.edu). Reprints can be ordered at https://www.ajph.org by clicking the "Reprints" link.

PUBLICATION INFORMATION

Full Citation: Harkness A, Reyes N, Shrader C-H, et al. A strategic alliance as an implementation strategy to achieve ending the HIV Epidemic goals among Latino men who have sex with men: Florida and Puerto Rico, 2023. *Am J Public Health*. 2026;116(5):619–624.

Acceptance Date: December 14, 2025.

DOI: https://doi.org/10.2105/AJPH.2025.308390

ORCID iDs:

Audrey Harkness https://orcid.org/0000-0003-2290-9904

Nequiel Reyes https://orcid.org/0009-0001-8690-3125

Cho-Hee Shrader https://orcid.org/0000-0003-3500-8507

Nicole Altenberg https://orcid.org/0009-0001-1355-3531

Amanda Cruz Gerena https://orcid.org/0009-0000-8206-0282

Jahn Jaramillo https://orcid.org/0000-0002-7395-6551

Ron Ledain https://orcid.org/0009-0003-4077-2312

Souhail M. Malavé Rivera https://orcid.org/0000-0003-3446-4869

Carlos E. Rodríguez-Díaz https://orcid.org/0000-0001-6333-0654

Edda I. Santiago Rodriguez https://orcid.org/0000-0001-7076-6907

Eric W. Schrimshaw https://orcid.org/0000-0003-2755-1796

CONTRIBUTORS

A. Harkness, N. Reyes, C.-H. Shrader, and M. Tidd wrote the original draft. A. Harkness, N. Reyes, C.-H. Shrader, S. M. Malavé Rivera, S. A. Safren, E. I. Santiago Rodriguez, and E. W. Schrimshaw developed the methodology. A. Harkness, N. Reyes, N. Altenberg, G. Carrasquillo Sánchez, S. M. Malavé Rivera, O. Martinez, C. E. Rodríguez-Díaz, R. Saber, S. A. Safren, E. I. Santiago Rodriguez, and E. W. Schrimshaw conducted the investigation. A. Harkness, N. Reyes, N. Altenberg, G. Carrasquillo Sánchez, S. M. Malavé Rivera, O. Martinez, R. Saber, S. A. Safren, E. I. Santiago Rodriguez, and E. W. Schrimshaw administered the project. A. Harkness, S. M. Malavé Rivera, C. E. Rodríguez-Díaz, S. A. Safren, E. I. Santiago Rodriguez, and E. W. Schrimshaw conceptualized the article. A. Harkness, S. A. Safren, E. I. Santiago Rodriguez, and E. W. Schrimshaw acquired funding. N. Reyes, C.-H. Shrader, and M. Tidd conducted the formal analysis. C.-H. Shrader created the visualizations. All authors reviewed and edited the article.

ACKNOWLEDGMENTS

This project was made possible by the National Institute of Mental Health, National Institutes of Health (NIH; grants P30MH133399, F31MH135828, T32MH126772) and the National Institute of Minority Health and Health Disparities, NIH (grant K23MD015690).

We would like to acknowledge the contributions of all members of SOMOS Alianza (San Juan, Orlando, Miami Organizational Strategic Alliance) to this project.

This article was originally submitted as part of the *AJPH* Supplement issue on "HIV Prevention, Care Continuum, and Health Outcomes Among Hispanic People in the US and Puerto Rico."

Note. The content is solely the responsibility of the authors and does not necessarily represent the official views of the NIH.

CONFLICTS OF INTEREST

The authors have no conflicts of interest to report.

HUMAN PARTICIPANT PROTECTION

This project was deemed not human participant research by the University of Miami institutional review board.

REFERENCES

1. McCree DH, Walker T, DiNenno E, et al. A programmatic approach to address increasing HIV diagnoses among Hispanic/Latino MSM, 2010–2014. *Prev Med.* 2018;114:64–71. https://doi.org/10.1016/j.ypmed.2018.06.007
2. Fauci AS, Redfield RR, Sigounas G, Weahkee MD, Giroir BP. Ending the HIV epidemic: a plan for the United States. *JAMA.* 2019;321(9):844–845. https://doi.org/10.1001/jama.2019.1343
3. Powell BJ, Waltz TJ, Chinman MJ, et al. A refined compilation of implementation strategies: results from the Expert Recommendations for Implementing Change (ERIC) project. *Implement Sci.* 2015;10:21. https://doi.org/10.1186/s13012-015-0209-1
4. Holley J. *Network Weaver Handbook: A Guide to Transformational Networks.* Portland, OR: Network Weaver Publishing; 2012.
5. Centers for Disease Control and Prevention. Changes in HIV preexposure prophylaxis awareness and use among men who have sex with men—20 urban areas, 2014 and 2017. *MMWR Morb Mortal Wkly Rep.* 2019;68(27):597–603. https://doi.org/10.15585/mmwr.mm6827a1
6. Sullivan PS, Mouhanna F, Mera R, et al. Methods for county-level estimation of pre-exposure prophylaxis coverage and application to the U.S. ending the HIV epidemic jurisdictions. *Ann Epidemiol.* 2020;44:16–30. https://doi.org/10.1016/j.annepidem.2020.01.004
7. Pew Research Center. Puerto Rican population by county. August 14, 2019. Available at: https://www.pewresearch.org/race-and-ethnicity/feature/puerto-rican-population-by-county. Accessed April 2, 2025.
8. Cheatham A, Roy D. Puerto Rico: a U.S. territory in crisis. January 8, 2025. Available at: https://www.cfr.org/backgrounder/puerto-rico-us-territory-crisis. Accessed March 24, 2022.
9. Harris PA, Taylor R, Thielke R, Payne J, Gonzalez N, Conde JG. Research electronic data capture (REDCap)—a metadata-driven methodology and workflow process for providing translational research informatics support. *J Biomed Inform.* 2009;42(2):377–381. https://doi.org/10.1016/j.jbi.2008.08.010
10. Shannon P, Markiel A, Ozier O, et al. Cytoscape: a software environment for integrated models of biomolecular interaction networks. *Genome Res.* 2003;13(11):2498–2504. https://doi.org/10.1101/gr.1239303
11. Metz A, Jensen T, Farley A, Boaz A, Bartley L, Villodas M. Building trusting relationships to support implementation: a proposed theoretical model. *Front Health Serv.* 2022;2:894599. https://doi.org/10.3389/frhs.2022.894599
12. Rapport F, Smith J, Hutchinson K, et al. Too much theory and not enough practice? The challenge of implementation science application in healthcare practice. *J Eval Clin Pract.* 2022;28(6):991–1002. https://doi.org/10.1111/jep.13600
13. Damschroder LJ, Reardon CM, Widerquist MAO, Lowery J. The updated Consolidated Framework for Implementation Research based on user feedback. *Implement Sci.* 2022;17(1):75. https://doi.org/10.1186/s13012-022-01245-0

An American Health Dilemma 25 Years Later

Theodore M. Brown, PhD

ABOUT THE AUTHOR

Theodore M. Brown is professor emeritus of history and public health sciences, University of Rochester, Rochester, NY, and an AJPH associate editor emeritus.

See also An American Health Dilemma 25 Years Later, pp. 628–656.

W. Michael Byrd and Lynda A. Clayton published two major volumes in 2000 and 2002, respectively: *An American Health Dilemma: A Medical History of African Americans and the Problem of Race, Beginnings to 1900*[1] and *An American Health Dilemma: Race, Medicine, and Health Care in the United States, 1900–2000*.[2] Reflecting retrospectively on the Byrd and Clayton volumes, the featured section in this *AJPH* issue is both a timely evaluation of important current issues and a retrospective apology. When the jointly written Byrd and Clayton volumes appeared a quarter of a century ago, they were reviewed with considerable enthusiasm in major journals, including the *Journal of Health Politics, Policy, and Law*,[3] the *New England Journal of Medicine*,[4] and the *Journal of the American Medical Association*.[5,6] But neither of Byrd and Clayton's volumes was reviewed in *AJPH* because at the time *AJPH* reviewed no books at all.

AJPH has since decided to review books again, but its policies restrict its reviews to recently published books. To make proper amends and in the spirit of the *New York Times*'s "Overlooked No More" obituaries (begun in March 2018 to pay respect to individuals who were inappropriately overlooked by the *Times* when they passed away), *AJPH*'s featured section in this issue collects articles and editorials about Byrd and Clayton's important two-volume book now. As announced earlier,[7] the articles and editorials have been solicited from prominent historical scholars to assess key features of the Byrd and Clayton volumes in ways that evaluate both what those authors claimed and what their claims look like in the light of contemporary scholarship.

The following summarizes the topics and authors in this featured section. The first two are history essays, and the next four are history editorials. The section also includes an Editor's Choice (p. 567) authored by Alfredo Morabia, *AJPH* former editor-in-chief, and Georges Benjamin, American Public Health Association chief executive officer, who offer a deeply respectful but probing set of reflections on this collection of essays and editorials and on Byrd and Clayton's two volumes.

Fett (p. 649) claims that Byrd and Clayton were right about a great deal, but the suffering of enslaved people leading to the destruction of Black lives before Emancipation and the "slave health deficit" transmitted to posterity was even greater than that captured in the mortality data the authors rely on. The etiology of injury was broader than physical brutality, horrific living and working conditions, and the exploitation of enslaved women as profitable

Continued on page 626...

HISTORY CORNER

10 YEARS AGO

Outstanding Services to Negro Health

Historian Samuel Kelton Roberts has argued that in the mid-20th century Black public health practitioners, influenced by their exclusion from the mainstream field and by their connections with other Black professionals, held an "expansive" view of public health that "allowed them to link a variety of social and political problems to health in ways not normally contemplated by White professionals." Indeed, for [Dr. Dorothy Boulding] Ferebee and [Dr. Virginia] Alexander public health sat at the intersection of their medical, social, and political concerns. . . . Ferebee believed that Black women had a "responsibility for promoting the physical, mental, and spiritual advance of the race." . . . In 1930, [Alexander] renovated her residence to open the Aspiranto Health Home, a three-bed private hospital used primarily for maternity care but also for convalescent care and minor surgery. She considered Aspiranto a teaching center for the provision of health education and birth control. She also wanted to link the facility to broader social concerns. Alexander saw Aspiranto as a refuge from the racism pervasive in Philadelphia hospitals.

From *AJPH*, Aug. 2016, pp. 1398–1401

breeding machines. Enslaved people and their descendants suffered an enormous burden of psychiatric trauma as well as physical injury. In addition, the "slave health subsystem," which in self-help fashion tried to mitigate enslaved people's suffering, was more important than Byrd and Clayton suggest, and its care should not be denigrated as inferior by comparison with the care episodically provided by practitioners trained in Western medicine.

Parallel to Fett's focus on slavery as the big pre-1900 issue, Adolphson and Hoffman (p. 643) focus on modern hospital care and access to it as the big post-1900 issue. They endorse Byrd and Clayton's framing of hospitals as "contested spaces" as well as their judgment that racial justice cannot be achieved in a medical system that is thoroughly embedded in an economic system that places profits before people. Adolphson and Hoffman also endorse Byrd and Clayton's analysis of hospitals' role in contributing to US medical racism by perpetuating inequities, initially through formal legal segregation and later, ironically, via new funding streams that pulled patients away from Black hospitals that originally arose as a survival necessity. The demise of Black hospitals was also influenced by social and economic factors such as suburbanization, White flight, government austerity measures and disinvestment in public services, and the rise of profit-driven hospital care. Like Fett, Adolphson and Hoffman chide Byrd and Clayton for their physician-centric focus, which made them less attentive than they should have been to the role of community advocacy and political mobilization.

Hogarth (p. 635) uses a medieval image to reflect on the deep-seated and stubbornly persistent belief in the innate biological differences between Black and White people, a central theme of Byrd and Clayton's first volume and an important lingering presence in the second. Byrd and Clayton pointed to Blackness as a proxy for innate difference and, Hogarth argues, 25 years later that connection is still with us. In the medieval era, even when race was marked by Black skin, the color did not always signify a derogatory Other. It was not the same after 1500, when associations between Blackness, sub-Saharan Africa, and slavery hardened, that Blackness was regularly treated as something biologically different and inferior to Whiteness.

Cooper Owens (p. 639) reinforces Byrd and Clayton's account of J. Marion Sims, the often heralded "founder of modern gynecology," and confirms their sense of his disregard for Black patients and their comfort and safety. Such callous indifference was made possible by slavery and has contributed over the years to Black–White maternal and infant mortality differences and other disparities.

An expert on the history of US medical education, Ludmerer (p. 628) generally endorses the overall contours of Byrd and Clayton's account of Black struggles for and achievements in US medical education. But he makes it clear that the Flexner Report, even if it embedded racist assumptions, was welcomed by leading Black medical educators at the time it was published and was not a major quantitative factor in suppressing the number of Black individuals receiving formal medical training. By comparison with women medical graduates of all races, the number of Black men allowed to earn

Continued on page 627...

HISTORY CORNER

19 YEARS AGO

Warm Springs, Tuskegee, and the March of Dimes

In 1946 Harry Weaver, newly appointed as director of research at the National Foundation . . . wrote to virologist Thomas Francis asking about research on race and polio: "I have been under the impression that most people believed that there was less poliomyelitis among Negroes than Whites." No, Francis told Weaver, "the incidence by race . . . was essentially the same"; poor statistical collection had previously skewed the statistics and "there has been a tendency in the past not to seek out colored cases as well as White." . . . This new science of polio, however, did not counter pervasive customs of medical racism. Thus, in May 1954, the month that the Supreme Court announced its Brown v. Board of Education decision, Black children in Montgomery, Ala, had to wait to receive their Salk shots on the front lawns of local White public schools. They were forbidden to use the restrooms inside.

From *AJPH*, March 2007, pp. 792–793

medical degrees was limited because of prejudice in admissions and the low number of qualified prospective students in the pipeline.

Gamble (p. 632) claims that Byrd and Clayton's books are an important, major contribution but that they leave out Black women physicians. Gamble tells shortened versions of the exemplary stories of Rebecca Crumpler, MD (1864), and Rebecca Cole, MD (1867), the first two US trained Black women physicians. Byrd and Clayton never mention Crumpler or Cole even though they discuss the challenges faced by contemporary White women physicians such as Elizabeth Blackwell. The scholarship on Black women physicians is now growing, but much work still needs to be done. AJPH

CORRESPONDENCE

Correspondence should be sent to Theodore M. Brown, Department of History, University of Rochester, Rochester, NY 14627 (theodore_brown@urmc.rochester.edu). Reprints can be ordered at https://www.ajph.org by clicking the "Reprints" link.

PUBLICATION INFORMATION

Full Citation: Brown TM. An American Health Dilemma 25 years later. *Am J Public Health.* 2026;116(5):625–627.

Acceptance Date: February 10, 2026.

DOI: https://doi.org/10.2105/AJPH.2026.308480

ORCID iD:
Theodore M. Brown https://orcid.org/0009-0000-9146-7412

CONFLICTS OF INTEREST

The author has no conflicts of interest to disclose.

REFERENCES

1. Byrd WM, Clayton L. *An American Health Dilemma: A Medical History of African Americans and the Problem of Race, Beginnings to 1900.* New York, NY: Routledge; 2000.
2. Byrd WM, Clayton LA. *An American Health Dilemma: Race, Medicine, and Health Care in the United States, 1900–2000.* New York, NY: Routledge; 2002.
3. Smith DB. *An American Health Dilemma: Race, Medicine, and Health Care in the United States, 1900–2000* [book review]. *J Health Polit Policy Law.* 2002;27(5):873–876. https://doi.org/10.1215/03616878-27-5-873
4. Washington HA. *An American Health Dilemma. Vol. 1. A Medical History of African Americans and the Problem of Race: Beginnings to 1900* [book review]. *N Engl J Med.* 2002;346(6):458. https://doi.org/10.1056/NEJM200202073460621
5. Johnson KA. *An American Health Dilemma: A Medical History of African Americans and the Problem of Race—Beginnings to 1900* [book review]. *JAMA.* 2001;285(9):1219. https://doi.org/10.1001/jama.285.9.1219
6. Johnson KA. *An American Health Dilemma: Race, Medicine, and Health Care in the United States 1900–2000, vol 2* [book review]. *JAMA.* 2002;287(22):3009. https://doi.org/10.1001/jama.287.22.3009-JBK0612-3-1
7. Brown TM. An American health dilemma 25 years later. *Am J Public Health.* 2025;115(6):862–863. https://doi.org/10.2105/AJPH.2025.308132

Black Struggles for Medical Education and Postgraduate Training

Kenneth M. Ludmerer, MD

ABOUT THE AUTHOR

Kenneth M. Ludmerer is with the Department of Medicine, School of Medicine, and the Department of History, Faculty of Arts and Sciences, Washington University, St. Louis, MO.

See also An American Health Dilemma 25 Years Later, pp. 625–656.

Twenty-five years ago, W. Michael Byrd and Linda A. Clayton published their monumental, two-volume study, *An American Health Dilemma*,[1,2] examining the role race played in determining health inequality in the United States. Vast in scope and detail, the book provided a comprehensive historical and sociocultural analysis of how race relations affected African American health. In this account, physicians and medical education are only two of several important themes. Indeed, for most of the first volume, formally educated doctors are notably scarce, except for their recurrent role in propagating racial fallacies about the intellectual and biological inferiority of Black people. But one contribution of the Byrd and Clayton volumes is their taking folk healing among slave populations seriously—exploring what these medical practices meant to African Americans and how they affected enslaved persons' health, beliefs, and fortitude—rather than simply writing them off as quackery.

EARLY BLACK PHYSICIANS AND MEDICAL EDUCATION

There were a small number of formally trained African American doctors, even during the antebellum period when folk medicine dominated Black health care. Byrd and Clayton tell this story well in appropriate parts of the study, particularly at the end of volume 1 and the beginning of volume 2. *An American Health Dilemma* begins its recounting of Black doctors by examining such early luminaries as James McCune Smith, Martin Robeson Delaney, David John Peck, and Alexander Thomas Augusta. Smith earned an MD degree at the University of Glasgow; Augusta, at Trinity Medical College in Toronto. Delaney, like most doctors of the era, was trained through the apprenticeship system. Later he tried to obtain a medical degree at Harvard Medical School, but in 1850 the school dismissed him, along with two other Black medical students, because the White students at Harvard objected to sharing classrooms with Black students. Peck, a protégé of Delaney, became the first African American to earn an MD degree from a US medical school (Rush Medical College, 1847). *An American Health Dilemma* recounts the staggering levels of professional and personal discrimination, obstruction, and frustration these individuals encountered. The commitment of these pioneering Black doctors to racial uplift and to providing medical care to the needy of all races also stands out.

As the socioeconomic position of some African Americans improved after emancipation, and as opportunities for Blacks to enter US society expanded, increasing numbers of formerly enslaved persons and other African Americans began to seek careers in medicine. Byrd and Clayton discuss prominent figures such as Nathan F. Mossell, Robert F. Boyd, and Daniel Hale Williams. Volume 1 describes the creation and early struggles of Meharry Medical College and Howard University Medical College, drawing a fascinating contrast between the more cosmopolitan outlook of Howard and the more local commitment of Meharry. Together, the two schools graduated nearly 90% of the US Black doctors. Black physicians were also trained at Black proprietary medical schools such as Leonard Medical School and Louisville National Medical College.

A few Black medical students found their way into predominantly White medical schools outside the South. All the Black medical schools struggled mightily against huge financial, social, and political obstacles. Although some Black medical graduates, such as Robert F. Boyd in Nashville, developed large, high-quality practices, most Black doctors before 1890 found a small market for their services. Byrd and Clayton called them "sundown doctors."[3] Unable to support themselves and their families by practicing medicine exclusively, they held other jobs during the day, seeing patients only after sundown.

GROWTH OF THE BLACK MEDICAL PROFESSION

The period from 1890 to 1910 marked the emergence of a distinct Black medical profession. During this period, the number of African American doctors

AJPH May 2026, Vol. 116, No. 5

rose from 900 to 3409. The Black medical profession became organized. The National Medical Association was established in 1895; its journal, the *Journal of the National Medical Association*, published its first issue in 1909. Such institutionalization was necessitated by the exclusion of Black doctors from mainstream medical organizations and institutions, most notably the American Medical Association—events that the authors accurately detail.

MEDICAL EDUCATION AFTER THE *FLEXNER REPORT*

Volume 2 examines the crisis in Black medical education that followed the publication of the *Flexner Report* in 1910. The report prompted all US medical educators to reorganize along university medical school lines, following the example of the Johns Hopkins Medical School. Dozens of proprietary schools, White and Black alike, were forced to close because of their inability or unwillingness to keep up with modern standards. The reforms were especially hard on the financially precarious Black medical schools, which had been struggling against difficult challenges to succeed in the scientific era. In 1900, 10 Black medical schools existed, and in 1910, seven. However, only two—Howard and Meharry—survived the Flexnerian era. Thereafter, the percentage of African Americans in medicine stabilized at around 2% of all physicians, compared with a general population that was 10% Black. The significant underrepresentation of African Americans in medicine has continued to the present.

In volume 2, other important subsequent events pertaining to the medical education of African Americans are examined. Most notably, the strengthening of Howard and Meharry during the second quarter of the 20th century is discussed, as is the rise of affirmative action programs in the 1970s and the subsequent obstacles these programs encountered following major legal challenges and the waning of enthusiasm for affirmative action at the end of the decade.

In both volumes 1 and 2, the overall discussion of Black medical education is accurate, thorough, and reliable. One great strength is that the authors delve into the lived experiences of African American medical students and doctors, providing a vivid account of the enormous prejudices, insults, exclusions, and dangers they experienced. External obstacles to success are clearly depicted, but so is the agency of many Black doctors who had the strength, character, and grit to persevere. The book is thus well balanced between its depiction of both the structural impediments of poverty, prejudice, and lack of educational opportunity and the strength of many individuals to rise against the odds. Both volumes 1 and 2 make good use of the writings of Herbert Morais,[4] Todd Savitt,[5] W. Montague Cobb,[6] Midian O. Bousfeld,[7] and Vanessa Northington Gamble,[8] and many others. The breadth and depth of the scholarship is impressive.

In the 25 years since the study's publication, the underrepresentation of Black people, particularly Black men, in US medicine has continued. This problem demands exploration; fortunately, *An American Health Dilemma* proves useful for that task. Some recent authors have maintained that the shortage of African American doctors, past and present, directly resulted from the closure of five of the seven Black medical schools in the aftermath of the *Flexner Report*. As one recent essay declared, the closure of these schools caused "enduring setbacks for racial diversity in medicine."[9] However, such claims do not withstand scrutiny. They overlook the fact that the National Medical Association, acknowledging that educational and professional standards needed to be raised everywhere to accommodate modern practices, endorsed the *Flexner Report*.[10] They do not account for the observation that Meharry and Howard were already producing roughly 85% of the country's Black physicians, making the closure of the remaining Black schools relatively unimportant quantitatively. Most important, this assertion ignores the compelling argument of *An American Health Dilemma* of the crucial importance of structural racism.

STRUCTURAL RACISM AND THE MEDICAL PIPELINE

Regarding structural racism, the imposition and continuation of educational segregation proved more powerful than the report of any one person. Flexner—like virtually all medical educators of the era—viewed the Black medical schools as primarily responsible for the education of Black doctors. No White medical educator of the era argued for integrating medical education. In the South, where one third of the nation's medical schools were located, no medical school admitted an African American student until 1948, whereas medical schools elsewhere were collectively admitting and graduating between 10 and 15 a year nationwide.[11] One study estimated that if every medical school during World War I had admitted just one Black student each year, the total number of Black medical graduates could have immediately doubled.[12] African American leaders of the era recognized the powerful effect that could occur for Black representation in medicine if White medical schools were to open their doors even a little to Black students.[13]

It is instructive to compare the position of African Americans with that of women in medicine. In 1910, there were three women's medical colleges. Only Woman's Medical College of Pennsylvania survived. However, 80% of women physicians were already graduates of coeducational schools, not separate women's schools. The closure of all but one women's medical colleges had little discernible effect on the number of women doctors.[14] Thus, the position of African Americans who hoped to enter medicine was more precarious than that of aspiring women doctors since for women integration in medical education (i.e., coeducation) had already occurred. Of course, the numbers of women doctors did not rise significantly until the feminist movement of the early 1970s, and Victorian mores often did not give women physicians during the reform era (1890s–1920s) an easy time or equal opportunity. However, because of coeducation, gender proved less of a barrier to entry than race.

Structural racism also impeded the entry of Blacks into medicine in other ways. The stricter post-Flexner admission requirements affected all prospective medical students, but none more so than Black youths, who far too often were educationally deprived. Black medical educators during World War I praised the more rigorous entrance requirements to medical school but lamented the inadequate pipeline of adequately prepared African American students—a problem, they contended, that began at the very bottom of the educational system. "The trouble here is often at the very bottom,—the fundamentals have been neglected. Not sufficient attention has been paid to the elementary education,—the grammar school."[15] The National Medical Association conducted its own survey of Black medical colleges in 1910 to investigate the problems of African Americans entering medicine. Several factors were identified, but of singular importance was poor preliminary education, coupled with early home environments that generally lacked books, magazines, and an intellectual atmosphere.[16]

Poverty aggravated the problems of poor educational preparation. During the reform era, the gradually increasing costs of medical education, coupled with an ever more demanding course of study, made it increasingly difficult for poor students to work their way through medical school. These trends affected all students from lower socioeconomic backgrounds, but Black students, who disproportionately came from low-income families, were especially vulnerable. Structural obstacles such as poverty and inadequate educational opportunities have impeded efforts to increase the pool of qualified African American applicants ever since. They remain as relevant to the present and future as they did to the past.

For those interested in improving educational opportunities in medicine for African Americans, there is much more that could be said about the impediments of structural and institutional racism. The difficulties that afflict potential Black doctors today reflect less the consequence of the racism in the *Flexner Report*, which is appropriately criticized by the authors, and more the deep-seated structural racism and prejudice that continue to afflict US society. These observations serve as a reminder that medical education is not the autonomous, self-regulating, altruistic activity that it is often thought to be. Medical schools have always depended on the financial support and good will of the public.[17] Similarly, attitudes, values, and prejudices exhibited by medical educators did not arise from within medicine or personal idiosyncrasy alone; rather, they reflected the impact of US culture and social mores on their own personal beliefs and actions. Ultimately, for African Americans to achieve greater opportunities in medicine, there is much that medical educators can and should do. But just as important, equity for Blacks in medical education will depend on achieving a more just society, not simply on the actions and decisions of professional leaders. AJPH

CORRESPONDENCE

Correspondence should be sent to Kenneth M. Ludmerer, Washington University School of Medicine, Department of Medicine, 660 South Euclid Ave, Campus Box 8066, St. Louis, MO 63110 (e-mail: kludmere@wustl.edu). Reprints can be ordered at https://www.ajph.org by clicking the "Reprints" link.

PUBLICATION INFORMATION

Full Citation: Ludmerer KM. Black struggles for medical education and postgraduate training. *Am J Public Health*. 2026;116(5):628–631.

Acceptance Date: January 31, 2026.

DOI: https://doi.org/10.2105/AJPH.2026.308454

ACKNOWLEDGMENTS

The author is grateful to the Gordon and Betty Moore Foundation for funding his research on this subject; to Harvey V. Fineberg, president of the Moore Foundation, for his encouragement and support; and to Theodore M. Brown for careful commentary and suggestions on an earlier draft of this article.

CONFLICTS OF INTEREST

The author has no conflicts of interest to report.

ENDNOTES

1. W. M. Byrd and L. A. Clayton, *An American Health Dilemma: A Medical History of African Americans and the Problem of Race: Beginnings to 1900* (New York, NY: Routledge, 2000).
2. W. M. Byrd and L. A. Clayton, *An American Health Dilemma: Race, Medicine, and Health Care in the United States, 1900–2000* (New York, NY: Routledge, 2002).

3. Byrd and Clayton, *American Health Dilemma: Beginnings to 1900*, 405.
4. H. M. Morais, *The History of the Negro in Medicine* (New York, NY: Publishers Company, 1967).
5. T. L. Savitt, *Medicine and Slavery: The Diseases and Health Care of Blacks in Antebellum Virginia* (Urbana: University of Illinois Press, 1987); *Race and Medicine in Nineteenth- and Early-Twentieth-Century America* (Kent, OH: Kent State University Press, 2007).
6. W. M. Cobb, *Medical Care and the Plight of the Negro* (New York, NY: National Association for the Advancement of Colored People, 1947); *Progress and Portents for the Negro in Medicine* (New York, NY: National Association for the Advancement of Colored People, 1948).
7. M. O. Bousfield, "An Account of Physicians of Color in the United States," *Bulletin of the History of Medicine* 17 (1945): 61–84.
8. V. N. Gamble, *Making a Place for Ourselves: The Black Hospital Movement, 1920–1945* (New York, NY: Oxford University Press, 1995).
9. N. Anderson, M. Nguyen, K. Marcotte, et al., "The Long Shadow: A Historical Perspective on Racism in Medical Education," *Academic Medicine* 98, suppl. 2 (2023): S28–S36, S31, https://doi.org/10.1097/ACM.0000000000005253
10. "Medical Education," *Journal of the National Medical Association* 3 (1911): 235; "Organized Effort," *Journal of the National Medical Association* 2 (1910): 192; "Medical Education Statistics for 1913," *Journal of the National Medical Association* 6 (1914): 66.
11. Morais, *History of the Negro in Medicine*, 94.
12. L. E. Miller and R. M. Weiss, "Revisiting Black Medical School Extinctions in the Flexner Era," *Journal of the History of Medicine and Allied Sciences* 67, no. 2 (2012): 217–243, https://doi.org/10.1093/jhmas/jrq084
13. Bousfield, "Account of Physicians of Color," esp. 83–84.
14. Council on Medical Education and Hospitals, "Medical Education in the United States," *Journal of the American Medical Association* 95 (1930): 504.
15. "Better Preparation for Practitioners of Medicine," *Journal of the National Medical Association* 11 (1919): 108.
16. Gamble, "Report on Medical Education," *Journal of the National Medical Association* 2, no. 1 (1910): 23–29, https://doi.org/10.1001/jama.1910.02550500034019
17. K. M. Ludmerer, *Learning to Heal: The Development of American Medical Education* (New York, NY: Basic Books, 1985); *Time to Heal: American Medical Education From the Turn of the Century to the Era of Managed Care* (New York, NY: Oxford University Press, 1999).

"A Wide Field Is Open Before Her, and Many of Her Sisters": Discovering Early African American Women Physicians

Vanessa Northington Gamble, MD, PhD

ABOUT THE AUTHOR

Vanessa Northington Gamble is with George Washington University, Washington, DC.

See also An American Health Dilemma 25 Years Later, pp. 625–656.

AJPH May 2026, Vol. 116, No. 5

On March 2, 1864, when 33-year-old Rebecca Lee Crumpler (1831–1895), a former nurse, received her medical degree from Boston, Massachusetts's New England Female Medical College, she became the first African American woman physician. At the commencement ceremony, several speakers highlighted Crumpler's trailblazing accomplishment. One "rejoiced that among the graduation was one of another color other than those who had hitherto received the honors of medical school." Another proclaimed, "In one respect this was peculiarly a *Commencement*—in sending out the first graduated Doctress of the African race . . . A wide field is open before her, and many of her sisters."[1] Yet, the conferral of a gender-specific degree and the speaker's identification of Crumpler's race underscored the fact that she would not just be a physician, let alone a woman physician, but a Black woman physician. Such a distinction would describe the generations of African American women who followed in Crumpler's professional footsteps, including this author.

THE ERASURE OF BLACK WOMEN PHYSICIANS IN MEDICAL HISTORY

It is, nonetheless, surprising how little historical consciousness there is today about the path Crumpler began to clear more than a century and a half ago. Her journey comes to mind in reading W. Michael Byrd and Linda A. Clayton's authoritative, exhaustively researched, encyclopedic two-volume *An American Health Dilemma*.[2] Since its publication in 2000 and 2002, there has not been any work that has come close to its ambitions or breadth. One of the authors' major contributions is revealing the critical work of Black physicians in improving the health of Black Americans and in fighting for health equity. They write, "This book is the first to chronicle in such detail, the courage, leadership, ingenuity of African American physicians . . . who struggled against great odds to build a responsive health system that would meet the needs of those living in a segregated society, often in great poverty."[3] They also make plain that the narratives of Black physicians are either frequently entirely absent from the historical record or relegated to the margins as peripheral and unimportant. Byrd and Clayton further acknowledge their debt to the men (Black and White) who were "foundation stones of intellect and inspiration" and who "laid the building blocks in the quest for justice and equity in health care for all people in the United States beginning in the 19th century."[4] These men included Black physicians such as James McCune Smith, John A. Kenney, and Charles Victor Roman. Their list, however, does not include any African American women physicians, whose endeavors, as the distinguished historian Darlene Clark Hine has argued, "would facilitate black survival by keeping black babies and their mothers alive and healthy."[5]

In both volumes of *An American Health Dilemma,* Byrd and Clayton mostly overlook the stories and accomplishments of African American women physicians. When they do make an appearance, examination of these pathbreakers is cursory and brief. The authors' detailed analysis of pioneering 19th-century Black physicians is illustrative. Crumpler is never mentioned, though Byrd and Clayton provide important biographical information about James McCune Smith who in 1837 became the first male African American physician. Racial discrimination forced Smith to attend medical school at the University of Glasgow. Upon his return to the United States, he gained prominence as a physician, abolitionist, and intellectual. *An American Health Dilemma* also traces the career of David Jones Peck, the first Black graduate of an American medical school. Ten years after Smith, he received his degree from Chicago, Illinois's Rush Medical

School. Moreover, although Byrd and Clayton neglect to include Crumpler, they do discuss the challenges faced by two White women, Elizabeth Blackwell and Harriot Hunt, in their pursuit of medical degrees. In 1849, Blackwell became the first woman physician in the United States when she graduated from the Geneva Medical College in New York. The following year, racial and sexual discrimination prompted Harvard Medical School to expel Hunt, along with three Black men. An analysis of the careers of the first two African American women physicians, Crumpler and Rebecca Cole (1846–1922), would enrich this story. Indeed, an examination of their lives is essential to a wider and more complete understanding of the history of African American physicians in medicine and public health.

THE CONTRIBUTIONS OF AFRICAN AMERICAN WOMEN PHYSICIANS

After Crumpler's 1864 medical school graduation, she practiced briefly in Boston before heading to Canada for additional training. Three years later, she moved to Richmond, Virginia, where she became one of the few African American doctors employed in the Medical Division of the Freedmen's Bureau. A deeply religious woman and an "indefatigable church worker," she found that taking care of recently emancipated slaves in the former capital of the Confederacy allowed her to practice "real missionary work."[6] She gained expertise in the diseases of women and children, taught Black midwives, and treated many indigent freedpeople who desperately needed medical care. However, despite her medical degree, the Freedmen's Bureau classified her as a nurse.[7] After her time in Richmond, Crumpler returned to Boston where she established a medical practice that focused primarily on women and children. In 1883, she published *A Book of Medical Discourses in Two Parts* and dedicated it "to Mothers, Nurses, and All Who May Desire to Mitigate the Afflictions of the Human Race."[8] Her primary objective was to provide women with practical advice to care for themselves and their children. But the book's broad scope offered an incisive critique of postbellum medical theories that attributed the poor health of African Americans to inherent biological inferiority and that predicted the extinction of the race. Crumpler detailed the impact of socioeconomic factors such as tenement housing on health.[9] She illuminated the influence of poor work conditions on Black women, many who worked as domestics and laundresses. "Our women work hard," she wrote, "and many of them against a heavy tide; nor does there ever seem to be an end to their toils. Especially do some of the laboring women of my race appear to work under heavy disadvantages."[10] In *Medical Discourses,* Crumpler emphasized the "possibilities of prevention," thus rebuking fatalistic theories about African American health. She instead presented a more optimistic view that contended that disease and mortality rates could be reduced in Black Americans.[11]

In 1867, three years after Crumpler became a physician, Cole received her medical degree from the Woman's Medical College of Pennsylvania (now Drexel University College of Medicine). During her 40-year career, she combined medicine, racial justice, and health equity activism. However, her accomplishments only warranted a single sentence in *An American Health Dilemma.* The book acknowledges her distinction as the second African American woman physician only in a caption to an illustration of a lecture held at a women's medical school in New York City, noting that Cole was one of the attendees.[12] After graduation, Cole moved to the city to work as a resident physician and sanitary visitor at the New York Infirmary for Women and Children, founded by Elizabeth Blackwell. Her responsibilities included visiting indigent women in their homes and instructing them in the basics of hygiene. Cole later served on the staffs of medical and social agencies in Philadelphia, Pennsylvania, and Washington, District of Columbia, that primarily assisted poor Black women. She also emerged as a staunch advocate for racial justice. In 1873, she protested the establishment of two racially separate women's committees in Philadelphia to celebrate the nation's upcoming centennial.[13]

Like Crumpler before her, Cole underscored the social and economic factors such as racism, inadequate medical care, and poor housing as the major contributing factors to the health of African Americans. Active in the National Association of Colored Women, in 1896, she wrote an article in the inaugural issue of its journal, *The Woman's Era*, that offered a stinging critique of theories that posited that African Americans were naturally susceptible to tuberculosis. She also used the piece to criticize sociologist W. E. B. Du Bois's preliminary research for his seminal work, *The Philadelphia Negro.* Du Bois argued that tuberculosis struck Black people in disproportionate amounts. Cole, however, challenged the accuracy of his statistics and questioned whether the rates were exaggerated. She did not have "implicit faith in these statistics" because the data had been collected by men "who are so warped by that strange American disease, colorphobia." She also wrote,

> On the point of deaths from consumption, I would say this: hosts of the poor are attended by young, inexperienced white physicians. They have inherited the traditions of their elders, and let a black person cough, they immediately have visions of tubercles, let him die, and he writes 'tuberculosis,' and heaves a great sigh of relief that one more source of contagion is removed.

At the same time, Cole recognized that African Americans suffered from tuberculosis and she was committed to stopping the spread of the disease. She advocated the expansion of hygiene education to African Americans and the application of political pressure on public officials to enact legislation to combat overcrowding at the hands of "soulless landlords" who packed people "like cattle" in tenements.[14]

In the years since Byrd and Clayton first published *An American Health Dilemma,* scholarship in the history of African American women physicians has grown, though the topic remains underresearched.[15] This new work removes them from history's shadows and recognizes their accomplishments, activism, and valuable contributions to medicine, public health, and the African American community. It makes plain that African American women physicians should have pride of place as "foundation stones of intellect and inspiration" in the fight for health equity. AJPH

CORRESPONDENCE

Correspondence should be sent to Vanessa Northington Gamble, MD, PhD, The George Washington University, Phillips Hall, Suite 412E, 801 22nd St NW, Washington, DC 20052 (e-mail: vngamble@gwu.edu). Reprints can be ordered at https://www.ajph.org by clicking the "Reprints" link.

PUBLICATION INFORMATION

Full Citation: Gamble VN. "A wide field is open before her, and many of her sisters": discovering early African American women physicians. *Am J Public Health*. 2026;116(5):632–634.

Acceptance Date: January 28, 2026.

DOI: https://doi.org/10.2105/AJPH.2026.308451

ACKNOWLEDGMENTS

I wish to thank Kiana Wilkerson for research and editorial assistance in the preparation of this essay and Ellen F. Fitzpatrick, PhD, for providing astute comments and suggestions.

CONFLICTS OF INTEREST

The author has no conflicts of interest to declare.

ENDNOTES

1. "New England Female Medical College," *Boston Daily Evening Traveller*, March 9, 1864, New England Female Medical College, Scrapbook, 1847–1865, Francis A. Countway Library of Medicine, Harvard University, Boston, MA, https://nrs.lib.harvard.edu/urn-3:hms.count:592799 (accessed November 26, 2025).
2. W. Michael Byrd and Linda A. Clayton, *An American Health Dilemma: Volume I: A Medical History of African Americans and the Problem of Race, Beginnings to 1900* (New York, NY: Routledge, 2000) and W. Michael Byrd and Linda A. Clayton, *An American Health Dilemma, Volume II: Race, Medicine, and Health Care in the United States, 1900–2000* (New York, NY: Routledge, 2002).
3. Byrd and Clayton, *An American Health Dilemma, Volume I,* xv.
4. Byrd and Clayton, *An American Health Dilemma, Volume I,* xix.
5. Darlene Clark Hine, "Taking Care of Bodies, Babies, and Business: Black Women Health Professionals in South Carolina, 1895–1954," in Elizabeth Anne Payne, ed., *Writing Women's History: A Tribute to Anne Firor Scott,* (Jackson, MS: University Press of Mississippi, 2011), 118.
6. "Sets in Colored Society," *Boston Daily Globe*, June 22, 1894, 29; and Rebecca Crumpler, *A Book of Medical Discourses in Two Parts* (Boston, MA: Cashman, Keating & Co, 1883), 2.
7. *Report of Persons and Articles Hired for July 1867*, NMAAHC.FB.M1913, Records of the Field Offices for the State of Virginia, Bureau of Refugees, Freedmen, and Abandoned Lands, 1865–1872, National Museum of African American History and Culture, Washington, DC, 4 (image 2), https://edan.si.edu/slideshow/viewer/?eadrefid=NMAAHC.FB.M1913_ref73_part2 (accessed March 12, 2026). My thanks to Wangui Muigai, PhD, for supplying this reference
8. For more extensive analysis of Crumpler's book see Adele Logan Alexander, *Homelands and Waterways: The American Journey of the Bond Family, 1846–1926* (New York, NY: Pantheon, 1999), 276–281; Susan Wells, *Out of the Dead House: Nineteenth Century Women Physicians and the Writing of Medicine* (Madison, WI: University of Wisconsin Press, 2001), 51–54; Perri Klass, "'To Mitigate the Afflictions of the Human Race'—The Legacy of Dr. Rebecca Crumpler," *The New England Journal of Medicine* 384, no. 13 (April 1, 2021): 1186–1189, https://doi.org/10.1056/NEJMp2032451; and Patrick S. Allen, "'We Must Attack the System': The Print Practice of Black 'Doctresses,'" *Arizona Quarterly* 74, no. 4 (Winter 2018): 87–113.
9. Crumpler, *A Book of Medical Discourses,* 99.
10. Crumpler, *A Book of Medical Discourses,* 115.
11. Crumpler, *A Book of Medical Discourses,* 83.
12. Byrd and Clayton, *An American Health Dilemma, Volume I,* 194.
13. "Radical Club," *The Philadelphia Inquirer*, May 29, 1873, 2.
14. Rebecca J. Cole, "First Meeting of the Women's Missionary Society of Philadelphia," *The Woman's Era,* 3 (October/November 1896), 4–6.
15. These works include Darlene Clark Hine, "The Corporeal and Ocular Veil: Dr. Matilda A. Evans (1872–1935) and the Complexity of Southern History," *Journal of Southern History* 70: (February 2004): 3–34, https://doi.org/10.2307/27648310; Vanessa Northington Gamble, "'Outstanding Services to Negro Health': Dr. Dorothy Boulding Ferebee and Dr. Virginia M. Alexander and Black Women Physicians' Public Health Activism," *American Journal of Public Health,* 106:8 (August 2016): 1397–1404, https://doi.org/10.2105/AJPH.2016.303252; Diane Kiesel, *She Can Bring Us Home: Dr. Dorothy Boulding Ferebee, Civil Rights Pioneer* (Lincoln, NE: University of Nebraska Press, 2015); Vanessa Northington Gamble, "'Sisters of a Darker Race': African American Graduates of the Woman's Medical College of Pennsylvania, 1867–1925," *Bulletin of the History of Medicine* 95, no. 2 (Summer 2021): 169–197, https://doi.org/10.1353/bhm.2021.0029; and Margaret Vigil-Fowler and Sukumar Desai, "'A Much Wider Field in Which to Operate': Early Black Women Physicians in Public Health," *Journal of the History of Medicine and Allied Sciences* 79, no. 2 (April 2024); 129–142, https://doi.org/10.1093/jhmas/jrad048

Of Miracles, Medicine, and the "Moor's" Leg: What Are We to Do With Race?

Rana A. Hogarth, PhD

ABOUT THE AUTHOR

Rana A. Hogarth is with the University of Pennsylvania, Philadelphia.

See also An American Health Dilemma 25 Years Later, pp. 625–656.

Origin stories are often complicated and contested. You can ask a historian of 19th-century America about the origins of the Civil War, and you will likely get a helpful answer that slavery was central to the conflict, but that will be the entry point into a larger, more complex discussion. Despite the roundabout way origin stories operate, historians remain committed to telling them. This, at least, accords with my own experience whenever I question the exact origin of race, as it refers to a category used to mark embodied difference (i.e., race as it might appear on the census, in medical records, and in clinical studies). Not satisfied with just one deceptively simple question, I also wonder why race continues to infiltrate our collective thinking about health and the human body when we know it has no significant biological meaning.

A DILEMMA AND THE NARRATIVE OF DISPARITIES

My line of questioning is of course informed by many things including the pioneering work done decades ago by two physicians, Michael W. Byrd and Linda A. Clayton, who investigated the origins of and reasons for the consistent "disparate health status and outcomes of African Americans" in comparison with Whites.[1] Their investigation culminated in *An American Health Dilemma: A Medical History of African Americans and the Problem of Race: Beginnings to 1900*. Weighing in at more than 600 pages (the second volume was even more lengthy), *An American Health Dilemma* tackled anti-Black racism in medicine with unflinching attention to history. They brought centuries of anti-Blackness in medical thought, practice, education, policy, and treatment under a magnifying glass for their readers. Byrd and Clayton's work might have been the first time audiences, removed from the academic orbits of history and African American studies, were made aware of the ways Black people's bodies had been pathologized, neglected, surveilled, and exploited in the name of medicine and science. Beyond that, they pointed to the obvious and consistent ways Blackness became wielded as a proxy for innate difference; they showed us how the tragedy of race did not unfold by chance, but by choice.

They did all of this roughly 25 years ago. Yet here we are, still bogged down by anti-Blackness, health disparities, and a continuing normalization of ideas of innate biological differences between Black and White people. But now we must contend with the ways in which fallacies of race and myths about Blackness continue to be reproduced from seemingly "neutral" and authoritative sources. More than just prescient, Byrd and Clayton's work remains a primer for those wishing to take a long view of the origin stories of Blackness as a biological entity. It has encouraged us to dig deeper and look even more carefully into the origins of race, no matter how thorny that process is.

THE PAST AND PROCESS

Questions about race are especially challenging because race is such a personal and political thing. Rather than looking for a singular explanation, I focus on the process of how people thought about race and its meanings. For many historians of the 18th and 19th century, a soft consensus on the origins of race has emerged. Many will tell you that our current understanding of race (the grouping of people into categories based on physical traits) originated sometime between the late 17th and 18th century.[2] But that soft consensus does not mean that topic is settled, or that correlated questions about how and why race came to carry biological meaning are easily settled, too.[3] Indeed, questions about the origins of race have sparked lively debates among early modern and medieval scholars, who suggest an earlier point of origin.[4] Race had not yet been consistently viewed as an embodied or anatomized characteristic in the medieval era. That said, features like Black skin were certainly recognized and noted. Textual and visual sources show us

AJPH May 2026, Vol. 116, No. 5

that even when race was marked by Black skin color in medieval contexts, the color did not always signify a derogatory Other, or anything that might be construed as biologically meaningful.[5] A person could be rendered Black in an image based on their character or for some socially constructed meaning. Even in cases where a person was depicted as Black, including skin and physiognomy, it might not connote something negative, as evidenced by the famed statue of Saint Maurice of Magdeburg found in the Magdeburg Cathedral in Germany (ca. 1240–1250). In this rendering of Saint Maurice, he appears as a venerated knight of Black African descent.[6]

The biological insignificance of race comes through quite well in the apocryphal medieval image, *The Miracle of the Black Leg*, taken from the *Golden Legend*, a 13th-century compilation of saints' lives (Figure 1).[7] Depictions of this miracle feature the martyred physician saints, Cosmas and Damian, performing a miraculous transplant surgery, in which they heal a sick White verger with a Black leg taken from a recently deceased "Moor" or Ethiopian. The contrast of skin color remains a fairly consistent detail in renditions of this painting.[8] And yet, art historians and medievalists have recognized that despite this very deliberate attention to the donor's non-White identity, and the deliberate emphasis on the difference in color of the transplanted leg and the transplant recipient, this miracle carried undertones of unity. In other words, it is not a story about embodied racial difference, even though it looks like one. This is at least how some art historians have understood images of the miracle before 1500. Despite the use of the word "moor" in the description of the miracle, the Black leg was likely taken from a Christian Ethiopian.[9] It is worth noting, that "moor" could mean a person who was African, or Muslim, or dark skinned. It was not until after 1500 when associations between Blackness, sub-Saharan Africans, and slavery hardened and took a permanently negative turn. Indeed, as the Atlantic slave trade in captive Africans boomed, so did the notion of treating Blackness as something inferior, anatomically peculiar and undesirable. This shift might arguably be palpable in renditions of *The Miracle of the Black Leg* created after the 1500s.[10]

SO MUCH FOR THE SOCIAL CONSTRUCT

This image leads me to think about what we are to do with the repeated statement we tell ourselves—namely, that race is a social construct, with no biological significance—a statement that was even en vogue when *An American Health Dilemma* first appeared. Relying on my untrained eyes, it appears as if the message behind this statement was apprehended centuries ago in the medieval painting. In the present moment, however, I have my doubts that the message is registering anymore. To be clear, the problem is not that we do not know that race is a social construct. We do. The problem is, we say it, but do not mean it. This disconnect is fairly glaring in how we present medical data. If you ask Google if race is a social construct, it will answer in the affirmative and tell you it is a category created by society rather than a biological reality. However, if one

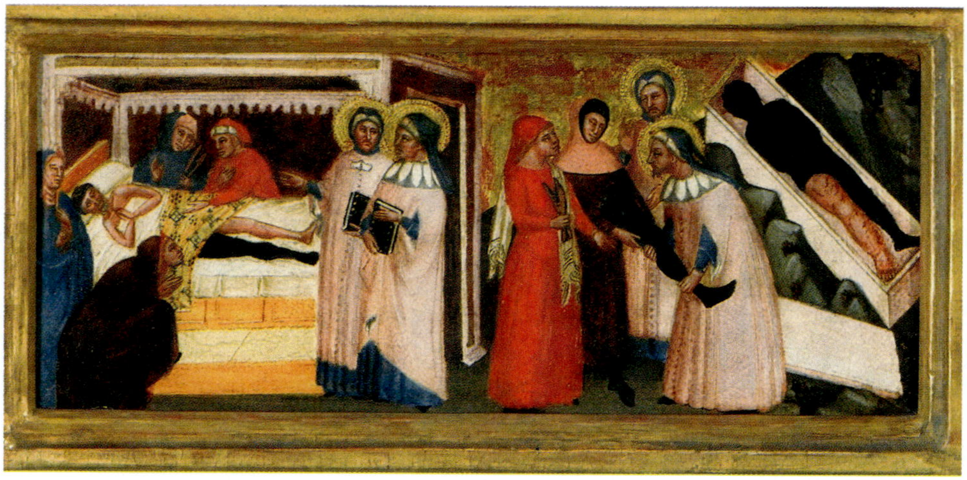

FIGURE 1— Saint Cosmas and Saint Damian (Detail of Lower Left Panel)

Note. Master of the Rinuccini Chapel (Matteo di Pacino), c. 1370–1375, tempera and gold leaf on panel, 79.4 × 135.6 cm (North Carolina Museum of Art, Raleigh).

asks Google, "Do Black people have denser bones than Whites?" Google will quickly give you an affirmative response generated by its artificial intelligence (AI) overview. AI knows race is a social construction, but AI does not care. Google will provide you with links to the studies that informed its affirmative answer. Some studies that might appear include, "Racial Differences in Bone Density Between Young Adult Black and White Subjects Persist After Adjustment for Anthropometric, Lifestyle, and Biochemical Differences."[11] That study, which constitutes part of the AI overview, provides no discussion that race is a social category.

Statements from the abovementioned study, published in 1997, include

> Many have hypothesized that genetically determined differences in skeletal metabolism account for racial differences in bone density; this hypothesis is supported by studies that show racial differences in calciotropic hormones and bone turnover markers. Compared with White persons, Black persons have lower urinary calcium excretion. . . .[12]

Such statements may leave readers convinced that being Black means having different biological functionality than being White.[13] Among the many things left unexplained in this study is how designations of racial groups were made. Was it self-identification or researcher-based identification? The study does not explain the relationship between genes and race, though it references genetics. Mixed-race people's bones are not mentioned in the study, which seems to have been devised with the premise that there is even such a thing as "pure races." The study's data are drawn from the United States, which means that the populations designated as Black likely have European admixture, because

> Researchers have found that a significant percentage of African-Americans, European Americans, and Latinos carry ancestry from outside their self-identified ethnicity. The average African-American genome, for example, is nearly a quarter European, and almost 4% of European Americans carry African ancestry.[14]

Thinking with the image of *The Miracle of the Black Leg* provides an instructive way for articulating the biological and medical insignificance of race. The image shows us clear racial contrast in a clinical setting, where race is embodied, but not biologically important. The miracle takes place at the bedside of a sick verger, not quite the "clinical setting" to which we are accustomed but, nevertheless, the place where the execution of a complex, albeit improbable transplant surgery took place. And while it is true that our clinical settings today are not sites for fantastical events, they are still home to fantastical notions about race, just as they were years ago when Byrd and Clayton published *An American Health Dilemma*. Now we know, based on systematic studies, that race is not only noted and acknowledged in our clinical settings of today, but it is given "magical" powers that allow it to explain differences in responses to drugs or pain.[15] Given our current approach to thinking about race and its deterministic applications, it is hard to know if we will ever get to a place where different races can be recognized superficially but not given biological weight. Perhaps it will take a miracle. AJPH

CORRESPONDENCE

Correspondence should be sent to Rana A. Hogarth, 303 Claudia Cohen Hall, 249 S 36th St, Philadelphia, PA 19104 (e-mail: rhogarth@sas.upenn.edu). Reprints can be ordered at https://www.ajph.org by clicking the "Reprints" link.

PUBLICATION INFORMATION

Full Citation: Hogarth RA. Of miracles, medicine, and the "Moor's" leg: what are we to do with race? *Am J Public Health*. 2026;116(5):635–638.

Acceptance Date: January 29, 2026.

DOI: https://doi.org/10.2105/AJPH.2026.308450

ORCID iD:
Rana A. Hogarth https://orcid.org/0009-0001-2222-5513

ACKNOWLEDGMENTS

The author wishes to thank Ted Brown.

CONFLICTS OF INTEREST

The author reports no conflicts of interest.

ENDNOTES

1. W. Michael Byrd and Linda A. Clayton, *An American Health Dilemma: A Medical History of African Americans and the Problem of Race: Beginnings to 1900* (New York, NY: Taylor & Francis Group, 2000), 31.
2. Henry Louis Gates Jr and Andrew S. Curran, eds., *Who's Black and Why? A Hidden Chapter From the Eighteenth-Century Invention of Race* (Cambridge MA: Harvard University Press, 2022).
3. Early iterations of race can be to the 15th century in Romance languages, where it was typically understood to explain "blood lines or pedigree"; Scott Netherolse, "Fra Angelico's *The Miracle of the Black Leg*: Skin Colour and the Perception of Ethiopians in Florence Before 1450," *Art History* 45, no. 2 (2022): 250–278, 252, https://doi.org/10.1111/1467-8365.12648
4. For more on growing pre-modern discussions of race see RaceB4Race, an ongoing symposium launched at Arizona State University in 2019, https://acmrs.asu.edu/RaceB4Race (accessed December 2, 2025).
5. Geraldine Heng reminds us that people in the medieval period could be depicted as Black because it corresponded to a "hermeneutic" Blackness—a social idea that might equate Blackness with something dark or some other meaning. That kind of Blackness was quite different from "physiognomic" Blackness (i.e., depicting figures with Black skin and African features). For more, see Geraldine Heng, *The Invention of Race in the European Middle Ages* (Cambridge, England: Cambridge University Press, 2018), 185; and Nethersole, "Fra Angelico's *The Miracle of the Black Leg*," 253.
6. Geraldine Heng, "An African Saint in Medieval Europe: The Black Saint Maurice and the Enigma of Racial Sanctity," in Molly H. Bassett, Vincent W. Lloyd, eds., *Sainthood and Race* (New York, NY: Routledge, 2014): 18–44, 21.
7. Alistair Minnis, "Proto-Surgery, Resurrection, and Race: Interpreting 'The Ethiopian's Leg Transplant' Miracle," *The Mediaeval Journal* (2021): 57–98, 59, https://doi.org/10.1484/J.TMJ.5.136463; Leth Chi'en, "*The Miracle of the Black Leg*," Smarthistory, https://smarthistory.org/miracle-black-leg (accessed November 21, 2025).

8. "Moor" could reference a Muslim or a person with dark skin. For more, see Leth Chi'en "*The Miracle of the Black Leg*"; Nethersole, "Fra Angelico's *The Miracle of the Black Leg*," 263.
9. Nethersole, "Fra Angelico's *The Miracle of the Black Leg*," 262; and Minnis, "Proto-Surgery, Resurrection, and Race," 79.
10 Minnis, "Proto-Surgery, Resurrection, and Race," 86.
11. Bruce Ettinger et al., "Racial Differences in Bone Density Between Young Adult Black and White Subjects Persist After Adjustment for Anthropometric, Lifestyle, and Biochemical Differences," *The Journal of Clinical Endocrinology and Metabolism* 82, no. 2 (1997): 429–434, https://doi.org/10.1210/jcem.82.2.3732
12. Ettinger et al., "Racial Differences in Bone Density," 429.
13. By the time the study was published, there had been ample academic discussion of race as a social construct; Barbara Jeanne Fields, "Slavery, Race and Ideology in the United States of America," *New Left Review* 181, no. 1 (1990): 95–118, https://doi.org/10.64590/cfe; and Richard Lewontin, "The Apportionment of Human Diversity," in E. Nathaniel Gates, ed., *The Concept of Race in Natural and Social Science* (New York, NY: Routledge, 2014), 7–24.
14. Lizze Wade, "Genetic Study Reveals Surprising Ancestry of Many Americans: Some African-Americans, European Americans, and Latinos Carry Genes That Don't Match Their Self-Identified Ethnicities," *Science* (December 18, 2014), https://www.science.org/content/article/genetic-study-reveals-surprising-ancestry-many-americans (accessed November 21, 2025).
15. Kelly M. Hoffman et al., "Racial Bias in Pain Assessment and Treatment Recommendations, and False Beliefs About Biological Differences Between Blacks and Whites, *Proceedings of the National Academy of Sciences of the United States of America* 113, no. 16 (2016): 4296–4301, https://doi.org/10.1073/pnas.1516047113. The now nearly 10-year-old study by Hoffman et al. published on racial bias in pain assessment is a case in point. That study made waves for some because it revealed that White residents (and laypeople, too) assumed Black people had thicker skins than Whites, had blood that coagulated more quickly than Whites, and were more likely to bear pain better.

Childbearing and Reproductive Health Under Slavery

Deirdre Cooper Owens, PhD

ABOUT THE AUTHOR

Deirdre Cooper Owens is with the Department of History and the Africana Studies Institute, University of Connecticut, Storrs Mansfield.

See also An American Health Dilemma 25 Years Later, pp. 625–656.

In 2000, the United States seemed gripped with fear about the impending close of another millennium. For many, the Y2K scare conjured up ideas about global computer systems shutting down and causing an unfathomable apocalypse. People responded to the imagined end of times by stockpiling provisions, purchasing firearms, and withdrawing their life savings. Yet for married physicians and public health scholars, Michael Byrd and Linda Clayton, who authored the magisterial two-volume set, *An American Health Dilemma: A Medical History of African Americans and the Problem of Race, Beginnings to 1900*[1] and *An American Health Dilemma: Race, Medicine, and Health Care in the United States, 1900–2000*,[2] the end of the 20th century signaled how terrifying it was for marginalized Americans, especially African Americans, given their fraught relationship with the US medical–industrial complex.

Instead of hoarding, as Y2K doomsdayers did, Byrd and Clayton released their arsenal of historical data that revealed the often abusive, exploitative, and unethical treatment meted out by an all-White medical establishment that stemmed from the United States' colonial past through the end of the 20th century. In the introduction, the authors proclaimed boldly and with righteous indignation that *An American Health Dilemma* was not meant to simply reveal the statistics that showed how drastic health disparities were for African Americans compared with White Americans: they intended the book to "devise analytical frameworks for examining social determinants of health."[3]

An American Health Dilemma forced many scholars of race, the history of medicine, and public health to create theoretical interventions that accurately named what had happened and what was happening to African Americans, women, poor people, and other racialized minorities via US medical practitioners. If Byrd and Clayton could offer up the "slave health deficit" as an intellectual point of origin for readers to fully understand the genealogy of "public health gaps between Blacks and others," I knew that I also had a responsibility to create frameworks that accurately defined how anti-Black medical practitioners had treated Black people historically. Nearly two decades later, when my monograph, *Medical Bondage: Race, Gender and the Origins of American Gynecology*,[4] was published, I coined the term "medical superbodies" to describe how White physicians transformed Black people's bodies into human sites capable of withstanding exploitative experimental surgeries, dangerous and physically violent procedures meant to cure imagined ailments, and objects instead of patients who needed care.

So, when the *AJPH* editorial staff approached me to write a long-overdue review of *An American Health Dilemma*, I jumped at the chance—largely because Byrd and Clayton's texts became sacred texts when I first started writing my dissertation 20 years ago but also because I now see how timely it still is regarding the ever-worsening racial health disparities between Black Americans and White Americans and, more specifically, the haves and the have-nots. I am a scholar of the history of early US gynecology, race, and slavery and a reproductive justice advocate with 15 years of experience. Thus, my review will focus primarily on what Byrd and Clayton wrote about childbearing and reproductive health under US slavery and the historical legacy that the United States continues to contend with in its current birthing crisis.

The authors detail the work of US gynecology's "founding fathers," such as Ephraim McDowell, who performed the first successful ovariotomy in 1809; John Richmond, who in 1827 is believed to have performed the first documented cesarean delivery west of the Allegheny Mountains in which both mother and child survived; and James Marion Sims, who in the mid- to late 1840s created the surgical technique that repaired obstetrical fistulas. Each of these doctors operated largely on Black women, both free and enslaved. In this chapter, Byrd and Clayton provide what they termed "a new perspective on a medical icon"[4(p1)]: James Marion Sims (whose colleagues regarded as "the father of American gynecology"[4(p1)] after his death because of his pioneering surgical work and institution building).

AJPH May 2026, Vol. 116, No. 5

Sims founded the first two US hospitals for women. The first dedicated women's hospital was for Alabaman enslaved women and was established in the 1840s. The second women's hospital was opened in 1855 Manhattan in New York City.

Byrd and Clayton describe Sims as deceitful and unethical. They claim Sims intentionally addicted his enslaved patients to opiates while they recovered from his surgery, cruelly provided no anesthetics to the women, and purposefully hid the racial identity of his enslaved experimental participants when he published his 1852 article, which detailed his pioneering surgical reparative work. All their notes in this section stem from secondary sources.[1] As you might imagine, I had to unpack some information and yet balance my critique of the book's mission, as outlined in the introduction.

The mythology of James Marion Sims contains both facts and fiction, like most mythologies. It is true that Sims was a slave-holding physician who used the system of slavery to have nearly unfettered access to enslaved people's bodies. He simply needed a fellow slave owner to grant him permission to treat a sick or "damaged" slave. The owners of the Black women who were Sims's first experimental gynecological patients granted him permission to reverse their condition so that their value as birthing property would be maintained or increased. Currency was at the heart of the economic system of US slavery. Thus, injuring or sterilizing reproductive age adolescent girls and women would be costly for Sims, who was neither a wealthy slave owner nor a physician.

Sims began experimenting on his enslaved patients nearly a year before dentist Samuel Morton first administered ether to a patient in October 1846. Furthermore, the branch of medicine that later came to be known as anesthesiology was not fully established until decades later. For instance, the term "anesthesiology" was coined in the early 1900s. Sims was not experienced enough to use ether or nitrous oxide on these women and might not have been exposed to surgeries in which anesthetics were used on gynecological patients.

It is also important to note that most, if not all, antebellum era surgeons did not fully understand the addictive nature of opiates. In Sims's earliest vesicovaginal fistula work, he administered opiate-based medicine to cause constipation so that his patients' sutures would remain unbroken. And lastly, Sims might not have been the illustrator of the White nurse and patient in the medical journal article that Byrd and Clayton mention in the chapter. The *American Journal of Medical Science*, which published Sims's 1852 article, hired professional medical illustrators. Also, the lithograph illustration of Sims's vesicovaginal operation supported with the assistance of a White nurse was drawn by J. B. Léveillé a quarter of a century later, in 1870 (Figure 1).[5]

Despite these errors, Byrd and Clayton's claims about Sims's anti-Black racism is accurate. They also rightly condemn his questionable and excessive actions regarding the public display of his enslaved patients before crowds (and later, in New York during the 1850s onward, how his medical theater antics of stuffing the hospital amphitheater with an unnecessarily large crowd of onlookers eventually caused his firing by the hospital's board of directors). Most notably, later in the chapter they ask how the "slave health deficit" resulted in the low birth weight or death of enslaved newborns. They call out the callous and dangerous treatment that enslaved women endured from their owners, who were more interested in these new mothers' work schedules than necessary postpartum care.[1(p283)] Byrd and Clayton provide tables and indices that show the high percentage of child mortality from the antebellum era through Jim Crow and how Black children's life expectancy remained lower than that of White children's from slavery to freedom.

Unsurprisingly, the statistics remain eerily similar for Black women and birthing people in the 21st century. In 2000, when *An American Health Dilemma* was published, the Black infant mortality rates in the United States were "2.4 times the non-Hispanic white rates."[6] Black mothers and birthing people fare no better in 2025 than their 19th-century predecessors. The current statistics show that the United States is the most dangerous high-income nation for a Black woman or birthing person to become pregnant and give birth. Most alarmingly, Black women and birthing people are three to four times more likely to die from pregnancy-related complications than are White women.[7]

Byrd and Clayton warn readers that until the United States addresses its practice of separate and unequal medical treatment of Black people, women, poor people, and other marginalized racialized groups of people, we will enter a new era with an even greater gap between Black people and White people in life expectancy, infant mortality and morbidity, maternal mortality and morbidity, and the number of marginalized Americans who do not receive adequate preventative care owing to limited access to life-saving and excellent medical treatment and care. The Black birthing crisis most starkly

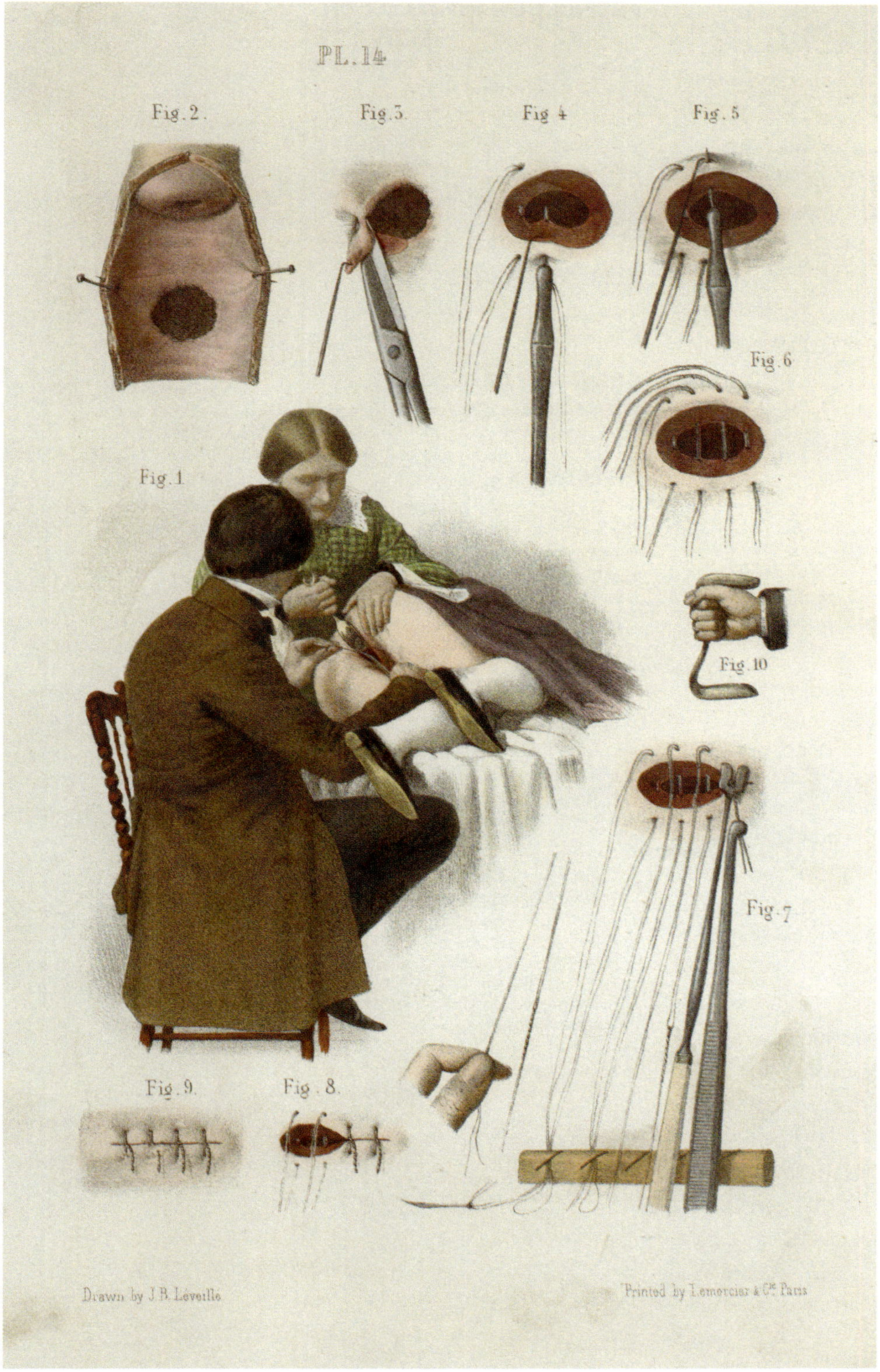

FIGURE 1— **Léveillé and Sims and Nurse Repairing a Vesico-Vaginal Fistula Patient: 1870**

Source. Savage.[5] Image Courtesy of the Hagströmer Medico-Historical Library, Karolinska Institute.

presents how much the continuation of medical racism affects Americans. Although reproductive justice was still in its infancy in 2000, Byrd and Clayton were also alluding to reproductive justice in their calls for unfettered access to equal and compassionate medical care.

In 1994, more than 10 Black women activists coined the term "reproductive justice" to push against a solely pro-choice abortionist political agenda popularized by White feminist activists.[8] According to Loretta Ross, one of the founding mothers of the reproductive justice movement:

> We were dissatisfied with the pro-choice language, feeling that it did not accurately encompass our twinned goals: Nor did the language of choice accurately portray the many barriers African American women faced when trying to make reproductive decisions.[8]

Byrd and Clayton's two-volume set was the perfect remedy for so many Americans focused on the wrong catastrophe. Y2K turned out to be nothing more than the culmination of fear unmanifested. Yet, the real terror Americans faced then and now, a quarter century later, especially with the current Black birthing crisis, is a legacy of medical racism that could easily be remedied. If we return to *An American Health Dilemma*, we might heed the authors' direction on eliminating a colonial era problem—racism—rooted in an ideology that serves no one. AJPH

CORRESPONDENCE

Correspondence should be sent to Deirdre Cooper Owens, 241 Glenbrook Rd, Unit 4103, Storrs Mansfield, CT 06269-4103 (e-mail: deirdre.cooper_owens@uconn.edu). Reprints can be ordered at https://www.ajph.org by clicking the "Reprints" link.

PUBLICATION INFORMATION

Full Citation: Owens DC. Childbearing and reproductive health under slavery. *Am J Public Health*. 2026;116(5):639–642.

Acceptance Date: January 31, 2026.

DOI: https://doi.org/10.2105/AJPH.2026.308455

ORCID iD:
Deirdre Cooper Owens https://orcid.org/0009-0008-7994-5037

ACKNOWLEDGMENTS

Thank you to Theodore Brown for his editorial advice.

CONFLICTS OF INTEREST

The author has no conflicts of interest to report.

REFERENCES

1. Byrd WM, Clayton L. *An American Health Dilemma: A Medical History of African Americans and the Problem of Race, Beginnings to 1900.* New York, NY: Routledge; 2000.
2. Byrd WM, Clayton LA. *An American Health Dilemma: Race, Medicine, and Health Care in the United States, 1900–2000.* New York, NY: Routledge; 2002.
3. Lewis & Wright Funeral Directors. Dr. W. Michael Byrd. March 4, 2021. Available at: https://www.lewisandwrightfuneraldirectors.com/obituaries/dr-w-byrd. Accessed March 7, 2026.
4. Cooper Owens DB. *Medical Bondage: Race, Gender and the Origins of American Gynecology.* Athens, GA: University of Georgia Press; 2017.
5. Savage H. *The Surgery, Surgical Pathology and Surgical Anatomy of the Female Pelvic Organs: in a Series of Coloured Plates Taken From Nature. With Commentaries, Notes, and Cases.* 2nd ed. London, England: J. & A. Churchill; 1870.
6. Centers for Disease Control and Prevention. QuickStats: infant mortality rates, by race and Hispanic ethnicity of mother—United States, 2000, 2005, and 2010. Available at: https://www.cdc.gov/mmwr/preview/mmwrhtml/mm6301a9.htm. Accessed March 7, 2026.
7. Howell EA. Reducing disparities in severe maternal morbidity and mortality. *Clin Obstet Gynecol.* 2018;61(2):387–399. https://doi.org/10.1097/GRF.0000000000000349
8. National Latina Institute for Reproductive Justice. 2026. What is reproductive justice? Available at: https://www.latinainstitute.org/resource/what-is-reproductive-justice-rj. Accessed March 7, 2026.

Hospitals and the History of Structural Racism in the United States

LeNie Adolphson, PhD, and Beatrix Hoffman, PhD

See also An American Health Dilemma 25 Years Later, pp. 625–656.

W. Michael Byrd and Linda A. Clayton's two-volume work *An American Health Dilemma* powerfully describes how racism has permeated every aspect of the US health delivery system. As part of commemorating *An American Health Dilemma* 25 years after its publication, this article discusses the place of hospitals in Byrd and Clayton's analysis. They argued that US hospitals have perpetuated health inequities through formal segregation, structural factors such as White flight and government disinvestment, and racist practices and ideologies that stigmatize African American patients as inferior or other. This article also seeks to integrate Byrd and Clayton's foundational work with recent scholarship on the history of community struggles against health disparities, including a new dissertation examining Chicago's Provident Hospital, the nation's first Black-run hospital. We demonstrate the enduring relevance of *An American Health Dilemma* and emphasize the need to recognize the role of hospitals in both maintaining and dismantling racial injustice. (*Am J Public Health*. 2026;116(5):643–648. https://doi.org/10.2105/AJPH.2026.308421)

AJPH May 2026, Vol. 116, No. 5

An American Health Dilemma, published by physicians W. Michael Byrd and Linda A. Clayton in 2000 and 2002, is a lengthy, ambitious analysis of health care inequality in the United States. In this two-volume work, Byrd and Clayton seek explanations for why Black Americans continue to suffer disproportionately poor health despite advances in medical technology and access to care. The authors' approach is multidisciplinary and, especially, historical: they posit that the roots of contemporary disparities lie in the enduring legacy of American racism. They emphasize that social determinants of health, including housing, education, and income inequality, are inseparable from structural racism, the enduring bias originating in the era of slavery. The authors underscore the continuity of racial health disparities, tracing a lineage from segregated hospital wards to current inequities in access, treatment, and outcomes.

An American Health Dilemma powerfully describes how racism has permeated every aspect of the US health delivery system. While Byrd and Clayton examine a multitude of events and institutions, this article discusses the place of hospitals in the American health dilemma. It is crucial to look deeply at hospitals because they have been, and remain, the "dominant health care institutions" in the United States.[1]

The two volumes tell the story of how hospitals have perpetuated health inequities through formal segregation, through structural factors such as White flight and government disinvestment, and through racist practices and ideologies that stigmatize African American patients as inferior or other. This article seeks to integrate Byrd and Clayton's foundational analysis with recent historical research, highlighting the enduring relevance of *An American Health Dilemma* today.

The early US hospital system, Byrd and Clayton write, operated along class lines, separating the worthy from the unworthy poor. In the context of slavery and American racism, Black patients in this system were rendered

> a particularly and peculiarly vulnerable and disadvantaged caste . . . African Americans were not only burdened with the stigma of low socioeconomic status and 'unworthiness,' but they also underwent health system abuse, exploitation, segregation, and discrimination on the basis of their race.[2]

As Jim Crow took hold in the South, hospitals reflected the dominant racial order; urban hospitals in Southern cities might have a "Jim Crow" ward (refusing admission to Black patients when those few beds were filled), but most hospitals refused Blacks altogether, leaving rural African Americans to rely on informal practitioners and folk remedies. In addition, the American Medical Association allowed local medical societies to exclude Black physicians, and most hospitals in both the North and South did not allow Black physicians to hold staff privileges.[3]

Formal hospital segregation in the South, the authors note, was underpinned by "codified legal practices separating the races and endorsing discrimination against African Americans."[4] The same was true of federally supported hospital expansion after World War II. The Hill–Burton Act, passed by Congress in 1946, allowed Southern hospitals to use taxpayer funds for "separate but equal" facilities. In fact, Byrd and Clayton assert,

> Hill-Burton provisions institutionalized segregation where it had not existed and often accentuated the plight of the racially excluded African American patients and doctors throughout the South for the first two decades of its existence.[5]

An American Health Dilemma emphasizes that hospital bias was never confined to the South. Hospitals in Northern cities such as Cleveland, Ohio, and Detroit, Michigan, also practiced racial discrimination and exclusion, especially after the Great Migration increased the demand for Black hospital care. In the North, "the formation of the 'Negro medical ghetto'" was one of the "natural by-products of Black ghetto formation" and the "institutionalization of Black/White economic differentials during an industrial age."[6] In other words, hospital discrimination was embedded in systemic racial inequities.

THE RISE AND FALL OF BLACK HOSPITALS

Byrd and Clayton also explicate how African Americans' distrust of the medical system was a rational response to hospital discrimination, to the well-known practices of medical experimentation targeting Black patients, and to the overt racial hostility of White practitioners. The absence of accessible and trusted medical care was the impetus for the Black Hospital Movement. Starting in the 1890s, Black physicians and activists founded more than 100 hospitals around the country to provide care to patients who were denied treatment in White institutions. Another key role of Black hospitals was to provide opportunities for Black physicians who were denied staff privileges in White hospitals, and to offer medical and nursing training for Black students. Despite chronically inadequate funding, these hospitals filled critical gaps in care and opportunity. Given the authors' cogent assessment of medical racism at the turn of the century, they clearly demonstrate that the Black Hospital Movement rose to save Black lives that were in peril.

Byrd and Clayton based their analysis of the Black Hospital Movement on extant secondary sources, particularly Vanessa Northington Gamble's now-classic *Making a Place for Ourselves.*[7] New scholarship utilizing primary research, such as LeNie Adolphson's 2024 dissertation on Provident Hospital in Chicago, Illinois, strengthens the contention of *An American Health Dilemma* that Black hospitals served as bulwarks against systemic racism. In addition, their leaders and staff were cognizant of and attempted to address racial health disparities.

Founded by Daniel Hale Williams on Chicago's South Side in 1891, Provident Hospital became both a pioneering medical center and a vital advocate for Black health. It trained Black nurses, offered staff privileges to Black physicians, and admitted patients who were turned away from White hospitals. Provident's role as a sanctuary for South Side residents was starkly evident during the 1919 race riot, when the hospital treated the wounded and provided shelter to those seeking refuge.[8]

Provident's leaders became aware that medical care alone could not meet the complex social needs of the Black patient population. The patients they served arrived not only with physical ailments but also with a complex web of social challenges. In such contexts, Provident found that treating a patient's immediate medical condition without addressing the underlying social factors that caused poor health proved insufficient and, at times, futile. As a result, the hospital evolved into a de facto social service agency. This expanded role reflected a recognition that health was not merely the absence of disease but a state of well-being shaped by structural conditions. Provident addressed social determinants of health by founding an infant milk station and a visiting nurse association. These nurses offered both medical care and social support, assisting with housing, employment, and food needs. By the 1930s, Provident formalized social work training, enabling staff to better address the systemic challenges facing their patients.[9]

One reviewer of *An American Health Dilemma* noted that Byrd and Clayton's analysis focused heavily on the role of Black physicians but gave scant attention to civil society organizations and nonprofessionals who fought against medical racism.[10] Yet historians Vanessa Gamble and Susan Smith had shown that Black churches and women's auxiliaries formed the backbone of the Black Hospital Movement.[11] Provident Hospital's creation and survival were deeply intertwined with the activism of Black women and the institutional support of Black churches. Emma Reynolds, a young Black woman who was denied admission to nursing schools because of her race, was a catalyst for the hospital's creation. Throughout Provident's history, Black women played a vital role in the hospital's development. Black women's clubs held countless dances, parties, and concerts to raise funds for Provident. Churches such as Quinn Chapel A. M. E. Church, Chicago's oldest Black congregation, and other churches mobilized their congregations to support Provident. Another Black institution that was essential to Provident was the *Chicago Defender* newspaper, which sponsored countless fundraisers and reported extensively on the hospital's achievements.[12]

Because Black hospitals "were handicapped by underfunding and spotty organization," Byrd and Clayton write, "they could not overpower the negative effects generated by the apartheid of a massive and generously funded mainstream health system."[13] Indeed, their existence allowed other hospitals to continue to discriminate. For example, in the 1930s, the University of Chicago established a clinical training program at Provident, supported by Rockefeller and Rosenwald funds, in part to keep its Black medical students out of its own hospital wards. In 1949, Provident threatened to close its clinics and emergency department if other hospitals in Chicago refused to relax their restrictive racial quotas. Rather than agree to admit more Black patients, segregated hospitals persuaded the county government to give Provident an infusion of cash to keep its doors open.[14]

Byrd and Clayton argue that the ultimate decline of Black hospitals had multiple causes. Starting in the 1950s, desegregation inadvertently undermined Black institutions that had been built out of necessity. The *Simkins v Cone* federal court decision in 1963, the mandates of the 1964 Civil Rights Act, and White hospitals' desire to receive Medicare funding finally forced integration, reducing the meager financial support that once sustained Black facilities. Furthermore, African American patients increasingly exercised their agency by opting for care at formerly White hospitals, a shift that reduced the patient base of Black-run hospitals.[15]

STRUCTURAL RACISM AND HEALTH DISPARITIES

Formal integration led to both the decline of the Black hospital and the exacerbation of de facto segregation. While government funds bolstered medical research and hospital growth, inner cities experienced "increasing residential and class segregation, White flight from central cities, and White suburbanization," Byrd and Clayton write. The public and "safety net" hospitals that remained to serve Black and poor communities had a lower quality of care and often treated Black patients as "'training material' for the medical school and research infrastructure." Medicaid, which pays doctors and hospitals at lower rates than private insurance, exacerbated "growing health services disparities between the mainstream and public care sectors."[16]

As health care spending soared in the 1970s and '80s, cost control became a higher priority than expanding care or providing coverage more equitably. Reagan-era Medicaid cuts and an increasing orientation toward market competition led to hospital mergers and acquisitions and the closing of unprofitable inner-city and rural hospitals. Private, nonprofit hospitals increasingly transferred uninsured and Medicaid patients to public safety-net hospitals, including patients with severe and life-threatening conditions. By 1986, this crisis of "patient dumping" was so severe that it led to the federal Emergency Medical Treatment and Active Labor Act that attempted to curb the practice. Both patient dumping and hospital closures disproportionately affected urban and rural communities of color.[17]

Byrd and Clayton assert that unequal access to hospitals is a crucial part of the puzzle of persistent racial health disparities in the United States. In their discussion of HIV/AIDS, for example, they argue that the United States failed to mobilize effectively against the epidemic because of its "'dual and unequal' health system," including the "outmoded, underfunded, understaffed public hospitals" in communities that were especially hard hit. Similarly, the COVID-19 pandemic exhibited the glaring and enduring racial and ethnic disparities in health outcomes and hospital care. Racial minorities were hospitalized for COVID-19 at rates disproportionately higher than their representation in the general population. Individuals from marginalized communities often entered hospitals with multiple comorbidities including diabetes, hypertension, asthma, and other chronic illnesses, further compounding the severity of their outcomes.[18]

COVID-19 patients who lived in communities with underfunded, understaffed hospitals were more likely to die than patients who were treated in more affluent hospitals. A *New York Times* report in 2020 found that 17% of COVID-19 patients at the prestigious Mount Sinai Hospital in Manhattan, New York, died; at the hospital's satellite campuses in Black and Latino neighborhoods in Brooklyn and Queens, New York, the percentages were double that.[19] Historian George

Aumoithe traces the origins of these shocking inequalities to the 1970s health system austerity measures discussed by Byrd and Clayton. Hospital consolidations and closings because of "underutilization," alongside White flight and the intensification of spatial segregation, left the remaining rural and inner-city hospitals not just understaffed but also with fewer emergency department facilities and intensive care units (ICUs). By 2020, Aumoithe notes, half of all inner-city residents in the United States lacked access to ICU beds.[20]

As well as laying bare the historical roots of deadly disparities, *An American Health Dilemma* highlights the medical professionals who have fought for more equitable hospital care. Black physicians' activism, and that of their professional organization the National Medical Association, shifted from support for separate Black hospitals and medical schools in the early 1900s to increasingly demanding integration later in the century. In the 1950s, doctors and activists created the Committee to End Discrimination in Chicago Medical Institutions, which targeted the city's hospitals that discriminated against Black physicians and patients. The Committee emphasized how racialized patient dumping was devastating to Black health, publicizing the

> recent deaths of African American children and adolescents due to delayed treatment of accidents and illnesses caused by inappropriate, discriminatory referrals.[21]

Byrd and Clayton's attention to physician activism did not extend to broader social movements against hospital discrimination. More recent scholarship has examined activism by patients, consumers, and community groups demanding equity, accountability, and justice from the hospital system. Historians are beginning to study multiracial social movements on behalf of hospital care, such as the decades-long struggle of residents of New York City's Lower East Side to prevent the closure of their local public hospital and to demand a new one, and community movements against hospital privatization.[22] In the 1960s and '70s, Black and Latino students and community members protested for better funding and staffing at safety-net hospitals such as Lincoln Hospital in the Bronx, New York, and Cook County Hospital in Chicago.[23] In the wake of the Watts Riots in Los Angeles, California, Black Power activists fought for, and won, a Black-led, publicly funded hospital, King–Drew Medical Center.[24]

Health justice advocates have also used legal strategies to attack hospitals' discrimination against poor and non-White patients. In 1970, African American Medicaid recipients won a class action lawsuit against 10 New Orleans, Louisiana, hospitals that regularly refused care for patients who were uninsured or on Medicaid. Antipoverty and welfare rights groups brought multiple lawsuits against hospitals for failing to meet the charity care and community service obligations required by Hill–Burton funding and nonprofit tax exemption laws. However, a handful of legal victories could make little headway because of government reluctance to enforce hospitals' obligations, and because of continuing and intensified systemic issues such as residential segregation and disinvestment.[25]

One the most prescient arguments in *An American Health Dilemma* is that racial justice cannot be attainable in a medical system that places profit before people. Byrd and Clayton insist that

> Reliance on monetary incentives to provide equitable health distribution to poor, often unemployed, medically high-risk populations in economically depressed areas is unproven, specious, counterintuitive, and fraught with difficulty.

In a statement that could have been written in 2025, they point out that "the United States is currently engaged in a massive radical social experiment in quasi-market-based, entrepreneurial, capitalistic health care," but unless "the health system's goals and objectives are geared toward serving the public, virtually no equitable or positive results with occur."[26]

Recent scholarship has begun to investigate how US hospitals—including in the so-called nonprofit sector—have become intensely market-driven since the 1980s and how this affects communities of color. Luke Messac in *Your Money or Your Life* examines how hospitals have adopted aggressive debt-collection practices against Black and poor patients, including garnishing wages and putting liens on property. Andrew Simpson's comparative study of the health care economies of Pittsburgh, Pennsylvania, and Houston, Texas, shows that as urban hospitals consolidated into multibillion-dollar economic engines, medical specialization and research flourished at the expense of communities' access to primary care. Inner-city residents paid another price for hospitals' growing wealth, historian Guian McKee demonstrates in his study of Baltimore, Maryland, as federal urban renewal funds were used to bulldoze entire Black neighborhoods to make room for medical center expansions. McKee and other scholars remind us that the US government pours taxpayer dollars into profit-seeking medical institutions without requiring significant accountability or public benefit in return.[27]

Case studies of individual hospitals or regions allow deeper understanding of how medical institutions are embedded in and help create economic change. Nic John Ramos analyzes the role of King–Drew Medical Center in Los Angeles's transformation into a low-wage service economy dependent on Black and immigrant labor. Gabriel Winant's history of the rise of the health care economy in the American Rust Belt shows how new "corporate health empires" intensified inequalities in both communities and workplaces. Brian Alexander tells the story of how a small-town hospital in Ohio struggled for decades against takeover by a corporate health system; such hospitals, serving communities ravaged by deindustrialization, unemployment, and chronic health problems, are "Band-Aid stations in a war," Alexander writes.[28]

If Byrd and Clayton were to write *An American Health Dilemma* today, they would benefit from an abundance of historical scholarship on hospitals that has been published since 2000. Deeply researched books by Keith Wailoo on Memphis, Tennessee; Samuel Kelton Roberts on Baltimore; Kevin McQueeny on New Orleans; and Catherine Mas on Miami, Florida, analyze the role of hospitals in maintaining and transforming local racial orders.[29] Scholars including Martin Summers and Kylie M. Smith are delving into the history of segregated psychiatric institutions, using rarely available patient records to examine individual patient experiences within an intensely racist mental health system.[30]

An American Health Dilemma was a pioneering work in its insistence on the multifaceted historical factors behind racial health disparities. US hospitals have been a critical such factor. However, there has yet to be a reckoning around hospital discrimination on a par with the 2008 apology by the American Medical Association for its historical exclusion of Black doctors. The American Hospital Association has issued no such apology.[31] Activists and health professionals have launched investigations of the historical legacies of racism at particular hospitals, which should provide important evidence and help educate the public and government officials about the role of hospitals in systemic disparities.[32] But such initiatives are being threatened by the attempts of the current administration to ban accurate depictions of US history and to quash research around race and health.[33]

By reframing hospitals as contested spaces rather than neutral sites of care, *An American Health Dilemma* challenged traditional narratives and, 25 years later, continues to invite scholars and activists to probe the hospital as an institution of social power and an integral factor in the reproduction of systemic racial disparities. In the past, institutions such as Provident Hospital demonstrated that healing cannot be confined to the examining room but needs to be a holistic endeavor rooted in dignity, equity, and collective action. Hospitals can also be part of the solution. AJPH

ABOUT THE AUTHORS

LeNie Adolphson is an instructor at City Colleges of Chicago, IL. Beatrix Hoffman is professor emeritus of history, Northern Illinois University, DeKalb.

CORRESPONDENCE

Correspondence should be sent to Beatrix Hoffman, Department of History, Northern Illinois University, DeKalb, IL 60115 (e-mail: bhoffman3@niu.edu). Reprints can be ordered at https://www.ajph.org by clicking the "Reprints" link.

PUBLICATION INFORMATION

Full Citation: Adolphson L, Hoffman B. Hospitals and the history of structural racism in the United States. *Am J Public Health*. 2026;116(5):643–648.

Acceptance Date: January 15, 2026.

DOI: https://doi.org/10.2105/AJPH.2026.308421

CONTRIBUTORS

L. Adolphson contributed original primary source research. B. Hoffman contributed historiographical summaries. Both authors participated equally in the writing and revision.

CONFLICTS OF INTEREST

The authors report no conflicts of interest.

ENDNOTES

1. W. Michael Byrd and Linda A. Clayton, *An American Health Dilemma: Race, Medicine, and Health Care in the United States, 1900–2000.* Volume 2. (New York, NY: Routledge, 2002), 499.
2. W. Michael Byrd and Linda A. Clayton, *An American Health Dilemma: A Medical History of African Americans and the Problem of Race: Beginnings to 1900.* (New York, NY: Routledge, 2000), 245.
3. Byrd and Clayton, *An American Health Dilemma*, Volume 2, 113–115.
4. Byrd and Clayton, *An American Health Dilemma*, Volume 2, 48.
5. Byrd and Clayton, *An American Health Dilemma*, Volume 2, 205.
6. Byrd and Clayton, *An American Health Dilemma*, Volume 2, 48.
7. Vanessa Northington Gamble, *Making a Place for Ourselves: The Black Hospital Movement, 1920–1940* (New York, NY: Oxford University Press, 1995).
8. LeNie Adolphson, "Guardians of the Community: A History of Provident Hospital, 1891–1950" (PhD diss., Northern Illinois University, 2024), 69–72.
9. Adolphson, "Guardians of the Community," 171.
10. Samuel Roberts, Review of *An American Health Dilemma*, Vol. 2, *Bulletin of the History of Medicine* 79 (2005), 349–351.
11. Gamble, *Making a Place for Ourselves*, 8, 25; Susan L. Smith, *Sick and Tired of Being Sick and Tired: Black Women's Health Activism in America, 1890–1950* (Philadelphia, PA: University of Pennsylvania Press, 1995).
12. Adolphson, "Guardians of the Community," 18–19.
13. Byrd and Clayton, *An American Health Dilemma*, Volume 2, 46.
14. Gamble, *Making a Place*; Adolphson, "Guardians of the Community," Chapters 4 and 6.
15. Byrd and Clayton, *An American Health Dilemma*, Volume 2, 207.
16. Byrd and Clayton, *An American Health Dilemma*, Volume 2, 206–207.
17. Byrd and Clayton, *An American Health Dilemma*, Volume 2, 500–502.
18. Centers for Disease Control and Prevention, "Risk for COVID-19 Infection, Hospitalization, and Death by Race/Ethnicity," May 25, 2023, https://archive.cdc.gov/www_cdc_gov/coronavirus/2019-ncov/covid-data/investigations-discovery/hospitalization-death-by-race-ethnicity.html (accessed July 17, 2025).

19. Brian M. Rosenthal et al., "A Stark Factor in Beating Covid: Which Hospital You Can Afford," *New York Times*, July 2, 2020 (accessed July 17, 2025).
20. George Aumoithe, "The Racist History That Explains Why Some Communities Don't Have Enough ICU beds," Made by History, *Washington Post*, September 16, 2020, 5, https://www.washingtonpost.com/outlook/2020/09/16/racist-history-that-explains-why-some-communities-dont-have-enough-icu-beds (accessed July 17, 2025).
21. Byrd and Clayton, *An American Health Dilemma*, Volume 2, 254.
22. Hongdeng Gao, "Community Struggles for a New Gouverneur: Tackling the Deeper Roots of the City's Unequal Hospital Care," The Gotham Center for New York History, January 5, 2021. https://www.gothamcenter.org/blog/community-struggles-for-a-new-gouverneur. Accessed July 17, 2025; Merlin Chowkwanyun, *All Health Politics Is Local: Community Battles for Medical Care and Environmental Health* (Chapel Hill, NC: University of North Carolina Press, 2022); George Aumoithe, "Dismantling the Safety-Net Hospital: The Construction of 'Underutilization' and Scarce Hospital Care," *Journal of Urban History* 49, no. 6 (2023): 1282–1311.
23. Johanna Fernandez, *The Young Lords: A Radical History* (Chapel Hill, NC: The University of North Carolina Press, 2020); Amy Zanoni, "Poor Health: Retrenchment and Resistance at Chicago's Public Hospital, 1950s–1990s" (PhD diss., Department of History, Rutgers University, 2020).
24. Nic John Ramos, *Health as Property: Racial Capitalism and Sexual Liberalism in Los Angeles* (Berkeley, CA: The University of California Press, 2025).
25. Beatrix Hoffman, "The American Hospital: Charity, Public Service, or Profit Center?" in Martin Gorsky, Margarita Vilar-Rodriguez, and Jeronia Pons-Pons, *The Political Economy of the Hospital in History* (Huddersfield, England: University of Huddersfield Press, 2020). The New Orleans lawsuit was *Cook v Ochsner* (1970). On attempts to curb "hospital flight" to the suburbs, see Beatrix Hoffman, *Health Care for Some: Rights and Rationing in the United States Since 1930* (Chicago, IL: University of Chicago Press, 2012), 151–152; David Barton Smith, *Health Care Divided: Race and Healing a Nation*, (Ann Arbor, MI: University of Michigan Press, 1999), 178–179, 183.
26. Byrd and Clayton, *An American Health Dilemma*, Volume 2, 582–583.
27. Luke Messac, *Your Money or Your Life: Debt Collection in American Medicine* (New York, NY: Oxford University Press, 2023); Andrew T. Simpson, *The Medical Metropolis: Health Care and Economic Transformation in Pittsburgh and Houston* (Philadelphia, PA: University of Pennsylvania Press, 2019); Guian McKee, *Hospital City, Health Care Nation: Race, Capital, and the Costs of American Health Care* (Philadelphia, PA: University of Pennsylvania Press, 2023). On the long history of market-driven medicine in the United States, see Nancy Tomes, *Remaking the American Patient: How Madison Avenue and Modern Medicine Turned Patients Into Consumers* (Chapel Hill, NC: University of North Carolina Press, 2016); on the often-hidden role of government subsidies in the US health system, see Rosemary A. Stevens, *The Public–Private Health Care State: Essays on the History of American Health Care Policy* (New York, NY: Routledge, 2017) and Colleen M. Grogan, *Grow and Hide: The History of America's Health Care State* (New York, NY: Oxford University Press, 2023).
28. Ramos, *Health as Property*; Gabriel Winant, *The Next Shift: The Fall of Industry and the Rise of Health Care in Rust Belt America* (Cambridge, MA: Harvard University Press, 2021), 219; Brian Alexander, *The Hospital: Life, Death, and Dollars in a Small American Town* (New York, NY: St Martin's Press, 2021).
29. Keith Wailoo, *Dying in the City of the Blues: Sickle Cell Anemia and the Politics of Race and Health* (Chapel Hill, NC: University of North Carolina Press, 2001); Samuel Kelton Roberts Jr, *Infectious Fear: Politics, Disease, and the Health Effects of Segregation* (Chapel Hill, NC: University of North Carolina Press, 2009); Kevin McQueeney, *A City Without Care: 300 Years of Racism, Health Disparities, and Health Care Activism in New Orleans* (Chapel Hill, NC: University of North Carolina Press, 2023); Catherine Mas, *Culture in the Clinic: Miami and the Making of Modern Medicine* (Chapel Hill, NC: University of North Carolina Press, 2022).
30. Martin Summers, *Madness in the City of Magnificent Intentions: A History of Race and Mental Illness in the Nation's Capital* (New York, NY: Oxford University Press, 2019); Kylie M. Smith, *Jim Crow in the Asylum: Psychiatry and Civil Rights in the American South* (Chapel Hill, NC: University of North Carolina Press, 2026).
31. AMA apology, https://www.ama-assn.org/sites/ama-assn.org/files/corp/media-browser/public/ama-history/ama-apology-african-americans.pdf (accessed July 17, 2025). The American Hospital Association did establish an Institute for Diversity and Health Equity in 2018.
32. For example, Tom Hall, Malarie Pinkard-Pierre, and Rob Sivak, "Hard Histories at Hopkins: Reckoning with Racism's Legacy," WYPR, March 30, 2022, https://www.wypr.org/show/midday/2022-03-30/hard-histories-at-hopkins-reckoning-with-racisms-legacy (accessed July 17, 2025); "Scholars Examine Duke's History of Unequal Medical Care for Black People," *Durham Reporter*, October 3, 2020, https://durhamreporter.com/duke-university-scholars-examine-dukes-history-of-unequal-medical-care-for-black-people (accessed March 1, 2026).
33. For example, Jessie Hellman, "Trump Cancels NIH Grants on Equity Research," *Roll Call*, March 24, 2025, https://rollcall.com/2025/03/24/trump-cancels-nih-grants-on-equity-research (accessed July 17, 2025).

Enslaved Health and Healing in *An American Health Dilemma*: A Retrospective Review

Sharla M. Fett, PhD

See also An American Health Dilemma 25 Years Later, pp. 625–648.

In *An American Health Dilemma* (2000), W. Michael Byrd and Linda A. Clayton synthesized historical scholarship to trace the devastating health impacts of chattel slavery, White supremacy, and racial science. Their study exposed disparate levels of death and illness experienced by generations of enslaved African Americans.

My retrospective review of *An American Health Dilemma* demonstrates how subsequent scholarship has reinforced Byrd and Clayton's analysis of the roots of African American health disparities but also illuminated some of the limitations of the authors' physician perspectives. By decentering biomedical frameworks and introducing new interdisciplinary approaches, historians of enslaved health and healing complicate the authors' conceptualization of the "slave health deficit" and challenge their assumptions about the "slave health subsystem."

New studies of slavery and capitalism, gender, reproduction, and disability expand the account of slavery's full impact on African American health. Furthermore, rather than viewing enslaved healers as members of a subsystem of superior Euro-American professional training, a new body of literature today explores the spiritual and intellectual worlds of Black healers grounded in Black mobility and the cultures of the African diaspora. (*Am J Public Health.* 2026;116(5):649–656. https://doi.org/10.2105/AJPH.2026.308422)

AJPH May 2026, Vol. 116, No. 5

Physicians W. Michael Byrd and Linda A. Clayton devoted much of their public health careers to uncovering the roots of persistent African American health disparities. Their sweeping study, *An American Health Dilemma: A Medical History of African Americans and the Problem of Race* (2000), synthesized a vast body of historical scholarship to trace the devastating health impacts of chattel slavery, White supremacist logics, and racial science.[1] Acknowledging a potentially controversial move into "uncharted territory," Byrd and Clayton coined the term "slave health deficit" (pp. 13, 194–197) to describe disparate levels of death, illness, and injury experienced by generations of enslaved Africans and their descendants. Any attempt to address the contemporary disparities of American health policy, they insisted, would have to contend with the legacies of this damning historical record. Importantly, Byrd and Clayton did not stop with their exposé of historically racialized medical treatment. They also chronicled the "slave health subsystem," composed of Black "hands-on" practitioners who supplied the bulk of enslaved health care (pp. 202–203). Recognizing a range of African-descended healers, *An American Health Dilemma* acknowledged traditions of care beyond Euro-American medical institutions and offered a prehistory for the entry of Black physicians into American professional medicine.

By decentering biomedical frameworks and introducing new interdisciplinary approaches, subsequent studies of medicine and slavery have both complicated the authors' conceptualization of the slave health deficit and challenged their assumptions about the slave health subsystem. Byrd and Clayton found evidence for the slave health deficit in historical patterns of mortality and morbidity and linked them to historical treatises on racial science. Recent literature reveals additional dimensions of enslaved health vulnerability with insights drawn from studies of slavery and capitalism, gender and reproduction, disability studies, and Black feminist theory.

Furthermore, Byrd and Clayton argued that Black practitioners' exclusion from Euro-American institutional medical training led to "untrained" enslaved practitioners serving as the primary source of enslaved medical care. This framing placed enslaved Black healers in a paradoxical position of simultaneously representing valued African traditions and serving as evidence of medical neglect. Scholars have subsequently challenged this view of the slave health subsystem with studies of the spiritual and intellectual worlds of enslaved healers grounded in Black mobility and the cultures of the African diaspora. A retrospective look at *An American Health Dilemma* from the vantage point of recent historiography thus underscores Byrd and Clayton's indictment of the historical roots of African American health disparities while highlighting some limitations of the authors' physician perspectives on the past.

FROM SLAVE HEALTH DEFICIT TO NEW HISTORIES

Byrd and Clayton's exploration of the slave health deficit emerged from a commitment to exploring African American health experiences through a "racial-historical analysis" (p. 9). Western physicians' role in the development of the idea of race, coinciding with the expansion of New World slavery and colonization, proved critical to understanding African American medical history. Byrd and Clayton took the long view, moving back into ancient Mediterranean and North African ideas about human taxonomy and medical treatment. Although sometimes painting with a broader brush than academic historians might, the authors outlined the epistemological foundations for scientific assertions of racial inequality that shaped the White medical profession's subsequent treatment of enslaved African Americans.

The first volume of *An American Health Dilemma*, covering "Beginnings to 1900," tells the story of African Americans as "both a people and a group of patients forced to receive health care in a system that since Colonial times has been largely hostile toward them" (p. 9). Hostility, expressed in the commodification of Black life, became evident not only in poor medical treatment but in the very system of chattel slavery rationalized by the ideology of race. The resulting slave health deficit manifested in comparatively higher mortality and morbidity, heightened infant and child mortality, shortened life expectancy, and exposure to malnutrition, injuries, and epidemics. The authors demonstrated how health disparities between White Europeans and captive Africans began in the "massive epidemiologic catastrophe" (p. 184) of the transatlantic slave trade. From traumatic capture to the unthinkable Middle Passage, the transatlantic trade exacted high mortality. European slave traders' economic investment created a "pathological relationship" (p. 194) between White shipboard physicians and the African captives they attended. Survivors of the passage disembarked carrying mental and physical trauma.

Once in North America, the legal codification of chattel slavery institutionalized the slave health deficit. As enslaved labor built the American nation, enslaved people bore the health impacts of extending the plantation "frontier" (pp. 279–289). Anticipating an expanded theme in later historical scholarship, Byrd and Clayton argued that the 1808 transatlantic slave trade ban increased enslavers' dependence on "domestic slave fertility and fecundability" with "profound adverse maternal and child health consequences" (p. 280). Enslavers aiming to control a resistant slave population enacted all manner of injury, sexual violation, and bodily mutilation on enslaved persons (p. 281). Although pre–Civil War historical records do not offer the type of comprehensive data available to modern public health scholars, Byrd and Clayton used US Census returns, state-level reports, and plantation records to show that enslaved and free African Americans' health metrics remained consistently worse relative to White people and actually declined in the pre–Civil War decades (pp. 286–287).

To make their case, Byrd and Clayton exhaustively surveyed the available historical scholarship on slavery, race, and medicine. Late twentieth-century studies primarily relied on social and economic history methods, demographic analysis, and retrospective diagnosis.[2] Richard Sheridan's 1985 study *Doctors and Slaves*, for example, used economic analysis and global ecology to chart the political economy of enslaved health and the disease environments of West Indian plantations.[3] Todd Savitt's 1978 *Medicine and Slavery*, a major source for *An American Health Dilemma*, used epidemiology, parasitology, nutrition, and other public health fields, to analyze evidence from Virginia's historical archives.[4]

In the 25 years since the volume's publication, scholars working on the history of enslaved health have turned to a "social constructivist" approach.[5] Delving into archives across the Atlantic World, recent studies illuminate historical dimensions of Black medical experience using insights from interdisciplinary fields such as Black feminism, critical geography, environmental studies, and disability studies. Subsequent scholarship on the transatlantic slave trade, for instance, has gone beyond quantitative mortality tables and lists of diseases to examine the embodied consequences of human commodification within the colonial political economy. Stephanie Smallwood's *Saltwater Slavery* (2007) interrogates the physical mechanisms and thought processes by which British slave traders routinized the commodification of captive Africans. European slavers specialized in "scaling life down" to the bare minimum of water, food, and air needed to transport bodies across the Atlantic.

By differentiating Africans as a group who could be acceptably (in European eyes) subjected to life-threatening conditions to increase the wealth of White elites, the routines of the transatlantic slave trade increased European callousness to African suffering and naturalized the concept of racial difference.[6] Sowande' Mustakeem's *Slavery at Sea* (2016) likewise scours ship logs and mortality lists to expose an "Atlantic human manufacturing process" that produced a "medical world of slavery at sea." The slave ship functioned as a sort of factory that produced both human commodities and the idea of race, while discarding the sick and disabled.[7] Nor did the toll on African lives end with the slave ship's journey. As Elise Mitchell demonstrates, smallpox and other epidemics imposed additional death and debility when captive Africans continued their "morbid crossings" on further intra-Caribbean voyages.[8]

Scholars informed by insights of Black feminist intersectional theory have built new understandings of how the system of transgenerational racial slavery emerged from European discourses on gender and reproduction in the early modern period. Jennifer Morgan's *Laboring Women* (2004) argues that gendered distinctions between White and Black women in colonial European discourse and law served to justify enslavement and assert racial difference. European observers propagated the belief that African women possessed a distinctive capacity (compared with European women) to simultaneously mother their infants and perform physical, productive labor.[9] An ensuing 1662 Virginia *partus sequitur ventrem* law broke from traditions of English patriarchy to institutionalize enslavement as hereditary by designating the child's status to follow that of the enslaved mother. The capitalist capture of enslaved women's childbearing also eviscerated notions of privacy and kinship for enslaved families, thus creating extreme vulnerability to sexual exploitation and familial trauma.[10] A wave of recent scholarship has examined enslaved women's reproductive health and fertility, experiences of motherhood and sexuality, and gynecological treatment and abuse by White medical practitioners—all with implications for today's Black maternal health crisis.[11]

Whereas *An American Health Dilemma* called the early American medical profession to account for treating racial difference as self-evident truth, decades of critical science studies have shown how thoroughly notions of racial difference permeated post-Enlightenment medical theory and practice.[12] Colonial plantation societies became the locus for White physicians who "medicalized [B]lackness," with devastating consequences for generations of African Americans to come.[13] Medical theories concerning Black people's insensibility to pain and White doctors' routine presumption of access to enslaved women's sexualized bodies created the broader context, excavated by Deirdre Cooper Owens, for infamous gynecological surgeries on enslaved women.[14] White physicians derived professional prestige from the predatory harvesting of enslaved and free Black people's corpses for medical school dissection and specimen museums.[15]

Far from being the exclusive specialty of a few Southern ideologues such as the often-cited physician Samuel Cartwright, White supremacist theories of polygenesis and other tenets of racial science pervaded elite medical school curricula and professional thought.[16] Enslaved practitioners sometimes assisted or practiced alongside White physicians while their own expertise was overlooked.[17] Only recently have we seen reparative gestures, such as the decommissioning of the J. Marion Sims statue in New York, the transfer of Harvard naturalist Louis Agassiz's exploitive photographs to a South Carolina museum, and the reckoning with research employing theories of racial science published in leading journals such as the *New England Journal of Medicine*.[18]

Interdisciplinary and theoretical interventions in the medical humanities have helped shed light on areas of enslaved health that were underdeveloped or even unrecognized in the scholarship at the time of *An American Health Dilemma*'s publication. Scholars working at the intersection of slavery studies and disability studies, for example, have shown how discussions of enslaved disability contributed to anti-Blackness both in the Caribbean and the US South. Emerging out of early modern cultural norms, Anglo-American legal and medical discourses depicted Blackness as a form of disfigurement and an attribute that impaired full humanity and citizenship. The system of chattel slavery depended on enslavers' power to inflict daily injury, violence, and trauma. Consequently, many enslaved people, as Stefanie Hunt-Kennedy has argued, existed and labored in the space between "fitness and death."[19] Medical historians' heavy focus on mortality rates, she argues, misses this vital aspect of enslaved health and daily life.

Varying studies estimate that between 4% and 10% of the enslaved in the antebellum United States lived with some form of embodied impairment.[20] Although enslavers' records often deemed such individuals worthless in terms of the market, Jenifer Barclay argues that enslaved men and women with disabilities in fact served as valued caregivers who "represented stability and continuity" within their enslaved communities.[21] Such studies offer insights into the lived experience of disability under slavery as well as the "historical intersections between racism and ableism."[22]

Mental health, another urgent area of unequal treatment today, has until recently not been sufficiently examined as a significant aspect of enslaved health vulnerability. Although Savitt's *Slavery and Medicine* devoted an entire chapter to "insanity," *An American Health Dilemma* remained notably silent on enslaved people's mental health. It is possible that neither Byrd nor Clayton considered mental health to lie within their fields of expertise. Perhaps, as Martin Summers has noted for late 19th-century African American physician–advocates, the complex etiology of mental illness did not carry the same "social urgency and political value" as infectious diseases did when advocating equal socioeconomic conditions as a civil right.[23]

Yet, as Summers's 2019 study of St. Elizabeths Hospital in Washington, DC, shows, physicians and asylum managers constructed the "[W]hite psyche" as the norm and the "[B]lack psyche as alien and fundamentally abnormal." From the 1850s onward, he argues, "This belief in distinctive racial psyches contributed to the persistent marginalization of mentally ill African Americans over the course of the development of American psychiatry."[24] White racist thought about Black inferiority extended from body to mind. Proslavery advocates used the 1840 Census figures for insanity among Northern free Blacks to argue that the "mental excitement" of modern life threatened free Black mental health. By extension, these propagandists argued for slavery's benevolent shielding effects on enslaved people's psyches.[25]

However, scholarship that is attentive to the full range of human affliction reveals that enslaved people living under the everyday trauma of chattel slavery did indeed suffer from mental illnesses of many kinds. Most mentally ill Americans in the antebellum era, including enslaved persons, received treatment (if any) in a domestic context.[26] Only a few institutions, such as Virginia's Eastern Lunatic Asylum, admitted enslaved Black patients when their enslavers paid the bill. If admitted at all, enslaved patients were housed in segregated facilities, some with supportive therapy (known as moral therapy) but others with only basic custodial care.[27] Slaveowners also abandoned or hired out mentally ill enslaved adults and children to avoid the burden of supporting them.[28] Furthermore, free and enslaved Blacks were consigned to the South's carceral spaces such as jails, poorhouses, and workhouses.[29] Punitive treatment of the enslaved mentally ill combined with scientific racist assertions about Black mental inferiority produced a legacy of "long-term connections between carceral logics and Black mental health."[30] Indeed, unequal access to mental health services remains a critical feature of contemporary American race and class health disparities.[31]

REVISITING THE SLAVE HEALTH SUBSYSTEM

Given the record of life-threatening conditions and unmet health needs, who supplied the health care for millions of enslaved Africans and their descendants? Byrd and Clayton's umbrella term "slave health subsystem" described the array of lay practitioners who provided health care to enslaved populations from the colonial through the antebellum period. Slaveowners and overseers as well as "traditional slave healers, herbalists, and midwives" attended to enslaved people in most cases (p. 184). Seeking to avoid White physicians' fees—and sometimes distrusting their competence—enslavers consulted domestic medicine manuals and brewed home remedies for the treatment of enslaved patients. Furthermore, the disorganized status of early 19th-century medical licensing across the country allowed a host of popular health practitioners to flourish. However, the ranks of "slave folk healers, root doctors, nurse-midwives, and bleeder-cuppers were the first line of defense for sick or injured slaves" (p. 315). Enslaved patients, archival evidence suggests, often preferred these enslaved or free Black healers with whom they shared some cultural and social affinity. Furthermore, Byrd and Clayton noted how the slave health subsystem, although present in North

America from early colonization, expanded and became more organized with the growth of the US plantation economy. They pointed to rudimentary sick houses and even slave hospitals on large estates where enslaved women worked in differentiated roles such as nurses, midwives, and "doctresses" (pp. 317–318).

An American Health Dilemma recognized a range of enslaved Black healers whose presence was only beginning to be taken seriously among late 20th-century scholars of slavery and medicine. Todd Savitt, for example, described a "dual system of health care" in which enslaved and free Black healers offered "their own brand of care" informed by "an ancient African heritage."[32] Deborah Gray White's path-breaking 1985 book, *Ar'n't I a Woman: Female Slaves in the Plantation South*, argued that Black midwives, nurses, and herbalists who attended to enslaved women's reproductive health needs promoted "cooperation and bonding" among networks of enslaved women.[33] By synthesizing such literature and emphasizing how scientific racism permeated White medical training, Byrd and Clayton outlined an entire arena of Black health care premised on enslaved communities' ethos of self-reliance. Significantly, the authors also acknowledged how enslaved communities cultivated African-based practices of "spiritual healers, conjure men, root doctors, and voodoo doctors" (p. 316). By portraying enslaved healers as critical participants in the slave health subsystem, *An American Health Dilemma* gave scholarly recognition to practices that some medical historians of their era deemed merely "superstitious" or "quackery."

Yet Byrd and Clayton's emphasis on the early medical profession also lent a note of ambivalence to their assessment of enslaved practitioners, who were, after all, positioned as a "subsystem," presumably underneath the normative (although racist) White male medical system. On one hand, enslaved healers were trusted, "popular and talented 'healer' chattel" informed by "an ancient African healing tradition" (p. 231). On the other hand, enslavers' reluctance to call White physicians "virtually guaranteed" dismal health outcomes for the enslaved (p. 231). The "obviously inferior" (p. 319) quality of the slave health subsystem could be primarily attributed to the racism and parsimony of White doctors, mistresses, and overseers. Yet, at other times, the authors connected the inferiority of enslaved health care and declining health outcomes to enslaved healers' lack of "formal" training, by which they meant institutional Euro-American medical schooling (pp. 319, 316, 399). Indeed, historian Samuel Roberts, in his 2005 review of the second volume of *An American Health Dilemma*, observes how the authors' "physician's-eye view" sometimes caused them to underestimate the full contributions of nonprofessional practitioners.[34]

Within the past quarter of a century, successive generations of slavery scholars have employed critical approaches outside biomedical frameworks to demonstrate that "western medicine was just one among many healing cosmologies" used by enslaved Africans.[35] As Fett's 2002 study *Working Cures* argued, "biomedical approaches are not well equipped to analyze the experiential or political dimensions of health. Nor are they conducive to serious analysis of popular or indigenous healing knowledge embedded in alternative epistemologies."[36] More recent scholars aim to understand African ideas about affliction and healing on their own terms and as resources for survival under starkly unequal power relations.

With a conceptual shift toward questions about the relationship of health and healing to community, culture, labor, and resistance, enslaved healers—and often enslaved women—move into clearer focus as primary health care providers in planter households, slave quarters, slave hospitals, and even mental asylums.[37] Struggles over appropriate forms of care politicized healing interactions as enslaved sufferers sought modes of healing outside the imperatives of slave market soundness.[38] A primary example is that of Black midwives, the most frequent attendants of enslaved childbirth, who often found themselves in contests over the location and methods of birth as White physicians began to assert medical expertise in obstetrics and gynecology.[39]

Scholars of Black diasporic healing today understand enslaved healers as empiricists and knowledge producers in the Black Atlantic and Pacific worlds, as well as in the development of Western medical thought. Examples abound. Jack Waldburg, an herbalist enslaved in coastal Georgia attributed his knowledge to his African-born grandmother, a midwife.[40] Galen, an African adolescent enslaved by a Scottish Jamaican physician, acquired doctoring skills through an apprenticeship with another White physician while tending to White militia men and enslaved Africans.[41] Domingos Álvares carried his training as a Sakpata priest from his Benin birthplace across the water to Brazil, where he continued to serve as a ritual specialist and healer.[42] Marta, an African woman enslaved in the New Granada city of Quibdó, was well-known enough to be summoned to prepare remedies for the lieutenant governor's household.[43] Enslaved barbers and bloodletters (*sangradores*) from West Africa working on Brazilian ships with clients in Bahia used botanical and spiritual therapies that reflected "African-oriented medical hybridity."[44]

Practitioners such as these generated important evidence-based knowledge about bodies and the natural world while working under conditions of extreme alienation and suffering.[45] Seen in this light, enslaved practitioners existed as more than a stopgap in the absence of Euro-American physicians. They created important knowledge about healing, the body, and therapies by innovating with available materials. Importantly, the African roots of their practice lay not only in distant ancient traditions but in more immediate West African therapies and conceptions of affliction with specific routes through the transatlantic slave trade.

Even after emancipation opened the door to the education and licensing of African American physicians, practitioners fostered by enslaved communities played an important role in Black health care. *An American Health Dilemma*'s final chapter emphasized the importance of Howard, Meharry, and other historically Black medical schools that trained the first generations of African American physicians. Byrd and Clayton cite liberally the work of historian Herbert Morais and physician–anthropologist William Montague Cobb, both of whom compiled important histories of early African American physicians.[46] However, recent scholarship also encourages us to broaden the framing of postemancipation period health care to encompass a wider array of Black practitioners. In *Doctoring Freedom* (2012), Gretchen Long argues that freed people viewed both access to health care and the ability to practice medical knowledge learned under slavery as important constituents of realizing freedom. For some formerly enslaved healers such as the Austin, Texas, herbalist John Donalson, who had been recognized in his community as a doctor, claims of efficacy could not surmount the absence of a state-sanctioned license.[47]

Nevertheless, many African American healing practices persisted even as Black medical schools and hospitals opened their doors and degreed Black physicians and nurses expanded their ranks. In both urban and rural neighborhoods, African Americans continued to seek the services of conjure doctors to address a wide range of afflictions.[48] Black lay midwives remained a vital resource to rural Black and White families, using skills passed down across generations.[49] In a context of persisting structural medical racism, these rich histories of African American doctoring offer important resources for promoters of more culturally responsive health programs. Reproductive justice advocates, for example, have explored the incorporation of African American historical birthing traditions into programs seeking to reduce Black maternal and infant health disparities.[50]

Overall, the retrospective view on *An American Health Dilemma* is a sobering one. A quarter century later, disparities in life expectancy, maternal mortality, and other measures of Black health vulnerability persist and, in some cases, have worsened.[51] The wealth of information now available on American health and racial injustice poses a critical question. Will greater knowledge lead to better policy, as Byrd and Clayton first proposed at the turn of the century? If anything, the current assault on federal health care programs, community-level funding, and public health research seems bent on moving the agenda for US health justice backward. *An American Health Dilemma* identified a historical pattern of Black community self-help in the face of scientific discourses that blamed both biology and behavior for health outcomes actually produced by structural racism. Although the historical literature has shifted our understanding of enslaved health and healing considerably beyond biomedical framing, the political call issued by Byrd and Clayton to confront the nation's health dilemma is now more urgent than ever. AJPH

ABOUT THE AUTHOR

Sharla M. Fett is a professor in the History Department, Occidental College, Los Angeles, CA.

CORRESPONDENCE

Correspondence should be sent to Sharla M. Fett, History Department, 1600 Campus Rd, Los Angeles, CA 90041 (e-mail: sfett@oxy.edu). Reprints can be ordered at https://www.ajph.org by clicking the "Reprints" link.

PUBLICATION INFORMATION

Full Citation: Fett SM. Enslaved health and healing in *An American Health Dilemma*: a retrospective review. *Am J Public Health*. 2026;116(5):649–656.

Acceptance Date: January 16, 2026.

DOI: https://doi.org/10.2105/AJPH.2026.308422

ORCID iD:

Sharla M. Fett https://orcid.org/0009-0006-4495-0827

ACKNOWLEDGMENTS

Thank you to the two generous anonymous readers of this article and to the cherished members of my writing group: Emily Abel, Carla Bittel, Charlotte Borst, Janet Farrell Brodie, Nina Gelbart, Janet Golden, and Alice Wexler.

CONFLICTS OF INTEREST

There were no conflicts of interest in the writing of this essay.

HUMAN PARTICIPATION PROTECTIONS

No human participants were involved in the research for this essay.

REFERENCES

1. W. Michael Byrd and Linda A. Clayton, *An American Health Dilemma: A Medical History of African Americans and the Problem of Race, Beginnings to 1900* (New York, NY: Routledge, 2000).
2. Eric Herschthal, "Slavery, Health, and Healing Now: The State of the Field," *Journal of the History of Medicine and Allied Sciences* 77, no. 1 (January 2022): 1–23. https://doi.org/10.1093/jhmas/jrab042
3. Richard B. Sheridan, *Doctors and Slaves: A Medical and Demographic History of Slavery in the British West Indies, 1680–1834* (New York, NY: Cambridge University Press, 1985).
4. Todd L. Savitt, *Medicine and Slavery: The Diseases and Health Care of Blacks in Antebellum Virginia* (Urbana, IL: University of Illinois Press, 1978).
5. Herschthal, "Slavery, Health, and Healing Now," 3; Charles E. Rosenberg, "Disease in History: Frames and Framers," *Milbank Quarterly* 67, suppl. 1 (1989): 1–15.
6. Stephanie E. Smallwood, *Saltwater Slavery: A Middle Passage From Africa to American Diaspora* (Cambridge, MA: Harvard University Press, 2007), 43.
7. Sowande' M. Mustakeem, *Slavery at Sea: Terror, Sex, and Sickness in the Middle Passage* (Urbana, IL: University of Illinois Press, 2016), 14, 132; Marcus Rediker, *The Slave Ship: A Human History* (New York, NY: Viking, 2007), 9–10.
8. Elise A. Mitchell, "Morbid Crossings: Surviving Smallpox, Maritime Quarantine, and the Gendered Geography of the Early Eighteenth-Century Intra-Caribbean Slave Trade," *William and Mary Quarterly* 79, no. 2 (2022): 177–210. https://doi.org/10.1353/wmq.2022.0021
9. Jennifer L. Morgan, *Laboring Women: Reproduction and Gender in New World Slavery* (Chapel Hill, NC: University of North Carolina Press, 2004).
10. Jennifer L. Morgan, "Partus Sequitur Ventrem: Law, Race, and Reproduction in Colonial Slavery," *Small Axe* 22, no. 1 (March 2018): 1–17.
11. Marie Jenkins Schwartz, *Birthing a Slave: Motherhood and Medicine in the Antebellum South* (Cambridge, MA: Harvard University Press, 2006); Deirdre Cooper Owens, *Medical Bondage: Race, Gender, and the Origins of American Gynecology* (Athens, GA: University of Georgia Press, 2017); Sasha Turner, *Contested Bodies: Pregnancy, Childrearing, and Slavery in Jamaica* (Philadelphia, PA: University of Pennsylvania Press, 2017); Katherine Paugh, *The Politics of Reproduction: Race, Medicine, and Fertility in the Age of Abolition* (New York, NY: Oxford University Press, 2017); Deirdre Cooper Owens and Sharla Fett, "Black Maternal and Infant Health: Historical Legacies of Slavery," *American Journal of Public* Health 109, no. 10 (October 2019): 1342–1345. https://doi.org/10.2105/AJPH.2019.305243; Wangui Muigai, "Framing Black Infant and Maternal Mortality," *Journal of Law, Medicine & Ethics* 50, no. 1 (2022): 85–91. https://doi.org/10.1017/jme.2022.12; Shannon C. Eaves, *Sexual Violence and American Slavery: The Making of a Rape Culture in the Antebellum South* (Chapel Hill, NC: University of North Carolina Press, 2024).
12. Suman Seth, *Difference and Disease: Medicine, Race, and the Eighteenth-Century British Empire* (Ithaca, NY: Cornell University Press, 2018); Sandra Harding, *Whose Science? Whose Knowledge? Thinking From Women's Lives* (Ithaca, NY: Cornell University Press, 2016).
13. Rana A. Hogarth, *Medicalizing Blackness: Making Racial Difference in the Atlantic World, 1780–1840* (Chapel Hill, NC: University of North Carolina Press, 2017).
14. Owens, *Medical Bondage*, 42–72, 108–114.
15. Stephen C. Kenny, "'A Dictate of Both Interest and Mercy'? Slave Hospitals in the Antebellum South," *Journal of the History of Medicine and Allied Sciences* 65, no. 1 (January 2010): 1–47. https://doi.org/10.1093/jhmas/jrp019; Stephen C. Kenny, "The Development of Medical Museums in the Antebellum American South: Slave Bodies in Networks of Anatomical Exchange," *Bulletin of the History of Medicine* 87, no. 1 (2013): 32–62. https://doi.org/10.1353/bhm.2013.0016; Daina Ramey Berry, *The Price for Their Pound of Flesh: The Value of the Enslaved From Womb to Grave in the Building of a Nation* (Boston, MA: Beacon Press, 2017), 148–193.
16. Christopher D. E. Willoughby, *Masters of Health: Racial Science and Slavery in US Medical Schools* (Chapel Hill, NC: University of North Carolina Press, 2022); Christopher D. E. Willoughby, "Running Away From Drapetomania: Samuel A. Cartwright, Medicine, and Race in the Antebellum South," *Journal of Southern History* 84, no. 3 (2018): 579–614. https://doi.org/10.1353/soh.2018.0164
17. Owens, *Medical Bondage*, 38–39; Elise A. Mitchell, "The 'Practitioner of Physick and Surgery' and the Enslaved 'Doctor': Medicine, Slavery, Race, and Patriarchy in the Eighteenth-Century Jamaica," *Journal of Irish and Scottish Studies* 11, no. 2 (2024): 155–182. https://doi.org/10.57106/jiss.v11i2.170
18. P. R. Lockhart, "New York Just Removed a Statue of a Surgeon Who Experimented on Enslaved Women," *Vox*, April 18, 2018; Scott Simon, "After Six Years, Harvard Relinquishes Images of Enslaved Ancestors to Their Descendant," *NPR*, May 31, 2025; David S. Jones, Evelynn Hammonds, Joseph P. Gone, and David Williams, "Explaining Health Inequities—the Enduring Legacy of Historical Biases," *New England Journal of Medicine* 390, no. 5 (2024): 389–395. https://doi.org/10.1056/NEJMp2307312
19. Stefanie Hunt-Kennedy, *Between Fitness and Death: Disability and Slavery in the Caribbean* (Urbana, IL: University of Illinois Press, 2020), 11–12; Dea H. Boster, "'Unfit for Ordinary Purposes': Disability, Slaves, and Decision Making in the Antebellum American South," in *Disability Histories*, ed. Michael Rembis and Susan Burch (Champaign, IL: University of Illinois Press, 2014), 201–217.
20. Jeff Forret, "'Deaf & Dumb, Blind, Insane, or Idiotic': The Census, Slaves, and Disability in the Late Antebellum South," *Journal of Southern History* 82, no. 3 (August 2016): 503–548. https://doi.org/10.1353/soh.2016.0219
21. Jenifer L. Barclay, *The Mark of Slavery: Disability, Race, and Gender in Antebellum America* (Urbana, IL: University of Illinois Press, 2021), 36–63; Jenifer L. Barclay, "Mothering the 'Useless': Black Motherhood, Disability, and Slavery," *Women, Gender, and Families of Color* 2, no. 2 (2014): 115–140. https://doi.org/10.5406/womgenfamcol.2.2.0115
22. Hunt-Kennedy, *Between Fitness and Death*, 3; Dea H. Boster, *African American Slavery and Disability: Bodies, Property, and Power in the Antebellum South, 1800–1860* (New York, NY: Routledge, 2013).
23. Martin Summers, "Diagnosing the Ailments of Black Citizenship: African American Physicians and the Politics of Mental Illness, 1895–1940," in *Precarious Prescriptions: Contested Histories of Race and Health in North America*, ed. Laurie B. Green, John Mckiernan-González, and Martin Summers (Minneapolis, MN: University of Minnesota Press, 2014), 108.
24. Martin Summers, *Madness in the City of Magnificent Intentions: A History of Race and Mental Illness in the Nation's Capital* (Oxford, UK: Oxford University Press, 2019), 17–18.
25. Savitt, *Medicine and Slavery*, 248; Elodie Edwards-Grossi, *Mad With Freedom: The Political Economy of Blackness, Insanity, and Civil Rights in the US South, 1840–1940* (Baton Rouge, LA: Louisiana State University Press, 2022), 45–66.
26. Peter McCandless, *Moonlight, Magnolias, & Madness: Insanity in South Carolina From the Colonial Period to the Progressive Era* (Chapel Hill, NC: University of North Carolina Press, 1996), 143–162.
27. Wendy Gonaver, *The Peculiar Institution and the Making of Modern Psychiatry, 1840–1880* (Chapel Hill, NC: University of North Carolina Press, 2018); Summers, *Madness in the City*, 49–53; McCandless, *Moonlight, Magnolias, & Madness*, 75–77.
28. Forret, "'Deaf & Dumb,'" 538, 547; Summers, *Madness in the City*, 36–38.
29. Forret, "'Deaf & Dumb,'" 527–528; McCandless, *Moonlight, Magnolias, & Madness*, 21–23, 156–158, 176; Summers, Madness in the City, 35–37.
30. Elodie Edwards-Grossi and Christopher D. E. Willoughby, "Slavery and Its Afterlives in US Psychiatry," *American Journal of Public Health* 114, suppl. 3 (2024): S251. https://doi.org/10.2105/AJPH.2023.307554.
31. Linda Villarosa, *Under the Skin: The Hidden Toll of Racism on American Lives* (New York, NY: Knopf Doubleday, 2022), 116–140; Supriya Misra et al., "Structural Racism and Inequities in Incidence, Course of Illness, and Treatment of Psychotic Disorders Among Black Americans," *American Journal of Public Health* 112, no. 4 (2022): 624–632. https://doi.org/10.2105/AJPH.2021.306631; Lonnie R. Sowden, "Health and Mental Health Policies' Role in Better Understanding and Closing African American–White American Disparities in Treatment Access and Quality of Care," *American Psychologist* 67, no. 7 (2012): 524–531. https://doi.org/10.1037/a0030054
32. Savitt, *Medicine and Slavery*, 171–184.
33. Deborah Gray White, *Ar'n't I a Woman? Female Slaves in the Plantation South* (New York, NY: W. W. Norton, 1985), 115–116, 124–128.
34. S. Roberts, *An American Health Dilemma*, vol. 2, *Race, Medicine, and Health Care in the United States, 1900–2000* (review), *Bulletin of the History of Medicine* 79, no. 2 (Summer 2005): 349–351.
35. Sean Morey Smith and Christopher D. E. Willoughby, "Introduction," in *Medicine and Healing in the Age of Slavery*, ed. Sean Morey Smith and Christopher D. E. Willoughby (Baton Rouge, LA: Louisiana State University Press, 2021), 5.
36. Sharla M. Fett, *Working Cures: Healing, Health, and Power on Southern Slave Plantations* (Chapel Hill, NC: University of North Carolina Press, 2002), 11.
37. Herschthal, "Slavery, Health, and Healing Now," 17–22; Gonaver, *Peculiar Institution*, 51–81.
38. Fett, *Working Cures*, 15–35.
39. Turner, *Contested Bodies*, 112–150; Cooper Owens, *Medical Bondage*, 80–81; Schwartz, *Birthing a Slave*, 146–153; Fett, *Working Cures*, 51, 111–141.

40. Fett, *Working Cures*, 76.
41. Mitchell, "The 'Practitioner of Physick and Surgery,'" 172–176; Christopher M. Blakely, "'I Have Been Obliged to Send Nassaw': An Enslaved Healer's Medical Labour and Skill in Eighteenth-Century Virginia," *Medical History* 65, no. 2 (2021): 121–139. https://doi.org/10.1017/mdh.2021.1
42. James H. Sweet, *Domingos Álvares, African Healing, and the Intellectual History of the Atlantic World* (Chapel Hill, NC: University of North Carolina Press, 2011).
43. Bethan Fisk, "Black Knowledge on the Move: African Diasporic Healing in Caribbean and Pacific New Granada," *Atlantic Studies* 18, no. 2 (2021): 244–270. https://doi.org/10.1080/14788810.2020.1839282
44. Mary E. Hicks, *Captive Cosmopolitans: Black Mariners and the World of South Atlantic Slavery* (Williamsburg, VA: Omohundro Institute of Early American History and Culture, 2024), 267–324, 296.
45. Pablo F. Gómez, *The Experiential Caribbean: Creating Knowledge and Healing in the Early Modern Atlantic* (Chapel Hill, NC: University of North Carolina Press, 2017); Kalle Kananoja, *Healing Knowledge in Atlantic Africa: Medical Encounters, 1500–1850* (New York, NY: Cambridge University Press, 2021); Karol K. Weaver, *Medical Revolutionaries: The Enslaved Healers of Eighteenth-Century Saint-Domingue* (Urbana, IL: University of Illinois Press, 2006); Susan Scott Parrish, "Diasporic African Sources of Enlightenment Knowledge," in *Science and Empire in the Atlantic World*, ed. James Delbourgo and Nicholas Dew (New York, NY: Routledge, 2007), 281–310; Londa Schiebinger, *Secret Cures of Slaves: People, Plants, and Medicine in the Eighteenth-Century Atlantic World* (Stanford, CA: Stanford University Press, 2017); Carolyn Roberts, "Pharmaceutical Captivity, Epistemological Rupture, and the Business Archive of the British Slave Trade," *Business History Review* 97, no. 2 (2023): 283–305; Jim Downs, *Maladies of Empire: How Slavery, Imperialism and War Transformed Medicine* (Cambridge, MA: Harvard University Press, 2021).
46. Herbert M. Morais, *The History of the Negro in Medicine* (New York, NY: Publishers Company, 1967); W. Montgomery Cobb's remarkable biographical series on early pioneering Black physicians (all men) appeared during the 1950s in the Journal of the National Medical Association.
47. Gretchen Long, *Doctoring Freedom: The Politics of African-American Medical Care in Slavery and Emancipation* (Chapel Hill, NC: University of North Carolina Press, 2012).
48. Yvonne P. Chireau, *Black Magic: Religion and the African American Conjuring Tradition* (Berkeley: University of California Press, 2003); Katrina Hazzard-Donald, *Mojo Workin': The Old African American Hoodoo System* (Urbana, IL: University of Illinois Press, 2013).
49. Margaret Charles Smith and Linda Janet Holmes, *Listen to Me Good: The Life Story of an Alabama Midwife* (Columbus: Ohio State University Press, 1996); Deborah Anne Susie, *In the Way of Our Grandmothers: A Cultural View of Twentieth-Century Midwifery in Florida* (Athens, GA: University of Georgia Press, 1988).
50. Elizabeth Mollard, Anabelle Elya, Cydney Gaines, et al., "Reclaiming Narratives of Empowerment around Black Maternal Health: A Strengths-Based, Community-Informed Focus Group Study," *Ethnicity & Health* 29, no. 6 (2024): 703–719. https://doi.org/10.1080/13557858.2024.2359384; Kacie C. A. Blackman, Urmeka Jefferson, Wyconda Cotton-Curtis, Detrich Galloway, "Story Circles of Black Doulas, Cultural Brokers for Birthing People in Healthcare," *Qualitative Health Research* 35, no. 8 (2025): 932–945. https://doi.org/10.1177/10497323241280828
51. Georges C. Benjamin, Jennifer DeVoe, Francis Amankwah, et al., eds., *Ending Unequal Treatment: Strategies to Achieve Equitable Health Care and Optimal Health for All* (Washington, DC: National Academies Press, 2024).

Designed for Disparity: The Structural Origins of Migrant Farmworker Health Inequities in Maryland, 1900–1950

Elise Ferrer, MA, Thurka Sangaramoorthy, PhD, MPH, and Devon Payne-Sturges, DrPH, MPH, MEngr

See also Markowitz, p. 582.

The COVID-19 pandemic has renewed attention to farmworker health disparities, prompting scholars to examine the structural determinants of agricultural worker health. Through analysis of archival materials, government documents, and period newspapers, we trace the evolution and institutionalization of migrant farm labor on Maryland's Eastern Shore from 1900 to 1950. We identify four key periods of transformation: the postemancipation agricultural adjustment (1900–1915), the rise of seasonal commodity agriculture (1915–1930), the response to mass displacement (1930–1940), and wartime labor management (1940–1950). At each stage, we demonstrate how agricultural industry interests deliberately cultivated conditions of racial stratification, worker precarity, and social isolation to establish and maintain the migrant labor system. Although contemporary public health frameworks often treat these conditions as independent social determinants of health, this history reveals them as essential, deliberately produced features of the migrant labor system itself. Understanding this historical context is crucial for public health practitioners working to address persistent health disparities in agricultural work, particularly as the COVID-19 pandemic has heightened attention to farmworker vulnerability. (*Am J Public Health*. 2026;116(5):657–664. https://doi.org/10.2105/AJPH.2025.308362)

AJPH May 2026, Vol. 116, No. 5

At the turn of the 20th century, the "migrant farmworker" did not exist as a distinct social or legal category. While agricultural labor had involved seasonal movement and racial exploitation, the systematic construction of a migrant labor force emerged through specific political, economic, and social transformations between 1900 and 1950 that positioned migrant and seasonal workers as central figures in American food production. Though this population has been subject to government intervention, advocacy, and research for decades, workers' plight gained renewed urgency amid the COVID-19 pandemic. Health scholars, confronted by farmworkers' disparate pandemic-related outcomes, sought to understand the root causes of such profound health inequities that mirror historical patterns of structural vulnerability.[1]

We examine how Maryland's Eastern Shore agricultural interests deliberately constructed a migrant labor system between 1900 and 1950, revealing how features often dismissed as "social determinants" of migrant health were essential ingredients that made migrant labor possible. Drawing on government records, commission reports, and media coverage from publications like the *Baltimore Afro-American*, we employ a critical archival method examining how specific actors—including Maryland Commissioner J. Knox Insley, the Farm Security Administration, workers refusing exploitative conditions, and Eastern Shore growers—deployed and contested bureaucratic documents as technologies of power. These sources simultaneously construct and naturalize social hierarchies while inadvertently preserving evidence of resistance and contradiction, revealing the mechanisms of control and the persistent struggles that challenged them.[2]

We situate this research within a framework of racial capitalism—a system where economic exploitation and racial hierarchy operate as mutually constitutive forces.[3] Following scholarship on how agricultural employers leveraged workers' legal status and racial positioning for labor control,[4]

we demonstrate how racialized vulnerability became essential to migrant labor systems. Building on work examining how immigrant bodies bear the disproportionate costs of agricultural production, how public health infrastructure reinforces racial hierarchies, and how structural violence shapes health outcomes for marginalized populations,[5] this study reveals how health disparities emerge from deliberately constructed systems rather than individual behaviors. Agricultural labor, when structured by racial capitalism, creates conditions where worker health becomes a calculated expenditure in pursuit of agricultural productivity—what scholars call racialized disposability.[6]

We argue that understanding this historical landscape fundamentally challenges contemporary frameworks that treat social determinants as modifiable elements to be addressed while leaving the underlying labor system intact. By examining how agricultural employers and state actors responded to successive economic and social crises, we reveal how racial stratification, economic precarity, and social isolation were not coincidental to migrant farm work but were deliberately cultivated as its defining and essential features.

1900–1915: DESIGNING FOR BELONGING

In the late 19th century, Maryland's postemancipation agricultural transformation established racial control patterns that would structure future labor systems. By 1900, three key characteristics defined the state's agricultural landscape. First, Maryland's Eastern Shore was dominated by grain production (wheat, corn, barley), truck crops (tomatoes, beans, potatoes), and seafood processing.[7] The region's peninsular geography, bounded by the Chesapeake Bay and Atlantic Ocean, created distinct microclimates suitable for diverse agricultural production while fostering economic dependence on seasonal labor patterns that would later structure migrant worker exploitation. Westward expansion had lessened Maryland's market position on these commodities, altering labor demands and forcing farmers to adapt their labor practices.[8] Though some farmers grew produce, it served local markets and subsistence needs.

Second, production operated through intricate land and labor arrangements. Those with "gainful employment in agricultural pursuits" included farmers and wage laborers, with farmers further subdivided as owners, part owners, owners and tenants, managers, cash tenants, or share tenants (those who paid a share of crops to live on the land).[9] Though agricultural space remained relatively constant since 1860 (+7%), farm numbers nearly doubled (+80%) while average acreage halved (−47%). This fragmentation reflected broader struggles over land control and labor power in the postemancipation period, as White landowners sought to maintain control through new forms of tenant farming and labor arrangements.

Third, the 1900 Census divided agricultural workers between "white and colored."[10] While 59% of approximately 68,000 White agricultural Marylanders held farmer status, Black farmers comprised 21% of overall Black agricultural workers and 13% of owners.[11] Their ownership was further constrained, controlling just 7% of acreage and 4% of farm property.[12] These stark inequities stemmed directly from postemancipation policies designed to limit Black economic independence.

As Maryland officials wrestled with agricultural economics at the beginning of the 20th century, questions of land and labor were inseparable from commitments to profit, racial hierarchy, and White settler colonialism. Believing that "a class of thrifty and desirable immigrants" could make "thousands of acres of land . . . the highest degree productive" and "add largely to the agricultural wealth and importance of the Commonwealth,"[13] Maryland established cooperatives to recruit workers from Western Europe.[14] These recruitment efforts aimed to maintain White control over agricultural land by offering European immigrants pathways to land ownership and permanent settlement that were systematically denied to Black workers, creating a buffer class that reinforced racial hierarchies while providing alternative labor when Black workers refused exploitative conditions.

These hiring initiatives explicitly blamed Black workers. White Eastern Shore farmers castigated Black workers as "worthless"[15] and "shiftless,"[16] masking anger over refused exploitation. The *Baltimore Afro-American* consistently documented these dynamics. A 1903 article noted, White tenant farmers

> want [Black] boys and girls to work for them for a few dollars and when they refuse they tell the owners the crop is not a success because [Black people] won't work.[17]

The writer pointedly asked, "Who is it that is doing all of the work in Talbot County?" Such accusations concealed White farmers' refusal to provide fair wages or working conditions.

The 1920 Census categorization formalized these racial hierarchies.[18] "Foreign-born" status applied only to White residents and could disappear within two generations. For those labeled "colored"—"Negro (Black and Mulatto), Indian, Chinese, Japanese, and all other"—there was no distinction between "native" and "foreign." Though officials acknowledged such groups could theoretically be foreign-born, "in the cases of these races, the distinction based on nativity has little significance."[19] This racial calculus—where the threat of borders could discipline dissidents and outsider status was permanent and racialized—would mirror and preempt forthcoming logics surrounding migrant farm work.

1915–1930: DESIGNING FOR PRECARITY AND POVERTY

Refrigerated transport in the 1910s enabled Maryland's shift to perishable "truck farm" commodities for distant markets.[20] This technological innovation became what geographer Don Mitchell identifies as agricultural Taylorism—using seasonality as pretext for reducing worker protections, justifying temporary housing, delayed wages, and disposable workforces rather than permanent infrastructure.[21] Mitchell identifies agricultural spaces as landscapes of vulnerability—geographic isolation, seasonal camps, and piece-rate systems that prevent worker organization.[22] This systematization marked a sharp departure from earlier labor patterns that had not yet crystallized into the migrant labor system that would emerge. For example, Polish laborers from Baltimore would move between locations throughout the year, harvesting agricultural produce or working in seafood industries. Black Eastern Shore workers seasonally tonged for oysters, a practice that, while "precarious, demanding, and occasionally dangerous," offered intermittent employment without requiring constant relocation.[23] These labor practices emerged from specific local economic needs rather than forming a systematic approach to migrant labor.

The new truck commodity agriculture institutionalized worker precarity through two core mechanisms. First, wages tied to hyper-extractive productivity made workers bear all "idle" time costs. Payment typically occurred through a metal or cardboard check system, with workers receiving compensation at the end of the season. In 1929, J. Knox Insley, Maryland Commissioner of Labor and Statistics, whose documentation legitimized these exploitative arrangements, noted,

> Payment is customarily made to the family as a group, and usually a metal or cardboard check is given for each piece of work accomplished. While, in some cases, these checks are accepted locally in exchange for purchases, they are generally held until the end of the season to be returned to the employer for cash money.[24]

Labor records documented farmers routinely withholding the entire season's worth of payments. Having time and money held hostage became standard practice.[25]

Though workers "technically" had more control over their free time, the economic reality was stark. Reports from the 1920s detailed how "on account of the scarcity of work . . . most families kept steadily at work."[26] Piece-rate wages meant workers were paid by basket, quart, or pound, with zero compensation for the inherent "idle" time of agricultural work. Wages were negligible. In one study, investigators revealed tomato pickers could earn

> 3 cents a box for strawberries, 25–30 cents for a bushel basket [approximately 24 pounds] of beans, and 4–5 cents for a five-eighths bushel of tomatoes.[27]

For families working 12-hour days, "daily earnings were low, seldom over $3 even for families of three or four members," and weather-related stoppages further cut into family earnings.[28]

Second, seasonality justified providing workers with minimum housing. Owners recruited workers from Baltimore who needed accommodations, claiming local labor could not meet demands. Housing was deemed a "necessary evil" and purely instrumental to agricultural production. Owners dismissed concerns about living conditions, excusing the "disgustingly inadequate" sanitation by claiming "the season, not more than eight weeks . . . is in the warm weather and so short that housing is of no importance."[29]

Government investigations documented systematic violations: 12 to 15 workers crowded into single 10-foot-by-12-foot rooms, with one water pump serving 75 to 100 workers and privies shared by 45 to 60 people.[30] Reports detailed poor sanitation and contaminated wells. When workers complained about disease outbreaks from these conditions, one farmer dismissed concerns, stating "he has too many expenses,"[31] revealing the fundamental devaluation of worker health and safety.

The shift to seasonal produce created a system where workers absorbed all agricultural uncertainty and hardship. Growers deliberately forced workers to bear costs and risks—their precarity was the foundation that made truck farming profitable. Seasonality became a mechanism for creating disposable workforces, transforming migration from survival strategy into a form of systematic displacement and extraction that fundamentally restructured human relationships to labor, land, and survival.

1930–1940: DESIGNING FOR MIGRANCY

The Great Migration, Great Depression, and Dust Bowl created unprecedented "roadside populations" across the United States. Although historical attention focuses on White settlers and urban laborers, Black workers faced equal displacement. Black workers fleeing Jim Crow terror found Maryland's Eastern Shore offering agricultural opportunities unavailable elsewhere, yet it came with its own forms of racial control. The mechanization of Southern agriculture displaced thousands of Black sharecroppers and tenant farmers, creating a population simultaneously pushed from traditional agricultural regions and pulled toward seasonal labor opportunities in border states like Maryland.

Federal intervention took shape through Roosevelt's 1935 Resettlement Administration, which was reorganized as the Farm Security Administration (FSA). The agency, funded at $5.5 million (in today's equivalent), sought to "resettle destitute or low-income families" and construct "migrant camps," revealing the government's emerging recognition of massive population displacements.[32] Federal commissions noted that "something fundamental has occurred to render the haphazard shifts of residence by the average American family a matter for national study and investigation."[33]

The New Deal altered Maryland's agricultural landscape through multiple interventions. The Agricultural Adjustment Act reduced crop production while displacing sharecroppers, the FSA constructed migrant camps, and the Works Progress Administration provided alternative employment. These federal programs created new mechanisms for managing agricultural labor while maintaining racial hierarchy by distinguishing between "removal migrants" who desired but could not obtain permanent residence and "constant migrants" who "makes his livelihood (whether by choice or compulsion) by casual or seasonal labor."[34] Yet this intervention revealed and reinforced racial and class hierarchies in how mobility was understood and managed.

The Tolan Commission, established in 1940, studied massive population movements during the Depression era.[35] While the Commission characterized unemployed White farmers as "normal, worthwhile American people" and "descendants of the oldest white families,"[36] Black migration was understood and responded to differently. White displacement signaled government failure to "anchor them to the soil," while newspapers and officials characterized unemployed Black workers as "loafing" and "idle."[37] This racialized framing presented Black unemployment as evidence of the state's failure to properly discipline and deploy available labor resources, justifying coercive interventions that would be unthinkable for White workers.

When Black workers resisted, Maryland agricultural interests mobilized legal and police power to force labor compliance and maintain labor control. Maryland Farm Bureau President P. C. Turner proposed a "compulsory farm labor law," a version of which was formally enacted by state officials.[38] Even before legislative approval, farmers coordinated with "the sheriff, the constable, the State's attorney and magistrate . . . to put [Black migrants] in jail or run them out of town" when they refused particular work arrangements.[39]

In the early 1940s, employers refined these mechanisms of control and exploitation. They would advertise extensively for workers, creating "a surplus of labor on hand . . . that keeps the wage rates down."[40] This intentional oversupply meant "there were too many pickers in each field to make any money." Work seasons could leave laborers so in debt that, rather than returning home, they were abandoned far from where they started, their transience only deepening. A 1941 story from the Eastern Shore epitomized these tactics:

> [A farmer] hired [workers from Baltimore] to come under the pretense that they would receive 30 cents an hour. When they arrived, they were told that they would receive 20 cents. The workers refused, and the Superintendent was forced to fly to Florida to get workers. They were promised 30 cents likewise. . . . When they arrived, they were given 20 cents, but without finances and being so far from home, they were forced to stay.[41]

The manufactured instability that fueled migrant labor produced devastating health outcomes. Earnings were often barely above a subsistence level.[42] Despite the abundant food that workers produced, malnutrition was common among both adults and children.[43] The constant search for work and shelter was a disabling process, and abysmal living conditions worsened disease spread.[44] The Tolan Commission reported the compounding health impacts:

> Diet changes caused by lack of sufficient funds have often resulted in the occurrence of rickets, pellagra, scurvy, secondary anemia, and other

> diseases of malnutrition which tend to make the patient susceptible to more serious diseases such as tuberculosis.[45]

Migration was not a choice, but a system of forced displacement. Each displaced worker represented not a failure of the economic system but its most ruthlessly efficient operation—a mechanism of control that transformed human beings into disposable labor. As the United States entered World War II, this carefully constructed system of worker vulnerability would face new challenges from wartime labor demands.

1940–1950: DESIGNING TO MINIMIZE AUTONOMY

World War II disrupted the carefully constructed labor surplus that had enabled systematic worker exploitation throughout the 1930s, presenting a brief moment of improved conditions for Maryland farmworkers. The reduced labor surplus gave workers unprecedented bargaining power for wages. During the mass displacements of the 1930s, there had been too few jobs for too many people, allowing employers to systematically drive down wages. As the country mobilized for war, underemployed laborers filled newly opened roles, and agricultural workers pushed for higher earnings.[46]

FSA's housing interventions represented a significant shift in conditions for some migrant workers. The FSA constructed camps in Maryland, providing federal oversight, basic sanitation facilities, communal kitchens, and self-governance structures that allowed workers to organize independently of employer control. These camps housed 200 to 300 workers each during peak season and included on-site health services, recreational facilities, and educational programs for workers' children.[47] The camps' democratic governance committees gave workers unprecedented autonomy to establish rules, resolve disputes, and coordinate with federal officials—a stark contrast to employer-controlled housing that had previously isolated and controlled workers.

This labor relations shift represents what historian Cindy Hahamovitch identified as the core dynamic of agricultural labor control during wartime mobilization:

> What occurred in the South during World War II was less a dearth of labor than a seismic shift in the balance of power between growers and farm laborers. Farm laborers hadn't vanished, but their reduced numbers gave them the courage to demand more for their services. And farmworkers'—especially black farmworkers'—ability to make demands infuriated employers, who refused to admit that the ground beneath them had shifted.[48]

Growers and agricultural industry leaders mobilized complex strategies to undermine worker power. Despite the availability of local labor, they publicly proclaimed severe worker shortages, a narrative that masked their true intentions. These tactics were deeply calculated and systemic. Local authorities were enlisted to exert coercive control over workers and agricultural interests worked to make farmworkers ineligible for military draft. They pushed through "labor piracy" laws that prevented workers from being recruited across jurisdictions, effectively trapping laborers in a localized system of control.[49] More significantly, they leveraged federal connections to import foreign workers, creating a labor pool even more vulnerable to exploitation.

In 1942, Bahamian and Jamaican workers were brought to Maryland to replace local workers supposedly unavailable or ill-equipped for agricultural labor. Federal agencies coordinated foreign labor importation, creating bureaucratic mechanisms that would outlast the war itself.[50] The US Employment Service established recruitment networks that channeled workers toward agricultural employers while the War Food Administration classified farm work as "essential," exempting agricultural workers from military service while simultaneously arguing that domestic labor was insufficient—a contradiction that revealed how these agencies functioned to maintain employer control rather than address labor shortages. The contracts promised specific standards of pay and housing, but these promises quickly unraveled. Newly imported foreign workers were subject to the same violent conditions as their predecessors as their status as foreign laborers made them ideal targets for exploitation.[51] Unable to return home, lacking local rights, and isolated from support networks, these workers were deliberately recruited because they were more amenable to control.[52]

This shift toward foreign labor marked a crucial transition in how the migrant labor system would operate in the postwar period. Native-born White migrant workers, particularly those displaced by the Dust Bowl and economic disruption, were increasingly viewed as temporarily displaced Americans who should be "settled" into permanent communities. Federal programs through the FSA prioritized their rehabilitation and reintegration into stable employment, offering pathways to land ownership, vocational training, and permanent settlement assistance. In contrast, Black workers and foreign laborers were categorized as naturally suited for permanent migrancy and seasonal labor—a racialized distinction that became embedded in federal policy by 1950.

As the war closed, the migrant labor system became increasingly institutionalized. Despite numerous government investigations documenting deplorable conditions, these official reports normalized the migrant labor system by treating worker vulnerability as an inevitable feature of agricultural production to be managed rather than a deliberately constructed system of exploitation to be dismantled, implicitly accepting that some workers would remain permanently transient and excluded from the protections available to other American workers.[53] While advocacy efforts and African American newspapers like the *Baltimore Afro-American* consistently exposed exploitation and worker resistance, their documentation was often co-opted by officials who used evidence of poor housing, low wages, and health disparities to justify minimal reforms that ultimately preserved the system's core functioning.

The wartime and postwar period did not represent a transformation of the migrant labor system but its ultimate consolidation. Workers' health became the reserve that kept the system running—an acceptable, if not calculated, expenditure in the pursuit of agricultural productivity and profit accumulation for agricultural elites. These decades of transformation reveal a systematic national approach to agricultural labor that extended far beyond Maryland. Each period—from postemancipation restructuring to wartime mobilization—demonstrated how racial capitalism continuously refined its mechanisms of worker control. Technological innovations, economic crises, and federal policies were not isolated events but interconnected strategies that progressively narrowed the possibilities for worker autonomy, particularly for Black and immigrant laborers.

CONCLUSION

The COVID-19 pandemic dramatically revealed migrant farmworkers' persistent vulnerabilities, exposing structural inequities that have historical roots. Scholars naming poverty and isolation as social determinants often treat these as independent factors addressable without challenging the underlying labor system. As scholars document, COVID-19 did not create new vulnerabilities among farmworkers but exposed the enduring legacy of deliberately constructed systems of worker disposability that originated in the early 20th century.[54]

Maryland's agricultural history demonstrates how poverty, racism, and isolation were not incidental conditions but deliberately produced features essential to the migrant labor system. These were active technologies of control and extraction, with agricultural interests consistently fighting interventions that threatened these foundational mechanisms of exploitation. The migrant labor system does not merely contain health determinants—it actively produces them. Workers' health serves as a calculated expenditure, a reserve that kept the system profitable. Each tuberculosis outbreak, instance of malnutrition, and premature death was not a failure of the system but its most efficient operation.

Contemporary debates about agricultural labor and health equity must reckon with this historical architecture of dispossession. Migrant workers continue to occupy a liminal space—essential yet disposable, visible yet systematically erased. To address migrant worker health, public health practitioners, policymakers, and researchers must move beyond reformist approaches and work toward dismantling systems that have historically transformed human beings into extractable resources.

Our analysis reveals that health equity demands a radical reimagining of labor, mobility, and human value. The history of migrant farmworkers remains an ongoing narrative of extraction and resistance, survival and struggle for dignity. AJPH

ABOUT THE AUTHORS

Elise Ferrer and Thurka Sangaramoorthy are with the Department of Anthropology, American University, Washington, DC. Devon Payne-Sturges is with the Department of Environmental Health Sciences, School of Public Health, University of Michigan, Ann Arbor, MI.

CORRESPONDENCE

Correspondence should be sent to Thurka Sangaramoorthy, PhD, MPH, Department of Anthropology, American University, Hamilton Hall, 4400 Massachusetts Ave NW, Washington, DC 20016 (e-mail: thurkas@american.edu). Reprints can be ordered at https://www.ajph.org by clicking the "Reprints" link.

PUBLICATION INFORMATION

Full Citation: Ferrer E, Sangaramoorthy T, Payne-Sturges D. Designed for disparity: the structural origins of migrant farmworker health inequities in Maryland, 1900–1950. *Am J Public Health*. 2026; 116(5):657–664.

Acceptance Date: October 17, 2025.

DOI: https://doi.org/10.2105/AJPH.2025.308362

ORCID iDs:

Elise Ferrer https://orcid.org/0009-0003-9225-4808

Thurka Sangaramoorthy https://orcid.org/0000-0002-8467-5907

Devon Payne-Sturges https://orcid.org/0000-0001-7343-2814

CONTRIBUTORS

E. Ferrer led the archival project from which these sources and analyses were pulled. E. Ferrer and

T. Sangaramoorthy conceptualized the article, contributed ideas, and critically edited, revised, and approved the final version. D. Payne-Sturges provided crucial insights throughout each step of the research and writing process.

ACKNOWLEDGMENTS

This work was supported by the National Institute of Environmental Health Sciences (award R01ES034303).

The authors extend their gratitude to the archivists, librarians, and research collaborators who contributed to this project, as well as the farmworkers, past and present, who inspire the pursuit of justice and dignity for all.

Additional references are available in the Appendix (available as a supplement to the online version of this article at https://www.ajph.org).

CONFLICTS OF INTEREST

We have no conflicts of interest to disclose.

ENDNOTES

1. Nick Juravich and Steve Striffler, eds., *The Pandemic and the Working Class: How US Labor Navigated COVID-19* (Champaign, IL: University of Illinois Press, 2021); Barbara Jeanne Fields, *Slavery and Freedom on the Middle Ground: Maryland During the Nineteenth Century* (New Haven, CT: Yale University Press, 1985).
2. Michel Foucault, *Discipline and Punish: The Birth of the Prison* (New York, NY: Vintage Books, 1977).
3. Cedric Robinson, *Black Marxism: The Making of the Black Radical Tradition* (Chapel Hill, NC: University of North Carolina Press, 2000); Whitney N. Laster Pirtle, "Racial Capitalism: A Fundamental Cause of Novel Coronavirus (COVID-19) Pandemic Inequities in the United States," *Health Education & Behavior* 47, no. 4 (2020): 504–508, https://doi.org/10.1177/1090198120922942
4. Cindy Hahamovitch, "Creating Perfect Immigrants: Guestworkers of the World in Historical Perspective," *Labor History* 44, no. 1 (2003): 69–94, https://doi.org/10.1080/0023656032000057010; Don Mitchell, *The Lie of the Land: Migrant Workers and the California Landscape* (Minneapolis, MN: University of Minnesota Press, 1996).
5. Paul Farmer, "An Anthropology of Structural Violence." *Current Anthropology* 45, no. 3 (2004): 305–325, https://doi.org/10.1086/382250; Seth Holmes, *Fresh Fruit, Broken Bodies: Migrant Farmworkers in the United States* (Berkeley, CA: University of California Press, 2013); Thurka Sangaramoorthy, *Landscapes of Care: Immigration and Health in Rural America* (Chapel Hill, NC: University of North Carolina Press, 2023).
6. Peter Benson, "El Campo: Faciality and Structural Violence in Farm Labor Camps," *Cultural Anthropology* 23, no. 4 (2008): 589–629, https://doi.org/10.1111/j.1548-1360.2008.00020.x
7. US Census Bureau, "[Bulletin] Agriculture: Maryland, Twelfth Census of the United States (1902)," Census Bulletin 151 (Washington, DC: Bureau of the Census, Department of Commerce, 1902), https://www2.census.gov/library/publications/decennial/1900/bulletins/agriculture/151-agriculture-md.pdf (accessed January 15, 2025).
8. Foucault, *Discipline and Punish.*
9. US Census Bureau, "Occupations of the Twelfth Census: States and Territories," Part 8 (Washington, DC: US Government Printing Office, 1900), https://www2.census.gov/library/publications/decennial/1900/occupations/occupations-part-8.pdf (accessed January 15, 2025).
10. *Ibid.*
11. US Census Bureau, "[Bulletin] Agriculture: Maryland, Twelfth Census of the United States (1902)."
12. *Ibid.*
13. "The Proud Old State of Maryland." *Denton Journal*, August 21, 1897, p. 2.
14. "The Promised Land: Maryland's Resources Set Forth in a Pamphlet of the State Bureau of Immigration," *Baltimore Sun*, September 30, 1896; Maryland Bureau of Immigration, *Maryland, Its Lands, Products and Industries; the Ideal Home for the Immigrant* (Baltimore, MD: Baltimore City Printing and Binding Company, 1915), https://hdl.handle.net/2027/uiug.30112062890238?urlappend=%3Bseq=1 (accessed February 1, 2025).
15. "Labor for Virginia," *Baltimore Sun*, January 26, 1903, p. 10.
16. "Make Him Work by Law: Dr. McConnell's Clear Statement and Wise Solution to the Negro Problem," *Brooklyn Eagle*, July 31, 1903, p. 4.
17. "Labor at a Premium in Easton Notwithstanding the Fact That Dr. McConnell Says Negroes Are Lazy and Will Not Work. . . ." *Baltimore Afro-American*, September 5, 1903, p. 1. ProQuest.
18. US Census Bureau, "Chapter 1: Color or Race, Nativity, and Parentage," In *1920 Census Published Tables*, Volume 2, Section 1, 15–20 passim (1920), https://usa.ipums.org/usa/resources/voliii/pubdocs/1920/Vol2/41084484v2ch01.pdf (accessed January 31, 2025).
19. *Ibid.*
20. William Jones, "Business and Industry: A Weekly Review of Labor and Business Farm," *Baltimore Afro-American*, October 31, 1925, p. 18.
21. Mitchell, *The Lie of the Land.*
22. Don Mitchell, *They Saved the Crops: Labor, Landscape, and the Struggle Over Industrial Farming in Bracero-Era California* (Athens, GA: University of Georgia Press, 2012), 45–67.
23. Juravich and Striffler, *The Pandemic and the Working Class*, p. 183.
24. J. Knox Insley, "Berry and Vegetable Pickers in Maryland: Child Labor in Vegetable Canneries in Maryland," Commissioner of Labor and Statistics, State of Maryland, Box 1, Folder 16, Baltimore Studies Archive, 1929, 7, https://archivesspace.ubalt.edu/repositories/2/archival_objects/64648 (accessed November 18, 2024).
25. Select Committee to Investigate the Interstate Migration of Destitute Citizens, *Preliminary Report of the Select Committee to Investigate the Interstate Migration of Destitute Citizens [The Tolan Commission]*, Report, 76th Congress, 3d Session, House of Representatives (1940), https://catalog.hathitrust.org/Record/102186977 (accessed August 2, 2024).
26. Alice Channing, "Child Labor on Maryland Truck Farms," United States Children's Bureau Publication 123 (May 1923): 25–29, 31, 40, 46, https://fraser.stlouisfed.org/title/child-labor-maryland-truck-farms-8405 (accessed July 31, 2024).
27. *Ibid.*
28. *Ibid.*
29. *Ibid.*
30. *Ibid.*
31. *Ibid.*
32. Franklin D. Roosevelt, "Executive Order 7027—Establishment of the Resettlement Administration" (Washington, DC: The White House, The American Presidency Project, 1935), https://www.presidency.ucsb.edu/documents/executive-order-7027-establishment-the-resettlement-administration (accessed August 5, 2024).
33. *Preliminary Report of the Select Committee to Investigate the Interstate Migration of Destitute Citizens,* p. 9.
34. *Ibid,* p. 23.
35. *Ibid.*
36. *Ibid,* p. 20.
37. "NJ Commission Urges Sending Jobless to Farm," *Baltimore Afro-American*, December 26, 1931, p. 9.
38. "'Work or Fight' Bill Signed by O'Conor; Doubts Legality," *Cumberland News*, April 2, 1943.
39. Ollie Stewart, "Here's How Work-Jail-or-Army Campaign Hits 100 Maryland Oakies: Ollie Stewart Spends Two Days with Migrant Oyster Shuckers Whom County Officials Would Impress for Farm Work at $8.75 a Week," *Baltimore Afro-American*, May 23, 1942.
40. Select Committee to Investigate the Interstate Migration of Destitute Citizens, *Final Report of the Select Committee to Investigate the Interstate Migration of Destitute Citizens [The Tolan Commission]*, 77th Congress, 1st Session, House Report 369 (1941): 101, 468, 562, https://catalog.hathitrust.org/Record/000952924 (accessed August 1, 2024).
41. Mary E. Cannon, "'The Acre': A Report of the Social Center at Bridgeville, Delaware from July 6th to August 31, 1940, H.P. Cannon Sons, Inc, Canner," Women's Council of Churches for Home Missions, Maryland Council of Churches Records, University of Baltimore Special Collections, 1941, 10–11.
42. *Final Report of the Select Committee to Investigate the Interstate Migration of Destitute Citizens.*
43. "Notes on Lower Virginia Peninsula Migration," Home Missions Council of North America, 1940, Maryland Council of Churches Records, University of Baltimore Special Collections.
44. *Final Report of the Select Committee to Investigate the Interstate Migration of Destitute Citizens.*
45. *Ibid,* p. 562.
46. Cindy Hahamovitch, "The Politics of Labor Scarcity," Center for Immigration Studies: Backgrounder, December 1999, https://cis.org/Report/Politics-Labor-Scarcity (accessed August 1, 2025).
47. Leslie Atkins, "The Other End of Democracy," *Greenbelt Cooperator*, November 14, 1941.
48. Cindy Hahamovitch, "Everything But a Gun to Their Heads: The Politics of Labor Scarcity and the Birth of World War II Guestworker Programs," In *No Man's Land: Jamaican Guestworkers in America and the Global History of Deportable Labor* (Princeton, NJ: Princeton University Press, 2011), p. 23.
49. "Maryland's Farm Labor Needs Given Priority – O'Conor Says," *Denton Journal*, June 23, 1944, p. 7.

50. Deborah Cohen, *Braceros: Migrant Citizens and Transnational Subjects in the Postwar United States and Mexico* (Chapel Hill, NC: University of North Carolina Press, 2011), 78–92; Cindy Hahamovitch, *The Fruits of Their Labor: Atlantic Coast Farmworkers and the Making of Migrant Poverty, 1870–1945* (Chapel Hill, NC: University of North Carolina Press, 1997), 156–178.

50. Hahamovitch, *The Fruits of Their Labor*.

52. Lowell Lomax, "Jamaican, Bahamian at Md. Camps List: Low Wages, Bad Food, No Recreational or Religious Facilities, No Hot Water and Sometimes No Work; Laborers Want Out," *Baltimore Afro-American*, July 22, 1944.

53. *Preliminary Report of the Select Committee to Investigate the Interstate Migration of Destitute Citizens*

54. Juravich and Striffler, *The Pandemic and the Working Class;* Caroline Keegan, "Essential Agriculture, Sacrificial Labor, and the COVID-19 Pandemic in the US South," *Journal of Agrarian Change* 23, no. 3 (2023): 611–621, https://doi.org/10.1111/joac.12522

Changes in All-Cause, Overdose, and Suicide Mortality Risk in the First 2 Years of Supported Housing, United States, 2017–2021

Jack Tsai, PhD, MSCP, Talya Peltzman, MPH, and Hind A. Beydoun, PhD, MPH

See also Hwang, p. 584.

Objectives. To examine whether there are reduced or elevated risks for all-cause, overdose, and suicide mortality after moving into supported housing.

Methods. A national retrospective cohort study compared a census of 60 888 veterans experiencing homelessness in the US Housing and Urban Development–Veterans Affairs Supportive Housing (HUD–VASH) program with a 1:1 propensity-score matched group of veterans experiencing homelessness from 2017 to 2021.

Results. Rates for all-cause mortality in the matched HUD–VASH group significantly increased after 6 months, and risk of all-cause mortality was slightly higher in the HUD–VASH group than the matched comparison cohort at 24-month follow-up. Overdose mortality risk was twice as high among the HUD–VASH cohort across all time points, and there was no significant group difference in suicide mortality risk across time.

Conclusions. Supported housing was associated with an initial lower risk of all-cause mortality that was not sustained over the course of 2 years. Veterans in supported housing were consistently more likely to die from drug overdose than were other veterans experiencing homelessness.

Public Health Implications. The timely provision of substance use treatment in supported housing could be important to prevent drug overdose deaths. (*Am J Public Health*. 2026;116(5):665–673. https://doi.org/10.2105/AJPH.2025.308371)

AJPH May 2026, Vol. 116, No. 5

Current evidence from the international literature indicates that adults experiencing homelessness are more susceptible to premature deaths than stably housed adults.[1–4] Specific causes of death have been examined, and homelessness has been shown to be associated with greater risks of dying from drug overdose[5,6] and suicide.[7–9] The time at which mortality risk is highest among adults experiencing homelessness as they receive homeless assistance and move into housing is unclear. Anecdotally, there are clinical reports that some individuals are at high risk for dying in their first year of supported housing. With the Housing First model being the predominant approach for supported housing,[10,11] some have theorized that the immediate transition from street homelessness into supported housing is a jarring experience accompanied by social isolation, psychological distress, and continued barriers to health care, all of which can adversely affect health and mortality risk.[12–14] Others have pointed to research that supported housing may not resolve substance misuse and that individuals in supported housing are at even greater risk for drug overdose because they are in their own apartments and not in a shelter or a public setting in which others can observe and intervene.[12–14] On the other spectrum of perspectives are those who have theorized various pathways for the positive impact of stable housing on health, including improved life stability, environment quality and safety, financial affordability, and neighborhood access.[15–17]

The US Department of Veterans Affairs (VA) operates the largest supported housing program in the country in partnership with the US Department of Housing and Urban Development (HUD) called the HUD–VA Supportive Housing (HUD–VASH) program.[18–20] Clinicians who determine veterans to be experiencing homelessness refer the veterans to the HUD-VASH program, and the HUD–VASH program serves thousands of veterans annually by seeking to rapidly house veterans experiencing homelessness. The HUD–VASH program provides a unique opportunity to examine mortality risks at different time points in a large sample of supported housing clients.

The current study used a national retrospective cohort design with propensity score matching to answer a critical question: are there reduced or elevated risks for all-cause, overdose, and suicide mortality in the first 2 years after moving into supported housing? For example, is there a period of improved health and reduced mortality risk when individuals first enter supported housing given the expected positive impacts of stable housing on health? We hypothesized that HUD–VASH participants would have lower all-cause mortality risk than their homeless counterparts over time, but that there would be an increased risk of drug overdose and suicide deaths among HUD–VASH participants, particularly during their first year in supported housing, because of social adjustment challenges, which would subside by the second year.

METHODS

In this retrospective cohort study, we relied on 3 linked databases—namely, VA's Corporate Data Warehouse (CDW) containing VA electronic health records populated by providers during clinical encounters; VA's Homeless Operations Management and Evaluation System (HOMES) containing data on veteran participation in VA homeless programs, populated by providers; and the Department of Defense/VA Mortality Data Repository (MDR) containing data from the National Death Index, including date of death, cause of death, state of death, date of birth, and sex of the decedent.[21,22] The linked CDW and HOMES databases were used to define national cohorts of veterans with an initial encounter between January 1, 2017, and December 31, 2019, who were followed between their initial encounter up to December 31, 2021, until censoring or death, using the National Death Index database. The census of all HUD–VASH participants during the study period was included, except individuals who did not meet the eligibility criteria described subsequently, had data that could not be linked, or were at VA Cerner facilities during 2021 (i.e., on a different data system). We extracted data elements from linked CDW, HOMES, and MDR databases to compare 2 distinct cohorts on all-cause, overdose, and suicide deaths occurring over a follow-up period of 2 years, and so the entire study period was from 2017 to 2021.

The first cohort consisted of veterans who entered HUD–VASH housing during the study period, and their baseline date was the day they moved into supported housing between January 1, 2017, and December 31, 2019. The second cohort consisted of veterans experiencing homelessness who met a VA operational definition of homelessness that included several indicators[23]—namely, *International Classification of Diseases, 10th Revision, Clinical Modification* (*ICD-10-CM*) diagnostic code Z59.0; clinic stop codes or HOMES records indicating use of VA homeless programs clinical encounters (excluding HUD–VASH); or a positive screen on an annual VA homeless screener (often administered in VA outpatient settings annually according to the veteran's last screening date). The second cohort's baseline date was defined as their first visit to the VA health care system between January 1, 2017, and December 31, 2019. Veterans who switched status between cohorts (i.e., exited HUD–VASH enrollment or enrolled in HUD–VASH, during the study period [2017–2021]) were excluded from the analysis.

Using the greedy method with a caliper size of 0.5, we compared the HUD–VASH and the homeless cohorts through 1:1 propensity score matching on baseline date, demographic, and clinical characteristics. Caliper size is recommended to be a fraction of the standard deviation of the logit of propensity scores with consideration of existing overlap between treated and control groups along with sample size needs.[24] Because both cohorts shared experiences with homelessness and overdose-specific and suicide-specific deaths are rare outcomes, we opted to use a caliper size of 0.5 to maximize the number of HUD–VASH enrollees matched to homeless veterans. We identified deaths by linking social security numbers from these cohorts to the MDR database whereby death status, cause, and date of death were ascertained for active-duty military and veterans for the study period (2017–2021).

Measures

We performed propensity score matched comparisons after matching HUD–VASH versus homeless cohorts on baseline date and a priori confounders for hypothesized relationships—namely, age, sex, race, marital status, combat service, VA service-connected disability rating, and Charlson Comorbidity Index score,[25] as well as diagnosed substance use (i.e., tobacco, alcohol, drug), and mental health (i.e., mood, psychotic, anxiety, stress-related, other) disorders.[26]

Using the MDR database, we identified all-cause deaths as well as deaths attributable to drug overdose and suicide based on the "underlying" cause of death only. We used *ICD-10-CM* codes to define drug overdose deaths, which comprised unintentional (X40–X44), homicide (X85), and undetermined intent codes (Y10–Y14). Suicide-specific deaths were identified by using *ICD-10-CM* codes focused on method-specific self-inflicted injury consistent with the 2023 Veteran Suicide Prevention Annual Report, which also included X60 to X64 codes that reflect a combination of overdose and suicide deaths.[27] As such, overdose deaths excluded any deaths identified as suicide deaths. We estimated overdose and suicide mortality rates (per 100 000 person-years) with 95% confidence intervals (CIs) by using the exact Poisson method for every 6 months within the first 2 years of follow-up. We performed survival analyses whereby all-cause, overdose, and suicide deaths were considered as events of interest. We defined the overall follow-up time for calculating mortality rates and survival analyses as time from baseline date until the occurrence of death or end of follow-up, within the first 2 years of follow-up (i.e., at 6, 12, 18, and 24 months of follow-up).

Data Analysis

We performed statistical analyses by using the SAS Enterprise Guide version 8.3 (SAS Institute, Cary, NC). Propensity score matching is a powerful tool for making causal inferences from observational studies by ensuring groups are comparable on prognostic characteristics affecting outcomes of interest.[28] Using the prematched sample, we confirmed that demographic and clinical characteristics were confounders of hypothesized relationships by being associated with both the outcomes (i.e., all-cause, overdose, and suicide-specific mortality risks among HUD–VASH and homeless veterans; Table A, available as a supplement to the online version of this article at https://ajph.org) and exposures of interest (i.e., HUD–VASH vs homeless veterans; Table B, available as a supplement to the online version of this article at https://ajph.org).

Second, we calculated propensity scores as predicted probabilities of "HUD–VASH versus homeless" for each veteran by defining "HUD–VASH versus homeless" as the outcome in a multiple logistic regression model, whereby baseline date, demographic, and clinical characteristics were entered as predictors.

Third, we used propensity scores of "HUD–VASH versus homeless" to generate a matched sample for the "HUD–VASH versus homeless" comparison, after verifying an overlap in propensity scores existed between comparison groups in the prematched samples (Table C, available as a supplement to the online version of this article at https://ajph.org). We assessed matching quality by examining differences in demographic and clinical characteristics between comparison groups in the matched sample (Table D, available as a supplement to the online version of this article at https://ajph.org).

Fourth, we examined differences in all-cause and cause-specific mortality risks between the HUD–VASH and homeless groups over a follow-up time of 24 months using the prematched and matched samples (Table E, available as a supplement to the online version of this article at https://ajph.org). All analyses described subsequently then used these matched cohorts for analysis. Given the retrospective cohort design and the fact that propensity score matching was performed for the exposure variable (HUD–VASH vs homeless), matching at the design stage did not modify the modeling strategy at the analysis stage.

For descriptive purposes, we used the matched samples to estimate all-cause, overdose, and suicide mortality rates (per 100 000 person-years) with 95% CIs over 6-month periods with a maximum follow-up time of 24 months. To examine changes in mortality rates within each group, nonoverlapping 95% CIs indicated statistically significant changes over time. We performed Cox regression modeling to examine differences in mortality risks between matched groups of HUD–VASH participants and nonparticipants over 6-month periods during a maximum follow-up time of 24 months.

RESULTS

As shown in Figure 1, a total of 7 176 577 veterans received VA health care between January 1, 2017, and December 31, 2021. Of these, 7 165 889 had records matching between linked CDW–HOMES and MDR databases and had known vital status. After excluding

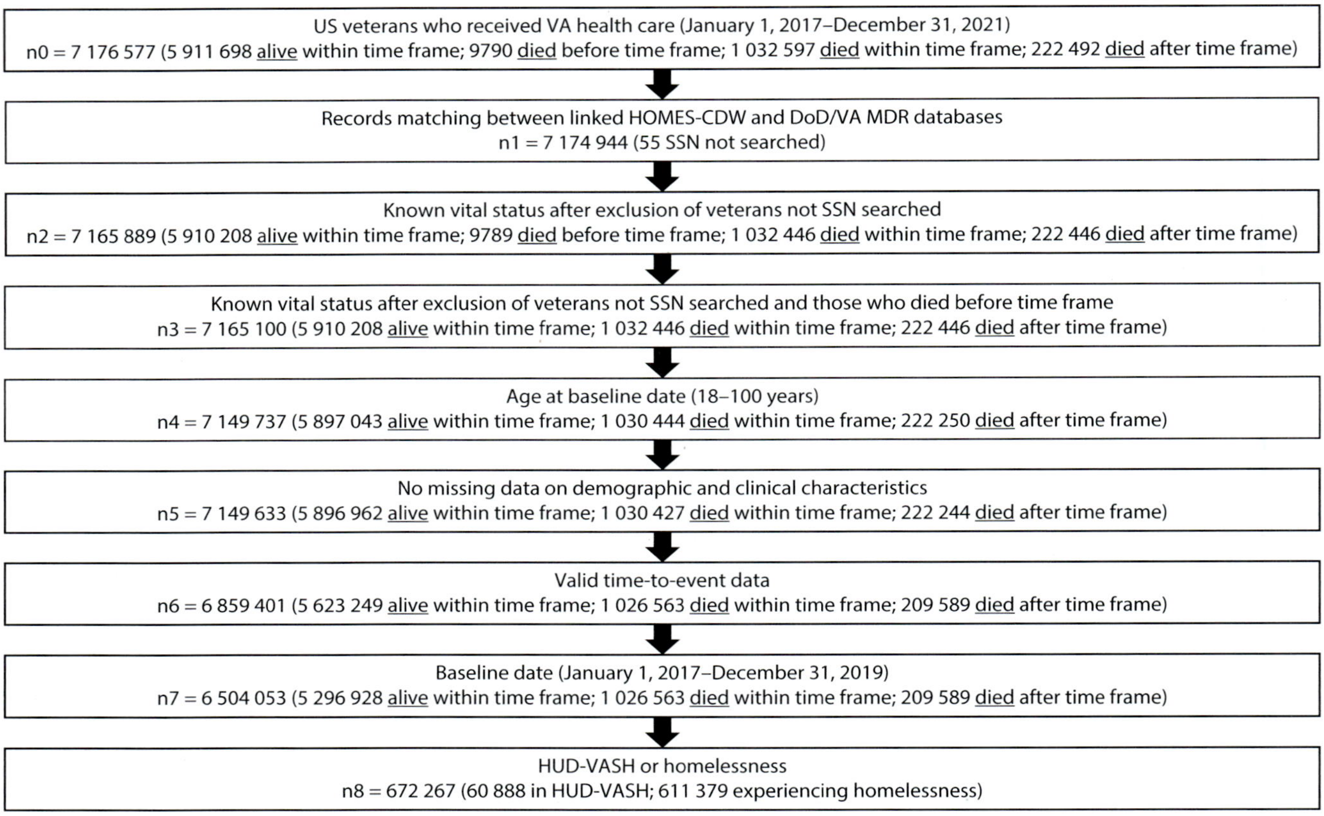

FIGURE 1— Study Flowchart for Changes in All-Cause, Overdose, and Suicide Mortality Risk in the First 2 Years of Supported Housing: United States, 2017–2021

Note. A total of 7 176 577 US veterans were initially identified through the Corporate Data Warehouse (CDW) database, but 1 032 597 died within the time frame, and 222 492 died after the time frame, based on Department of Defense (DoD)/VA Mortality Data Repository (MDR) data. Of those, 7 174 944 had records matching between linked Homeless Operations Management and Evaluation System (HOMES)–CDW and DoD/VA MDR databases using scrambled social security numbers (SSNs). After limiting the sample through several additional steps, the sample became 60 888 veterans who were in Housing and Urban Development–Veterans Affairs Supportive Housing (HUD–VASH) and 611 379 veterans who were homeless within the study period. Propensity score matching resulted in 60 888 in the HUD–VASH group and 60 888 in the homeless group.

HUD–VASH, homeless, or independently housed veterans who died before the time frame of interest, those younger than 18 years, those older than 100 years, those with missing data on demographic and clinical characteristics, and those with invalid time-to-event data (e.g., errors with their dates, missing dates), 6 859 401 veterans remained, of whom 6 504 053 veterans (60 888 in HUD–VASH, 611 379 homeless, and 5 831 786 presumed to be independently housed) had a baseline visit between January 1, 2017, and December 31, 2019. The final analytic samples consisted of 60 888 from the HUD–VASH cohort matched to 60 888 from the homeless cohort.

As shown in Table 1, comparisons on demographic and clinical characteristics between the HUD–VASH and homeless cohorts indicated that propensity score matching substantially reduced differences between matched groups on a priori confounders. Specifically, the standardized mean difference between propensity score matched comparison groups was 0.10 for propensity score and ranged between −0.26 and 0.04 for a priori confounders. Furthermore, the percentage reduction between unmatched and matched samples was 93.4% for the propensity score and ranged between 0.0% and 99.7% for a priori confounders, with variance ratios ranging between 0.76 and 1.37. Comparisons between the HUD–VASH group, the prematching homeless group, and the matched homeless group on demographic and clinical characteristics used in propensity score matching are available upon request from the corresponding author.

Table 2 presents all-cause and cause-specific mortality rates (per 100 000 person-years) among the matched

TABLE 1— Standardized Mean Difference Between Propensity Score Matched Comparison Groups (HUD–VASH vs Homeless Veterans), Percentage Reduction Between Unmatched and Matched Samples, and Variance Ratio for Log-Odds of Propensity Score and Matching Characteristics: United States, 2017–2021

	HUD–VASH vs Homelessness[a]		
	Standardized Mean Difference	Percentage Reduction	Variance Ratio
Log-odds propensity score	0.10	93.4	1.29
Baseline date	−0.07	95.1	0.81
Sex			
Male	0.01	91.4	1.01
Female (Ref)	0	. . .	. . .
Age, y			
18–49 (Ref)	0	. . .	. . .
50–59	−0.08	72.9	1.06
60–69	−0.04	53.6	1.04
70–79	0.01	95.6	0.91
80–100	−0.00	99.7	1.02
Race/ethnicity			
Non-Hispanic White (Ref)	0	. . .	. . .
Non-Hispanic Black	−0.03	84.3	1.01
Hispanic	0.00	97.0	0.99
Mixed race or other	0.01	91.4	0.97
Missing	0.04	0.0	0.89
Marital status			
Married (Ref)	0	. . .	. . .
Single or never married	0.03	86.5	0.98
Separated or divorced	−0.06	75.3	1.00
Widowed	−0.01	89.5	1.07
Missing	0.03	0.0	0.76
VA service-connected disability rating, %			
0 (Ref)	0	. . .	. . .
10–40	−0.03	79.2	1.04
50–100	−0.01	93.9	1.01
Combat service			
Yes	−0.00	93.9	1.04
No (Ref)	0	. . .	. . .
Charlson comorbidity index			
0 (Ref)	0	. . .	. . .
1	−0.11	0.0	1.37
2	−0.06	60.5	1.41
≥3	−0.04	81.8	1.31
Substance use disorder			
Yes	−0.21	44.3	1.12
No (Ref)	0	. . .	. . .

Continued

comparison groups. Across the 24-month follow-up period, the HUD–VASH cohort's all-cause mortality rate was 2155 to 2902 per 100 000 person-years, overdose mortality rate was 382 to 403 per 100 000 person-years, and suicide mortality rate was 46 to 88 per 100 000 person-years. In the comparison homeless cohort, the all-cause mortality rate was 2445 to 2756 per 100 000 person-years; overdose mortality was 168 to 225 per 100 000 person-years, and suicide mortality was 76 to 93 per 100 000 person-years. Within the HUD–VASH cohort, all-cause mortality rates significantly increased after 6 months and remained elevated for the remaining 24-month follow-up period (i.e., all-cause mortality rates at 12, 18, and 24 months were higher than at 6 months); this pattern was not observed in the comparison homeless cohort. There was also no significant change within either cohort in overdose or suicide mortality across the 24 months of follow-up.

Cox regression models directly compared the 2 cohorts on all-cause and cause-specific mortality over the 24 months of follow-up (Table 3). All-cause mortality risk was significantly lower among the HUD–VASH cohort than the homeless cohort at 6 months (hazard ratio [HR] = 0.88; 95% CI = 0.79, 0.98), but significantly higher among the HUD–VASH cohort than the homeless cohort at 24 months of follow-up, although the effect was small (HR = 1.05; 95% CI = 1.00, 1.10). Conversely, overdose mortality risk was consistently higher among the HUD–VASH cohort than the homeless cohort at 6 months (HR = 2.29; 95% CI = 1.65, 3.18), 12 months (HR = 2.22; 95% CI = 1.77, 2.79), 18 months (HR = 1.80; 95% CI = 1.51, 2.15), and 24 months (HR = 1.79; 95% CI = 1.54, 2.07) of

TABLE 1— Continued

	HUD–VASH vs Homelessness[a]		
	Standardized Mean Difference	Percentage Reduction	Variance Ratio
Mental health disorder			
Yes	−0.26	0.0	1.10
No (Ref)	0	. . .	. . .

Note. HUD–VASH = US Department of Housing and Urban Development and Veterans Affairs Supportive Housing; VA = US Department of Veterans Affairs.
[a]Of 672 267 veterans, 60 888 were in HUD–VASH housing and 611 379 were experiencing homelessness in the prematched sample. Propensity score matching yielded 60 888 HUD–VASH and 60 888 veterans experiencing homelessness.

follow-up. Suicide mortality risk was not significantly different between HUD–VASH and homeless cohorts at 6, 12, 18, or 24 months of follow-up.

DISCUSSION

This large retrospective cohort study examined how mortality risks changed over time in supported housing by following a national sample of veterans in the largest supported housing program in the United States. Answering our originally posed question, veterans who entered HUD–VASH had slightly lower risk of all-cause mortality 6 months after moving into supported housing compared with a matched comparison group. However, all-cause mortality rates in HUD–VASH increased after 6 months, and after 24 months, the HUD–VASH group had slightly higher risk of all-cause mortality than the comparison group. These findings ran contrary to our study hypothesis and suggest that mortality risk in supported housing may take time to manifest. That is, the effects of any social adjustment challenges experienced by veterans when they first move into supported housing may be delayed or occur later. Notably, the observed increase in all-cause mortality risk in the HUD–VASH group after 6 months could not be directly attributed to suicide or overdose because we did not detect any significant change in suicide or overdose death rates in either the HUD–VASH or comparison groups. In relation to the research literature, the higher mortality risk among individuals

TABLE 2— All-Cause and Cause-Specific Mortality Rates (per 100 000 Person-Years) With 95% Confidence Intervals Within Propensity-Score Matched Comparison Groups (HUD–VASH vs Homeless Veterans), at 6 Months, 12 Months, 18 Months, and 24 Months of Follow-Up: United States, 2017–2021

	HUD-VASH (n = 60 888)		Homeless (n = 60 888)	
	No. of Individuals (Person-Years)	Mortality Rate (95% CI)	No. of Individuals (Person-Years)	Mortality Rate (95% CI)
All-cause mortality, mo				
6	653 (30 298)	2 155 (1 993, 2 327)	740 (30 259)	2 445 (2 272, 2 628)
12	1 578 (60 187)	2 622 (2 494, 2 754)	1 502 (60 152)	2 497 (2 372, 2 626)
18	2 495 (89 617)	2 784 (2 676, 2 895)	2 397 (89 622)	2 674 (2 568, 2 783)
24	3 442 (118 584)	2 902 (2 806, 3 001)	3 271 (118 654)	2 756 (2 663, 2 853)
Overdose mortality, mo				
6	117 (30 298)	386 (319, 463)	51 (30 259)	168 (125, 222)
12	240 (60 187)	398 (350, 452)	108 (60 153)	180 (147, 217)
18	342 (89 617)	382 (342, 424)	190 (89 622)	212 (183, 244)
24	478 (118 584)	403 (368, 441)	268 (118 654)	225 (199, 254)
Suicide mortality, mo				
6	14 (30 298)	46 (25, 76)	23 (30 259)	76 (48, 114)
12	52 (60 187)	86 (64, 113)	51 (60 152)	85 (63, 111)
18	79 (89 617)	88 (70, 110)	78 (89 622)	87 (69, 109)
24	97 (118 584)	82 (66, 100)	110 (118 654)	93 (76, 111)

Note. CI = confidence interval; HUD–VASH = US Department of Housing and Urban Development and Veterans Affairs Supportive Housing.

TABLE 3— Cox Regression Models for Propensity-Score Matched Comparison Groups (HUD–VASH vs Homeless Veterans) as Predictors of All-Cause, Overdose, and Suicide-Specific Mortality Risks at 6 Months, 12 Months, 18 Months, and 24 Months of Follow-Up: United States, 2017–2021

	HUD-VASH vs Homeless, HR (95% CI)
All-cause mortality, mo	
6	0.88 (0.79, 0.98)
12	1.05 (0.98, 1.13)
18	1.04 (0.98, 1.10)
24	1.05 (1.00, 1.10)
Overdose mortality, mo	
6	2.29 (1.65, 3.18)
12	2.22 (1.77, 2.79)
18	1.80 (1.51, 2.15)
24	1.79 (1.54, 2.07)
Suicide mortality, mo	
6	0.61 (0.31, 1.18)
12	1.02 (0.69, 1.50)
18	1.01 (0.74, 1.39)
24	0.88 (0.67, 1.16)

Note. CI = confidence interval; HR = hazard ratio; HUD-VASH = US Department of Housing and Urban Development and Veterans Affairs Supportive Housing. Propensity score matching of 60 888 HUD-VASH versus 60 888 veterans experiencing homelessness on baseline date, sex, age, race, marital status, US Department of Veterans Affairs service-connected disability rating, combat service, Charlson comorbidity index, and substance use and mental health disorders.

experiencing homelessness compared with the general population is well-known,[5–9] but our findings newly contribute to knowledge about differences in all-cause and cause-specific mortality risk based on enrollment in supported housing and changes that occur over time.

Perhaps our most striking study finding was the consistently higher risk of overdose mortality (i.e., about 2 times higher risk) found in the HUD–VASH group compared with the comparison group throughout the 24 months of follow-up. The high risk of overdose mortality we found in HUD-VASH veterans is consistent with several studies of general adults experiencing homelessness, including nonveterans.[12,13] One study examining mortality rates among US adults in supported housing with the Housing First model found that participants experienced excess mortality compared with the general population and that mortality rates in supported housing were higher than those reported among general populations experiencing homelessness.[13] Similarly, a randomized trial in France found that 39% of deaths in a supported housing group occurred in the first 6 months compared with 18% in a treatment-as-usual group.[12] Strikingly, 35% of these deaths in supported housing were attributable to overdose compared with 0% in the treatment-as-usual group. Moreover, the high prevalence of substance use disorders in populations experiencing homelessness is well-documented,[29,30] as is the link between homelessness and fatal and nonfatal drug overdose.[31,32] The HUD–VASH program does not have any requirements regarding substance use treatment[10,11]; therefore, participants may have had active unresolved substance use problems that preceded the program and continued unabated in supported housing. The consistent risk of overdose deaths over the 2-year period in supported housing suggests the need for sustained substance use treatment and preventive interventions for drug overdose.

The finding that there was no significant difference in suicide mortality risk between and within the HUD–VASH and homeless cohorts is also informative as they may reflect the fact that suicide prevention is VA's top clinical priority with system-wide implementation of screening and referral procedures focused on suicide prevention across all service lines within the VA health care system, including in VA homeless services.[33,34] Veterans served across VA homeless programs, whether they are in supported housing or not, are regularly screened for suicide risk and referred for intervention when warranted. Targeted training and strategies to synergize VA homeless and suicide prevention activities have been undertaken.[35]

These study findings should be interpreted taking several limitations into consideration. First, data were limited to those available in the 3 linked administrative databases accessed for the study. Second, some individuals were excluded from the study sample because of missing data on background characteristics, and this may have resulted in selection bias. Third, although propensity score matching was applied, unmeasured differences in background characteristics between cohorts may have influenced the results of Cox regression analyses. Fourth, the temporal sequence of events in the study cannot be definitively ascertained because retrospective data from electronic health records were used. Finally, analyses were based on propensity-score matched groups of relatively small samples of veterans and, as such, replication and generalizability of study findings to all HUD–VASH veterans need further evaluation.

In conclusion, veterans who entered HUD–VASH housing had a significantly higher risk of all-cause mortality at 24-month follow-up than a matched comparison group of veterans experiencing homelessness, and HUD–VASH veterans showed consistently higher risk of overdose mortality at each time point throughout the 24 months. Further research is needed to examine how to mitigate this long-term risk while maximizing the potential benefits of supported housing.[15–17] These analyses were also limited by having no prehousing observation period, the use of administrative VA data, and the lack of data about case manager support; as such, more rigorous studies are needed. Nonetheless, the study findings indicate that greater clinical attention is needed for long-term supported housing clients, and there is a need for substance use treatment and overdose prevention interventions during critical time periods after individuals move into supported housing. AJPH

ABOUT THE AUTHORS

Jack Tsai and Hind Beydoun are affiliated with the Homeless Programs Office in the US Department of Veterans Affairs, Washington, DC, and with the School of Public Health at the University of Texas Health Science Center at Houston. T. Peltzman is affiliated with the US Department of Veterans Affairs, White River Junction Health Care System, White River Junction, VT.

CORRESPONDENCE

Correspondence should be sent to Jack Tsai, PhD, 810 Vermont Ave NW, Washington, DC 20420 (e-mail: jack.tsai2@va.gov). Reprints can be ordered at https://www.ajph.org by clicking the "Reprints" link.

PUBLICATION INFORMATION

Full Citation: Tsai J, Peltzman T, Beydoun HA. Changes in all-cause, overdose, and suicide mortality risk in the first 2 years of supported housing, United States, 2017–2021. *Am J Public Health*. 2026;116(5):665–673.

Acceptance Date: October 10, 2025.

DOI: https://doi.org/10.2105/AJPH.2025.308371

ORCID iD:

Jack Tsai https://orcid.org/0000-0002-0329-648X

CONTRIBUTORS

J. Tsai conceptualized the study and wrote the article. H. Beydoun led data analyses and helped write the article. T. Peltzman provided consultation on data analyses and helped write the article.

ACKNOWLEDGMENTS

This work was supported with in-kind support from the US Department of Veterans Affairs (VA) Homeless Programs Office.

We thank the VA Homeless Programs Office and Office of Mental Health and Suicide Prevention for their support of this study. The VA/Department of Defense Mortality Data Repository data were provided by the VA Office of Mental Health and Suicide Prevention; more information can be found here: https://www.mirecc.va.gov/suicideprevention/documents/VA_DoD-MDR_Flyer.pdf.

The data dictionary and statistical/analytic code can be made available from the lead author upon reasonable request.

Note. The views expressed in this article are those of the authors and do not reflect the official policy of the VA.

CONFLICTS OF INTEREST

None of the authors report any conflicts of interest with this work.

HUMAN PARTICIPANT PROTECTION

This project was conducted under the auspices of VA's Homeless Programs Office for quality improvement purposes and was exempt from the institutional review board.

REFERENCES

1. Aldridge RW, Menezes D, Lewer D, et al. Causes of death among homeless people: a population-based cross-sectional study of linked hospitalisation and mortality data in England. *Wellcome Open Res*. 2019;4:49. https://doi.org/10.12688/wellcomeopenres.15151.1
2. Courtepatte A, Dugan E, Pino EC. Differences in risks for recurrent injury and death among survivors of violence by homeless status. *J Urban Health*. 2023;100(5):972–983. https://doi.org/10.1007/s11524-023-00781-4
3. Hessol NA, Eng M, Vu A, Pipkin S, Hsu LC, Scheer S. A longitudinal study assessing differences in causes of death among housed and homeless people diagnosed with HIV in San Francisco. *BMC Public Health*. 2019;19(1):1440. https://doi.org/10.1186/s12889-019-7817-7
4. Slockers MT, Nusselder WJ, Rietjens J, van Beeck EF. Unnatural death: a major but largely preventable cause-of-death among homeless people? *Eur J Public Health*. 2018;28(2):248–252. https://doi.org/10.1093/eurpub/cky002
5. Booth RG, Shariff SZ, Carter B, et al. Opioid-related overdose deaths among people experiencing homelessness, 2017 to 2021: a population-based analysis using coroner and health administrative data from Ontario, Canada. *Addiction*. 2024;119(2):334–344. https://doi.org/10.1111/add.16357
6. Lowrie R, McPherson A, Mair FS, et al. Baseline characteristics of people experiencing homelessness with a recent drug overdose in the PHOENIx pilot randomised controlled trial. *Harm Reduct J*. 2023;20(1):46. https://doi.org/10.1186/s12954-023-00771-4
7. Henkind R, Carmichael H, Stearns DR, et al. Suicide among persons experiencing homelessness. *J Surg Res*. 2023;284:213–220. https://doi.org/10.1016/j.jss.2022.10.060
8. Kleinman RA, Morris NP. Suicide, homicide, and other violent deaths among people experiencing homelessness in the United States: a cross-sectional study. *Public Health Rep*. 2023;138(2):309–314. https://doi.org/10.1177/00333549221087228
9. Slesnick N, Brakenhoff B, Chavez LJ, et al. Suicide prevention for substance using youth experiencing homelessness: study protocol for a randomized controlled trial. *Trials*. 2024;25(1):174. https://doi.org/10.1186/s13063-024-07997-y
10. Tsai J. Is the Housing First model effective? Different evidence for different outcomes. *Am J Public Health*. 2020;110(9):1376–1377. https://doi.org/10.2105/AJPH.2020.305835
11. Baxter AJ, Tweed EJ, Katikireddi SV, Thomson H. Effects of Housing First approaches on health and well-being of adults who are homeless or at risk of homelessness: systematic review and meta-analysis of randomised controlled trials. *J Epidemiol Community Health*. 2019;73(5):379–387. https://doi.org/10.1136/jech-2018-210981
12. Tinland A, Loubiere S, Cantiello M, et al. Mortality in homeless people enrolled in the French Housing First randomized controlled trial: a secondary outcome analysis of predictors and causes of death. *BMC Public Health*. 2021;21(1):1294. https://doi.org/10.1186/s12889-021-11310-w
13. Henwood BF, Byrne T, Scriber B. Examining mortality among formerly homeless adults enrolled in Housing First: an observational study. *BMC Public Health*. 2015;15:1209. https://doi.org/10.1186/s12889-015-2552-1
14. Parpouchi M, Moniruzzaman A, Rezansoff SN, Russolillo A, Somers JM. The effect of Housing First on adherence to methadone maintenance treatment. *Int J Drug Policy*. 2018;56:73–80. https://doi.org/10.1016/j.drugpo.2018.03.012
15. Taylor LA. Housing and health: an overview of the literature. *Health Affairs Health Policy Brief*.

June 7, 2018. Available at: https://www.healthaffairs.org/content/briefs/housing-and-health-overview-literature. Accessed January 20, 2026.

16. Krieger J, Higgins DL. Housing and health: time again for public health action. *Am J Public Health.* 2002;92(5):758–768. https://doi.org/10.2105/ajph.92.5.758
17. Gibson M, Petticrew M, Bambra C, Sowden AJ, Wright KE, Whitehead M. Housing and health inequalities: a synthesis of systematic reviews of interventions aimed at different pathways linking housing and health. *Health Place.* 2011;17(1):175–184. https://doi.org/10.1016/j.healthplace.2010.09.011
18. Cusack M, Montgomery AE. Barriers and facilitators to housing access and maintenance in HUD-VASH: participant and staff perspectives. *Soc Work Health Care.* 2018;57(6):422–439. https://doi.org/10.1080/00981389.2018.1441213
19. Kertesz SG, Austin EL, Holmes SK, DeRussy AJ, Van Deusen Lukas C, Pollio DE. Housing First on a large scale: fidelity strengths and challenges in the VA's HUD-VASH program. *Psychol Serv.* 2017;14(2):118–128. https://doi.org/10.1037/ser0000123
20. Montgomery AE, Cusack M, Szymkowiak D, Fargo J, O'Toole T. Factors contributing to eviction from permanent supportive housing: lessons from HUD-VASH. *Eval Program Plan.* 2017;61:55–63. https://doi.org/10.1016/j.evalprogplan.2016.11.014
21. US Department of Veterans Affairs. Using data to prevent veteran mortality. 2017. Available at: https://www.mirecc.va.gov/suicideprevention/documents/VA_DoD-MDR_Flyer.pdf. Accessed June 5, 2025.
22. Hoffmire CA, Schneider AL, Gaeddert LA, et al. Harnessing national data systems to understand circumstances surrounding veteran suicide: linking Department of Veterans Affairs and National Violent Death Reporting System Data. *Inj Epidemiol.* 2025;12(1):6. https://doi.org/10.1186/s40621-024-00559-5
23. Tsai J, Szymkowiak D, Jutkowitz E. Developing an operational definition of housing instability and homelessness in Veterans Health Administration's medical records. *PLoS One.* 2022;17(12):e0279973. https://doi.org/10.1371/journal.pone.0279973
24. Lanza ST, Moore JE, Butera NM. Drawing causal inferences using propensity scores: a practical guide for community psychologists. *Am J Community Psychol.* 2013;52(3-4):380–392. https://doi.org/10.1007/s10464-013-9604-4
25. Sundararajan V, Henderson T, Perry C, Muggivan A, Quan H, Ghali WA. New *ICD-10* version of the Charlson comorbidity index predicted in-hospital mortality. *J Clin Epidemiol.* 2004;57(12):1288–1294. https://doi.org/10.1016/j.jclinepi.2004.03.012
26. Beydoun HA, Szymkowiak D, Kinney R, Beydoun MA, Zonderman AB, Tsai J. Is the risk of Alzheimer's disease and related dementias among US veterans influenced by the intersectionality of housing status, HIV/AIDS, hepatitis C, and psychiatric disorders? *J Gerontol A Biol Sci Med Sci.* 2024;79(8):glae153. https://doi.org/10.1093/gerona/glae153
27. US Department of Veterans Affairs. 2023 National Veteran Suicide Prevention Annual Report. 2023. Available at: https://www.mentalhealth.va.gov/docs/data-sheets/2023/2023-National-Veteran-Suicide-Prevention-Annual-Report-FINAL-508.pdf. Accessed June 5, 2025.
28. Williamson EJ, Forbes A. Introduction to propensity scores. *Respirology.* 2014;19(5):625–635. https://doi.org/10.1111/resp.12312
29. Tsai J, Kasprow WJ, Rosenheck RA. Alcohol and drug use disorders among homeless veterans: prevalence and association with supported housing outcomes. *Addict Behav.* 2014;39(2):455–460. https://doi.org/10.1016/j.addbeh.2013.02.002
30. Fazel S, Khosla V, Doll H, Geddes J. The prevalence of mental disorders among the homeless in Western countries: systematic review and meta-regression analysis. *PLoS Med.* 2008;5(12):e225. https://doi.org/10.1371/journal.pmed.0050225
31. Cano M, Oh S. State-level homelessness and drug overdose mortality: evidence from US panel data. *Drug Alcohol Depend.* 2023;250:110910. https://doi.org/10.1016/j.drugalcdep.2023.110910
32. Yamamoto A, Needleman J, Gelberg L, Kominski G, Shoptaw S, Tsugawa Y. Association between homelessness and opioid overdose and opioid-related hospital admissions/emergency department visits. *Soc Sci Med.* 2019;242:112585. https://doi.org/10.1016/j.socscimed.2019.112585
33. Tsai J, Trevisan L, Huang M, Pietrzak RH. Addressing veteran homelessness to prevent veteran suicides. *Psychiatr Serv.* 2018;69(8):935–937. https://doi.org/10.1176/appi.ps.201700482
34. Holliday R, Hostetter T, Brenner LA, Bahraini N, Tsai J. Suicide risk screening and evaluation among patients accessing VHA services and identified as being newly homeless. *Health Serv Res.* 2024;59(5):e14301. https://doi.org/10.1111/1475-6773.14301
35. Tsai J, Cao X. Association between suicide attempts and homelessness in a population-based sample of US veterans and non-veterans. *J Epidemiol Community Health.* 2019;73(4):346–352. https://doi.org/10.1136/jech-2018-211065

Reasons for Choosing Telehealth Abortion Based on Food Insecurity Status: United States, 2021–2022

Courtney E. Williams, PhD, MPH, Andréa Becker, PhD, Leah R. Koenig, PhD, MSPH, Lisa Peters, MPH, and Ushma D. Upadhyay, PhD, MPH

Objectives. To determine differences in reasons for choosing telehealth abortion based on food insecurity status.

Methods. We analyzed data from the California Home Abortion by Telehealth (CHAT) Study, which included survey responses from patients who received medication abortion care between 2021 and 2022 from 1 of 3 virtual US clinics. Based on responses from 1726 survey participants, we used multivariable logistic regression to analyze differences in reported reasons for choosing telehealth abortion among individuals who experienced food insecurity versus those who did not.

Results. Compared with individuals in food-secure households, individuals who experienced food insecurity were more likely to choose telehealth abortion because of cost, challenges in finding transportation, challenges in finding child or dependent care, and concerns related to fear, judgment, and discrimination regarding care at an in-person clinic.

Conclusions. When seeking an abortion, individuals in food-insecure households consider many factors relevant to their abortion care preferences and reproductive health. Telehealth abortion, with its lower cost, may be particularly appealing to individuals who experience economic constraints. (*Am J Public Health*. 2026;116(5):674–682. https://doi.org/10.2105/AJPH.2025.308372)

AJPH May 2026, Vol. 116, No. 5

Abortion is an essential form of health care, and access to this service is paramount to ensuring reproductive justice. Yet even before the *Dobbs v Jackson Women's Health Org*. (No. 19-1392, slip op. at 5; US June 24, 2022) Supreme Court decision allowed states to completely ban abortion, people seeking an abortion in the United States combated economic barriers to accessing care. Costs are recognized as the greatest barrier to abortion care[1,2] and can severely restrict access to reproductive services. Individuals who seek an abortion also confront other economic hardships that exacerbate the challenge of paying for the service. For instance, an individual seeking an abortion who lives far from their nearest provider may incur exorbitant costs because of travel or dependent care.[3] Across the economic spectrum, people who seek an abortion describe these ancillary health expenses as hardships,[3] but abortion access may be even more challenging for individuals navigating economic adversity.[1]

Food insecurity is an indicator of economic hardship. Individuals who experience food insecurity face arduous economic constraints, are more likely to live in lower-income households,[4] and may forgo meals because of insufficient economic means.[5] Defined as "limited or uncertain availability of nutritionally adequate and safe foods,"[6(p1598)] food insecurity affected 10.2% of US households in 2021, increasing to 12.8% of households in 2022.[7] With respect to food insecurity and reproductive health care, research from 2018 related to economic hardship and abortion expenses in Texas[1] shows that 17% of patients in low-income positions delayed purchasing groceries to pay for their abortion service. Because people seeking clinician-provided abortions are disproportionately of low income[8] and consequently are more likely to experience food insecurity,[4] knowing more about reproductive decision-making among individuals in food-insecure households can illuminate economic disparities in abortion access.

Telehealth abortion can increase abortion access by delivering medication through the mail, providing preabortion counseling, and offering follow-up services.[9,10] Notwithstanding potential drawbacks of telehealth abortion for individuals who prefer in-person care,[11] telehealth abortion is patient-centered and as safe and effective as in-person care.[9,12] Increasingly utilized by people seeking an abortion, telehealth abortions accounted for 1 in 4 abortions by the end of 2024.[13] Although data from 2021 to 2022 suggest that a considerable proportion of people seeking clinician-provided abortions are low income or living below the federal poverty level,[8] the limited literature on people seeking abortion via telehealth before the *Dobbs* decision indicates that most had more than a high school education.[14] However, data from after the *Dobbs* decision show that telehealth provision is higher in counties with higher rates of poverty.[15]

When making decisions about their care, individuals seeking a telehealth abortion consider a multitude of factors. Several studies document that, alongside comfort, privacy, and convenience, the lower cost of telehealth abortion is a top reason for choosing the service.[11,14,16,17] These findings suggest that the economic aspects of telehealth services are critical for many people looking for an abortion. Thus, in our analysis, we sought to understand whether reasons for choosing telehealth abortion differed between patients in food-secure and those in food-insecure households.

Using food insecurity status as a measure of economic standing and a proxy for income level, we hypothesized that we would see significant differences in reasons for choosing a telehealth abortion based on food insecurity status. Relative to individuals in food-secure households, people who experience food insecurity will be more likely to choose a telehealth abortion because of cost and cost-related reasons (e.g., travel). Structural inequities can also contribute to distinct health care experiences[18]; therefore, compared to individuals in food-secure households, people who experience food insecurity will also be more likely to choose a telehealth abortion.

Our study fills a notable gap in public health research. By focusing on telehealth abortion—an underresearched topic in abortion scholarship—we extend conversations related to telemedicine, reproductive health care, and abortion access to new domains. Notwithstanding previous scholarship that documents myriad patient-reported benefits of a telehealth abortion,[11] it is unclear whether specific subgroups (i.e., people seeking a telehealth abortion who also experience food insecurity) prefer telehealth for distinct reasons. Considering increased utilization of telehealth abortion[13] and the millions of US households experiencing food insecurity,[7] more research on reasons for choosing telehealth abortion, and importantly differences in those reasons based on social characteristics (i.e., economic position), is needed. Given the dearth of empirical work in this field of scholarship, our study addresses a notable shortcoming in the public health literature, refines the understanding of economic disparities in health care, and expands knowledge on reproductive decision-making.

Increasingly restrictive abortion policies in the United States further substantiate the relevance of our study. In a post-*Dobbs* landscape, people who seek an abortion encounter high prices for medication abortion via in-person care[19] and lengthy travel times to brick-and-mortar abortion facilities.[20,21] Policies such as the Hyde Amendment (1976) prohibit federal funding of abortions via Medicaid except in extreme cases. Because a considerable portion of Medicaid enrollees experience food insecurity,[22] the Hyde Amendment exacerbates economic inequities in abortion access and threatens reproductive justice.[23] Amid a contentious US political climate that continues to expand abortion bans, our work elucidates important variation across food insecurity status in telehealth abortion preferences and reproductive decision-making.

METHODS

We used data from the California Home Abortion by Telehealth (CHAT) Study—a longitudinal analysis of the safety, effectiveness, and acceptability of telehealth abortion care from 3 virtual clinics in the United States (i.e., Abortion on Demand, Choix, and Hey Jane). The clinics offered fully remote medication abortion care to patients as either synchronous or asynchronous services. The price of services from the clinics ranged from $199 to $289. The median price for an in-person medication abortion was $568 in 2021.[19] Between April 2021 and January 2022, the CHAT Study collected electronic medical record data from all abortions provided by the participating facilities. Alongside electronic medical record data, patients were invited to complete 3 surveys at varying time intervals. In the first survey, administered at the time of abortion intake, survey participants were asked about initial reasons for choosing telehealth abortion and sociodemographic characteristics. Data in our study came from electronic medical records and the first survey. Our analytic sample included the 1726 participants with no missing data on our key study measures.

Measures

Our outcomes of interest included participants' reasons for choosing telehealth abortion. Participants were asked, "Please tell us some of the reasons you wanted an abortion where your abortion pills were sent to you through the mail instead of going to a clinic?" The research team developed a closed-ended list of 15 reasons for choosing a telehealth abortion. The list included 9 reasons that were guided by early empirical work on telehealth abortion[14] and 6 de novo items. Participants could select all the reasons that applied to their decision or "other" reasons. For further explanation, participants could also provide an open-ended response. If a participant's open-ended response aligned with 1 or more of the 15 closed-ended responses, it was recoded where appropriate. Otherwise, the open-ended response was recoded as "other" reason. Specifically, 4 open-ended responses were recoded as "I want to have my abortion as soon as possible," 4 open-ended responses were recoded as "other," and 1 open-ended response was recoded as "Couldn't take time off school or work." Two open-ended responses included multiple reasons and were recoded as appropriate.

Our primary independent variable was food insecurity status. Asking about income in survey research may lead to unreliable data because of factors such as sensitivity, recall, and inaccurate reporting.[24,25] Additionally, adolescents may not be aware of their family income. Hence participants were not asked to report their income level; rather, we assessed food insecurity status. The Household Food Security Survey is a validated survey assessment commonly used to screen for food insecurity status, but the complexity of the 18-item survey can restrict wide routine use.[26,27] To enhance efficiency and minimize respondent burden, the Hunger Vital Sign, a 2-item screening tool that draws from the Household Food Security Survey, was developed in 2010.[28] With high sensitivity (97%) and high specificity (83%), the Hunger Vital Sign identifies food-secure people using 2 questions and a 12-month recall period.[28] A study using the 2-item Hunger Vital Sign survey and a 30-day recall period also revealed high sensitivity at 93%.[27]

Like Makelarski et al.[27] we asked participants 2 questions and used a 1-month recall period. We asked participants first about the extent to which they were worried whether food purchased in the past month would run out before they had money to buy more and then whether the food purchased in the past month did not last and whether they did not have enough money to buy any more. For both questions, participants selected from 4 categorical responses: never, sometimes, often, or prefer not to answer. Following previous work,[29] we categorized participants as food-insecure if they responded "sometimes" or "often" to either question or food-secure if they responded "never" to both questions. We removed participants with missing responses or who responded "prefer not to answer" to either food insecurity question from the analysis (n = 53; 3% of the starting sample).

Because research documents relatively younger and multiracial people as more likely to utilize telehealth abortion services,[30] we adjusted for age, race, and ethnicity. We developed categorical measures for age at the time of the telehealth abortion (i.e., younger than 25 years, 25–29 years, 30–34 years, older than 34 years, and unknown age) using data from the electronic medical records. CHAT participants were also asked to self-report their race and ethnicity. The question included 5 response categories pertaining to racialized groups (i.e., Asian, Native Hawaiian, or Pacific Islander; Black or African American; American Indian or Alaska Native; Middle Eastern or North African; and White), 1 category for an ethnic group (Hispanic or Latinx/a/o), and a category for "other" race. Because of small sample sizes, we combined American Indian or Alaska Native with Middle Eastern or North African. Participants could select all racial and ethnic groups that applied. If participants selected 1 or more racial groups or included multiple racial groups in an open-ended response, we recoded them as "multiracial." We recoded participants who selected "prefer not to answer" or "don't know" or were missing data on race and ethnicity as "unknown." Following Hummer,[31] hereafter we refer to our categorical measure of race and ethnicity as ethnoracial.

Statistical Analysis

In our statistical analysis, we first described the characteristics of the entire analytic sample, both overall and stratified by food insecurity status. We then conducted difference-in-proportions tests to examine whether there were significant differences in sociodemographic characteristics and reasons for choosing a telehealth abortion among individuals who were categorized as food-insecure or food-secure. Next, we used multivariable logistic regression to assess the odds of a reason for choosing telehealth abortion. Each model adjusted for age at the time of the telehealth abortion and ethnoracial identity. We set the α level for all statistical tests at $P<.05$. We used Stata version 18.0 (StataCorp LP, College Station, TX) to conduct our statistical analyses.

RESULTS

Descriptive statistics are shown in Table 1. In all, 69% of the sample experienced food security, whereas 31% experienced food insecurity. Regarding the total study population, 52% of participants were racialized as White, 14% as multiracial, and 9% as Black; 13% identified ethnically as Hispanic or Latinx/a/o. Less than 10% of participants self-reported their ethnoracial identity as Asian, Native Hawaiian, or Pacific Islander (6%) and American Indian or Alaska Native or Middle Eastern or North African (1%). More than one fourth (26%) of participants were younger than 25 years, 24% were aged 25 to 29 years, 23% were between 30 and 34 years, and 19% were older than 34 years. Older participants and those who self-identified as Asian, Native Hawaiian, or Pacific Islander had a higher proportion in the food-secure category. Younger participants and those who self-identified as Hispanic or Latinx/a/o had a higher proportion in the food-insecure category.

Reasons for choosing telehealth abortion are reported in Table 2. In the overall sample, the most frequently reported reasons included being more comfortable at home (76%), wanting a more private and confidential abortion (59%), and finding telehealth less costly (57%). Notably, reasons for choosing telehealth abortion also varied by food insecurity status. Relative to their counterparts in food-secure households, respondents who experienced food insecurity reported higher proportions of choosing telehealth abortion because it was less costly (62% vs 54%; 95% confidence interval [CI] = 2.9%, 12.9%), they were worried about judgment or discrimination at a clinic (42% vs 34%; 95% CI = 2.5%, 12.5%), they were afraid of what would happen at the clinic (24% vs 16%; 95% CI = 4.2%, 12.6%), they did not have child or dependent care (17% vs 14%; 95% CI = 0.11%, 7.63%), or they lived a long-distance from the clinic or lacked transportation (11% vs 7%; 95% CI = 1.4%, 7.5%).

Conversely, individuals in food-insecure circumstances reported a relatively lower proportion of choosing telehealth

TABLE 1— Sample Size and Percentage Distribution by Participant Characteristics: California Home Abortion by Telehealth Study, 2021–2022

Sociodemographic Characteristics	Total Participants (n = 1726), No. (%)	Food Secure (n = 1193; 69%), No. (%)	Food Insecure (n = 533; 31%), No. (%)	95% CI[a]
Ethnoracial identity				
Asian, Native Hawaiian, or Pacific Islander	112 (6)	89 (7)	23 (4)	(0.86, 5.42)
Black or African American	153 (9)	107 (9)	46 (9)	(−2.54, 3.22)
Hispanic or Latinx/a/o	229 (13)	137 (11)	92 (17)	(2.09, 9.46)
American Indian or Alaska Native, Middle Eastern or North African	24 (1)	19 (2)	5 (1)	(−0.43, 1.74)
White	900 (52)	633 (53)	267 (50)	(−2.14, 8.07)
Multiracial	236 (14)	157 (13)	79 (15)	(−5.23, 1.91)
Unknown	72 (4)	51 (4)	21 (4)	(−1.68, 2.35)
Patient age at abortion intake,[b] y				
< 25	445 (26)	266 (22)	179 (34)	(6.63,15.94)
25–29	414 (24)	292 (24)	122 (23)	(−2.73, 5.91)
30–34	406 (23)	294 (25)	112 (21)	(−0.61, 7.87)
> 34	326 (19)	247 (21)	79 (15)	(2.09, 9.68)
Unknown	135 (8)	94 (8)	41 (8)	(−2.54, 2.92)

Note. CI = confidence interval.
[a]We drew 95% CIs from difference-in-proportions tests, comparing individuals in the food-secure group to individuals in the food-insecure group. For 95% CIs that do not cross zero, $P<.05$.
[b]Age is from electronic medical records (EMRs). EMR data were missing for 135 patients.

TABLE 2— Sample Size and Percentage Distribution by Participants' Reasons for Choosing Telehealth Abortion and Food Insecurity Status: California Home by Telehealth Abortion Study, 2021–2022

Reasons for Choosing Telehealth Abortion	Total Participants (n = 1726), No. (%)	Food Secure (n = 1193; 69%), No. (%)	Food Insecure (n = 533; 31%), No. (%)	95% CI[a]
More comfortable at home	1309 (76)	918 (77)	391 (73)	(−0.86, 8.04)
Wanted more private and confidential abortion	1022 (59)	709 (59)	313 (59)	(−5.73, 4.32)
Less costly	978 (57)	647 (54)	331 (62)	(2.87, 12.86)
I want to have my abortion as soon as possible and I'm concerned going to a clinic may add time	949 (55)	678 (57)	271 (51)	(1.10, 11.30)
Rather take care of own treatment	764 (44)	553 (46)	211 (40)	(1.74, 11.79)
Could not take time off school or work	651 (38)	458 (38)	193 (36)	(−7.02, 2.83)
Worried I'd be judged or discriminated against at a clinic	633 (37)	410 (34)	223 (42)	(2.49, 12.45)
I didn't want to see any clinic protesters	549 (32)	367 (31)	182 (34)	(−1.42, 8.19)
Liked the mission	535 (31)	375 (31)	160 (30)	(−3.28, 6.11)
Afraid of what happens at clinic	328 (19)	196 (16)	132 (24)	(4.20, 12.64)
Didn't have child or dependent care	255 (15)	162 (14)	93 (17)	(0.11, 7.63)
I didn't want tests	209 (12)	140 (12)	69 (13)	(−2.17, 4.60)
COVID-19 and other infection concerns	184 (11)	119 (10)	65 (12)	(−1.00, 5.48)
Distance or lack of transportation	141 (8)	81 (7)	60 (11)	(1.43, 7.51)
Didn't know where to go	83 (5)	57 (5)	26 (5)	(−2.30, 2.09)
Other	20 (1)	12 (1)	8 (2)	(−0.68, 1.67)

Note. CI = confidence interval.
[a]We drew 95% CIs from difference-in-proportions tests, comparing individuals in the food-secure group to individuals in the food-insecure group. For 95% CIs that do not cross zero, $P < .05$.

abortion because they were concerned that going to a clinic might add time (51% vs 57%; 95% CI = 1.1%, 11.3%) or they would rather take care of their own treatment (40% vs 46%; 95% CI = 1.7%, 11.8%). We found similar results in our multivariable logistic regression models in which we predicted the adjusted odds of choosing telehealth abortion by food insecurity status, controlling for potential confounders (Figure 1).

DISCUSSION

In this study, we drew on survey data collected in a pre-*Dobbs* context to show how reasons for choosing telehealth abortion varied between individuals who experienced food security versus those who experienced food insecurity. Our findings reveal significant differences across economic position, suggesting that individuals who experience food insecurity have distinct abortion preferences and likely engage in unique decision-making processes when making choices about their reproductive health care.

As expected, we found that individuals who experienced food insecurity were more likely to choose telehealth abortion because the option was less costly. We show that the lower cost of telehealth abortion is preferable for individuals who experience economic constraints. Offering telehealth to patients at no cost would make abortion more economically feasible. Indeed, some telehealth providers are offering abortion care to people in states with abortion restrictions for as little as $5.[32] Differences in cost-related reasons were also present. Relative to their food-secure counterparts, food-insecure individuals had a higher likelihood of choosing telehealth abortion because they were unable to travel to a clinic owing to distance, lacking transportation, or not having dependent care. Aligned with existing knowledge that out-of-state travel is often impossible for low-income individuals and other historically marginalized people seeking an abortion,[21] we found that individuals who experience food insecurity may prefer telehealth because it mitigates, or at best eliminates, economic constraints related to ancillary abortion costs.

Our analysis also presents novel insights into differences in reasons for choosing a telehealth abortion because of concerns about judgment and discrimination at an in-person clinic, fear, timing, and a desire to take care of

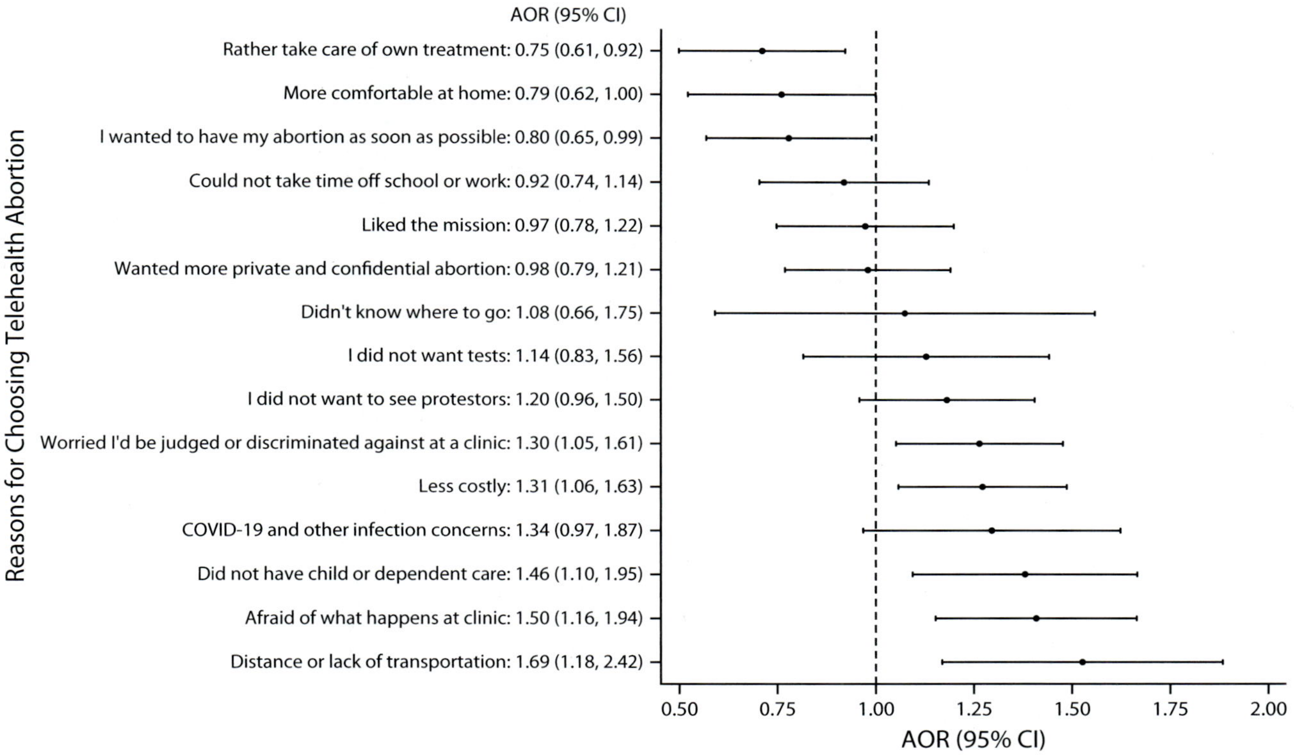

FIGURE 1— Associations Between Participants' Food Insecurity Status and Reasons for Choosing Telehealth Abortion: California Home Abortion by Telehealth (CHAT) Study, 2021–2022

Note. AOR = adjusted odds ratio; CI = confidence interval. Sample size was n = 1726. AOR > 1 indicates higher odds among participants in food-insecure households relative to participants in food-secure households. AOR < 1 indicates lower odds among participants in food-insecure households relative to participants in food-secure households. We excluded "other" reasons from the multivariable logistic regression models because of data limitations. The model adjusts for age at time of telehealth abortion and ethnoracial identity.

one's own treatment. Compared with their counterparts, individuals who experienced food insecurity were more likely to pursue telehealth abortion because this service kept them away from a brick-and-mortar clinic—an environment where they anticipated encountering judgment or discrimination. Relatedly, people from food-insecure households were more worried about what happens at a clinic, leading them to utilize telehealth abortion. Factors such as low-income stigma[18] may be salient deterrents to in-person abortion care for individuals in food-insecure households. When navigating the abortion care landscape, members of historically marginalized groups are likely acutely aware of discriminatory patterns in health care settings and may turn to alternative abortion care options, such as telehealth, to circumvent exposure to stigmatization.

The fact that individuals from food-insecure households were less likely to choose telehealth abortion for its promptness suggests that timing is a lower priority for individuals in this economic position. If people with lower incomes are likely to confront logistical hardships when seeking an abortion,[33] having fewer economic resources to cover abortion costs could also mean that logistical setbacks precluded people in food-insecure households from receiving an earlier abortion. Assuming members of food-insecure households anticipated logistical battles, these individuals may have wanted an abortion sooner but considered timeliness a trivial facet of telehealth abortion if concurrently preparing to combat other, more pressing needs. Although beyond the scope of this analysis, understanding cognitive schemas among individuals who experience food insecurity when pursuing telehealth services is an important next step for abortion scholarship.

Additional research is also needed to unravel our significant finding related to patient-led care. People in food-insecure households were less likely to pursue a telehealth abortion because this service provided opportunities to care for their own treatment—a reason possibly tethered to agentic beliefs.

Irrespective of economic constraints or type of abortion care, the ability to manage one's health care is essential. Yet many individuals in food-insecure circumstances are combating structural factors (i.e., unaffordable housing).[34] If months of food insecurity are coupled with structural obstacles that are perceived as uncontrollable, someone wanting a telehealth abortion might minimize their capacity for self-determination. Because acute attention has been given to telehealth abortion preferences, especially aspects of timing and agency, we draw attention to the novelty of our findings. We encourage researchers to expand on our study by using methodological approaches, such as qualitative analyses, that are well suited to exploring these complexities.

Although our study focused on variation in reasons for choosing a telehealth abortion, our findings have implications for research on telehealth abortion more broadly. Consistent with previous scholarship,[11,14,16,17] we lend empirical muscle by also showing comfort, privacy, confidentiality, and cost as top reasons for choosing a telehealth abortion—regardless of food insecurity status. Consider that more than 50% of individuals in food-secure households in our study utilized telehealth because of its lower cost. People experiencing food insecurity likely garner the greatest economic benefit from telehealth abortion, but we suggest that telehealth's affordability is attractive to a large swath of individuals. Increasing access to this highly desired form of care by reducing telehealth abortion costs would advance reproductive autonomy for people across the economic spectrum.

Limitations

Our findings should be considered alongside limitations. First, reasons for choosing a telehealth abortion may be shaped by previous exposure to discourse surrounding medication abortion or familiarity with receiving medication through the mail. Because of data limitations, we were unable to incorporate these potential confounders into our analyses. Second, we were unable to ascertain whether the lower price of telehealth abortion appeals to individuals who, in any other circumstance, would prefer an in-person abortion. Third, we recognize that the privileges associated with being in a food-secure position may vary by ethnoracial identity. However, given limited sample sizes in certain ethnoracial groups and subsequent statistical power issues, we were unable to estimate statistically meaningful interactions between ethnoracial identity and food insecurity status. Because experiences with classism are tethered to experiences of racism,[25] more research is required to understand the intersecting systems of oppression that reduce options for reproductive care.

Conclusions

Despite these limitations, our study provides new insights into economic inequities in abortion access and should be considered alongside policy implications. The Hyde Amendment is a restrictive federal policy that, in most states, curbs reproductive autonomy by leaving individuals with Medicaid without comprehensive coverage for abortion care. Approximately 23% of Medicaid enrollees are food insecure, and a considerable portion are Black, Indigenous, or other people of color, meaning mandates such as the Hyde Amendment have a disproportionate impact on people seeking an abortion from historically oppressed groups.[22,35] Repealing the Hyde Amendment is paramount for mitigating health inequity and advancing reproductive justice.

People seeking an abortion face costly prices for medication abortion via in-person care and exorbitant travel times to abortion facilities in a post-*Dobbs* landscape. Individuals in economically constrained situations prefer telehealth when striving to surmount cost-related barriers to abortion care and logistical complications. To ensure equitable access to reproductive health services, we must acknowledge the deeply entrenched economic inequalities in the United States, actively pursue efforts to uphold the fundamental tenets of reproductive justice, and strive to eliminate disparities in abortion access. AJPH

ABOUT THE AUTHORS

Courtney E. Williams is with the Population Research Center, University of Texas at Austin. Andréa Becker is with the Department of Sociology, Hunter College, City University of New York, NY. Leah R. Koenig was with Advancing New Standards in Reproductive Health (ANSIRH), Department of Obstetrics, Gynecology & Reproductive Sciences, University of California, San Francisco, and the Department of Epidemiology and Biostatistics, University of California, San Francisco at the time of this study. Lisa Peters and Ushma D. Upadhyay are with ANSIRH, Department of Obstetrics, Gynecology & Reproductive Sciences, University of California, San Francisco.

CORRESPONDENCE

Correspondence should be sent to Ushma Upadhyay, PhD, MPH, Advancing New Standards in Reproductive Health, University of California, San Francisco, 1330 Broadway, Suite 1100, Oakland, CA 94612 (e-mail: ushma.upadhyay@ucsf.edu). Reprints can be ordered at https://www.ajph.org by clicking the "Reprints" link.

PUBLICATION INFORMATION

Full Citation: Williams CE, Becker A, Koenig LR, Peters L, Upadhyay UD. Reasons for choosing telehealth abortion based on food insecurity status: United States, 2021–2022. *Am J Public Health*. 2026;116(5):674–682.

Acceptance Date: November 20, 2025.

DOI: https://doi.org/10.2105/AJPH.2025.308372

ORCID iDs:
Courtney E. Williams https://orcid.org/0000-0002-7173-8147

Andréa Becker https://orcid.org/0000-0002-7948-4276

Leah R. Koenig https://orcid.org/0000-0002-4982-8672

Lisa Peters https://orcid.org/0009-0006-5597-8876

Ushma D. Upadhyay https://orcid.org/0000-0002-2731-2157

CONTRIBUTORS

C. E. Williams conceptualized the analysis and wrote the initial draft of the article. C. E. Williams, A. Becker, L. R. Koenig, and U. D. Upadhyay interpreted the data. C. E. Williams and L. Peters analyzed the data. C. E. Williams and U. D. Upadhyay revised the article. A. Becker, L. R. Koenig, and L. Peters provided substantive input on article content. A. Becker, L. R. Koenig, and U. D. Upadhyay reviewed and contributed to drafting the article. L. R. Koenig, L. Peters, and U. D. Upadhyay contributed to data acquisition. All authors approved the final version of the article to be published.

ACKNOWLEDGMENTS

This research was supported by the BaSe Family Fund, Erik E. and Edith H. Bergstrom Foundation, Isabel Allende Foundation, Jess Jacobs, Kahle/Austin Foundation, Lisa and Douglas Goldman Fund, Preston-Werner Ventures, and a Resource Allocation Program award from the University of California, San Francisco National Center of Excellence in Women's Health. C. E. Williams was partially supported by the Eunice Kennedy Shriver National Institute of Child Health and Human Development via the Population Research Center at the University of Texas at Austin (grant P2CHD042849 and grant T32HD007081, Training Program in Population Studies). L. R. Koenig was funded in part by a training grant from the National Institute of Child Health and Human Development of the National Institutes of Health (NIH; award F31HD111277) for the duration of the study. U. D. Upadhyay's time was funded in part by the National Institute of Child Health and Human Development, NIH (grant R01HD110659).

An earlier version of this article was presented at the 2025 Annual Meeting of the American Sociological Association.

The authors appreciate contributions to data collection and management and other input and research partnership on the CHAT Study from Jennifer Ko, Karen Meckstroth, Maricela Cervantes, Ena Suseth Vallardes, Linda Shin, Kelly Song, Stephanie Sumstine-Felice, Sun Cotter, Francine Coeytaux, and Elisa Wells as well as the collective efforts of all from the University of California Global Health Institute's Center for Gender and Health Justice and California Latinas for Reproductive Justice. We thank Cindy Adam, Mark Adam, Kate Baron, Stephanie Bussmann, Leah Coplon, Lauren Dubey, Lindsay DuBois, Kiki Freedman, Gaby Izarra, Jamie Phifer, and Aisha Wagner for supporting data acquisition. We gratefully thank Christy L. Erving, Keif Godbout-Kinney, Ricardo H. Lowe, and Heather Rackin for their helpful comments, support, and detailed feedback.

Note. The funders had no role in study design, data collection and analysis, decision to publish, or preparation of the article.

CONFLICTS OF INTEREST

The authors do not have any competing interests to disclose.

HUMAN PARTICIPANT PROTECTION

The study was approved by the University of California, San Francisco institutional review board (#20-32951). All patients provided electronic consent.

REFERENCES

1. Dickman SL, White K, Sierra G, Grossman D. Financial hardships caused by out-of-pocket abortion costs in Texas, 2018. *Am J Public Health.* 2022;112(5):758–761. https://doi.org/10.2105/AJPH.2021.306701
2. Upadhyay UD, McCook AA, Bennett AH, Cartwright AF, Roberts SCM. State abortion policies and Medicaid coverage of abortion are associated with pregnancy outcomes among individuals seeking abortion recruited using Google Ads: a national cohort study. *Soc Sci Med.* 2021;274:113747. https://doi.org/10.1016/j.socscimed.2021.113747
3. Kimport K. Reducing the burdens of forced abortion travel: referrals, financial and emotional support, and opportunities for positive experiences in traveling for third-trimester abortion care. *Soc Sci Med.* 2022;293:114667. https://doi.org/10.1016/j.socscimed.2021.114667
4. Gundersen C, Ziliak JP. Food insecurity and health outcomes. *Health Aff (Millwood).* 2015;34(11):1830–1839. https://doi.org/10.1377/hlthaff.2015.0645
5. Wolfson JA, Leung CW. Food insecurity during COVID-19: an acute crisis with long-term health implications. *Am J Public Health.* 2020;110(12):1763–1765. https://doi.org/10.2105/AJPH.2020.305953
6. Anderson SA. Core indicators of nutritional state for difficult-to-sample populations. *J Nutr.* 1990;120(suppl 11):1555–1598. https://doi.org/10.1093/jn/120.suppl_11.1555
7. Reed-Jones M. Prevalence of US household food insecurity increased in 2022. October 25, 2023. Available at: https://www.ers.usda.gov/data-products/charts-of-note/chart-detail?chartId=107694. Accessed September 2, 2025.
8. Jones RK. Medicaid's role in alleviating some of the financial burden of abortion: findings from the 2021–2022 Abortion Patient Survey. *Perspect Sex Reprod Health.* 2024;56(3):244–254. https://doi.org/10.1111/psrh.12250
9. Chong E, Shochet T, Raymond E, et al. Expansion of a direct-to-patient telemedicine abortion service in the United States and experience during the COVID-19 pandemic. *Contraception.* 2021;104(1):43–48. https://doi.org/10.1016/j.contraception.2021.03.019
10. Upadhyay UD, Schroeder R, Roberts SCM. Adoption of no-test and telehealth medication abortion care among independent abortion providers in response to COVID-19. *Contracept X.* 2020;2:100049. https://doi.org/10.1016/j.conx.2020.100049
11. Koenig LR, Ko J, Valladares ES, et al. Patient acceptability of telehealth medication abortion care in the United States, 2021–2022: a cohort study. *Am J Public Health.* 2024;114(2):241–250. https://doi.org/10.2105/AJPH.2023.307437
12. Upadhyay UD, Koenig LR, Meckstroth K, Ko J, Valladares ES, Biggs MA. Effectiveness and safety of telehealth medication abortion in the USA. *Nat Med.* 2024;30(4):1191–1198. https://doi.org/10.1038/s41591-024-02834-w
13. Society of Family Planning. #WeCount report, April 2022 to December 2024. June 23, 2025. Available at: https://societyfp.org/research/wecount/wecount-december-2024-data. Accessed September 2, 2025. https://doi.org/10.46621/725961gzsnai
14. Raymond E, Chong E, Winikoff B, et al. TelAbortion: evaluation of a direct to patient telemedicine abortion service in the United States. *Contraception.* 2019;100(3):173–177. https://doi.org/10.1016/j.contraception.2019.05.013
15. Aiken ARA, Scott JG, Gomperts R. Provision of abortion medications using online asynchronous telemedicine under shield laws in the US. *JAMA.* 2025;334(15):1388–1390. https://doi.org/10.1001/jama.2025.11420
16. Aiken ARA, Starling JE, Gomperts R. Factors associated with use of an online telemedicine service to access self-managed medical abortion in the US. *JAMA Netw Open.* 2021;4(5):e2111852. https://doi.org/10.1001/jamanetworkopen.2021.11852
17. Godfrey EM, Fiastro AE, Thayer EK, Gomperts R, Orlando SM, Myers CK. No-test telehealth medication abortion services provided by US-based clinicians in 21 states and the District of Columbia, 2020–2022. *Am J Public Health.* 2025;115(2):221–231. https://doi.org/10.2105/AJPH.2024.307892
18. Ragosta S, Fix L, Forsberg H, Thompson TA. Opinions on public funding of abortion among Medicaid-eligible abortion patients in the United States. *Sex Res Soc Policy.* 2025. https://doi.org/10.1007/s13178-025-01145-0
19. Upadhyay UD, Schroeder R, Kaller S, Stewart C, Berglas NF. Pricing of medication abortion in the United States, 2021–2023. *Perspect Sex Reprod Health.* 2024;56(3):282–294. https://doi.org/10.1111/psrh.12280
20. Rader B, Upadhyay UD, Sehgal NKR, Reis BY, Brownstein JS, Hswen Y. Estimated travel time and spatial access to abortion facilities in the US before and after the Dobbs v Jackson Women's Health decision. *JAMA.* 2022;328(20):2041–2047. https://doi.org/10.1001/jama.2022.20424
21. Forouzan K, Friedrich-Karnik A, Maddow-Zimet I. The high toll of US abortion bans: nearly one in five patients now traveling out of state for abortion care. December 2023. Available at: https://www.guttmacher.org/2023/12/high-toll-us-abortion-bans-nearly-one-five-patients-now-traveling-out-state-abortion-care. Accessed September 4, 2025.
22. Hall C, Artiga S, Orgera K, Garfield R. Food insecurity and health: addressing food needs for Medicaid enrollees as part of COVID-19 response

efforts. August 14, 2020. Available at: https://www.kff.org/medicaid/food-insecurity-and-health-addressing-food-needs-for-medicaid-enrollees-as-part-of-covid-19-response-efforts. Accessed September 3, 2025.

23. Ross L, Solinger R. *Reproductive Justice: An Introduction.* Berkeley, CA: University of California Press; 2017. https://doi.org/10.1525/9780520963207

24. Prati A. Hedonic recall bias: why you should not ask people how much they earn. *J Econ Behav Organ*. 2017;143:78–97. https://doi.org/10.1016/j.jebo.2017.09.002

25. Williams DR, Collins C. US socioeconomic and racial differences in health: patterns and explanations. *Annu Rev Sociol.* 1995;21:349–386. https://doi.org/10.1146/annurev.so.21.080195.002025

26. Bickel G, Nord M, Price C, Hamilton W, Cook J. Guide to measuring household food security. Revised 2000. Available at: https://nhis.ipums.org/nhis/resources/FSGuide.pdf. Accessed January 25, 2026.

27. Makelarski JA, Abramsohn E, Benjamin JH, Du S, Lindau ST. Diagnostic accuracy of two food insecurity screeners recommended for use in health care settings. *Am J Public Health*. 2017;107(11):1812–1817. https://doi.org/10.2105/AJPH.2017.304033

28. Hager ER, Quigg AM, Black MM, et al. Development and validity of a 2-item screen to identify families at risk for food insecurity. *Pediatrics*. 2010;126(1):e26–e32. https://doi.org/10.1542/peds.2009-3146

29. Okafor M, Chiu S, Feinn R. Quantitative and qualitative results from implementation of a two-item food insecurity screening tool in healthcare settings in Connecticut. *Prev Med Rep*. 2020;20:101191. https://doi.org/10.1016/j.pmedr.2020.101191

30. Fiastro AE, Zheng Z, Ruben MR, Gipson J, Godfrey EM. Telehealth vs in-clinic medication abortion services. *JAMA Netw Open*. 2023;6(9):e2331900. https://doi.org/10.1001/jamanetworkopen.2023.31900

31. Hummer RA. Race and ethnicity, racism, and population health in the United States: the straightforward, the complex, innovations, and the future. *Demography*. 2023;60(3):633–657. https://doi.org/10.1215/00703370-10747542

32. Cambridge Reproductive Health Consultants. The MAP. 2025. Available at: https://www.cambridgereproductivehealthconsultants.org/map. Accessed November 10, 2025.

33. Foster DG, Kimport K. Who seeks abortions at or after 20 weeks? *Perspect Sex Reprod Health*. 2013;45(4):210–218. https://doi.org/10.1363/4521013 [Erratum in: *Perspect Sex Reprod Health*. 2019;51(3):185. https://doi.org/10.1363/psrh.12114]

34. Raskind IG. Hunger does discriminate: addressing structural racism and economic inequality in food insecurity research. *Am J Public Health*. 2020;110(9):1264–1265. https://doi.org/10.2105/AJPH.2020.305841

35. Pillai A, Hinton E, Rudowitz R, Artiga S. Medicaid efforts to address racial health disparities. July 1, 2024. Available at: https://www.kff.org/medicaid/issue-brief/medicaid-efforts-to-address-racial-health-disparities. Accessed March 8, 2025.

Societal Costs of Total Abortion Bans in 14 US States After *Dobbs*

Isabel S. Platt, PhD, Jennifer E. Starling, PhD, Emma Pendl-Robinson, BS, Sammie Chavez, MPH, Divya Vohra, PhD, and Kara Zivin, PhD, MS, MA, MFA

Objectives. To estimate societal costs, comprising personal and external costs, of total abortion bans in the first year of enactment for 14 states after *Dobbs* overturned the constitutional right to abortion.

Methods. We developed a model to estimate personal and external costs associated with total abortion bans in the first year after bans were enacted. We conducted a literature review to identify model inputs and included states with total abortion bans as of September 1, 2024.

Results. We estimated in the year after enacting abortion bans, 104 369 people could not access in-clinic abortion in 14 states with total abortion bans, costing $339.6 million. Specifically, travel to another state for in-clinic abortions cost $104.7 million (30.8%), pregnancies ending in miscarriage or stillbirth cost $1.7 million (0.5%), and carrying pregnancy to term cost $233.2 million (68.7%). Apart from these costs, we estimated $9.4 million in decreased costs attributable to changes in post-*Dobbs* abortion care delivery, including increased use of telemedicine.

Conclusions. Abortion bans are economically burdensome. Our findings provide compelling evidence that restoring and protecting abortion access would improve economic outcomes. (*Am J Public Health*. 2026;116(5):683–691. https://doi.org/10.2105/AJPH.2025.308411)

AJPH May 2026, Vol. 116, No. 5

On June 24, 2022, the US Supreme Court's decision in *Dobbs v Jackson Women's Health Organization* overturned *Roe v Wade*, eliminating federal constitutional protection for abortion and allowing states to ban or restrict abortion at any point in pregnancy.[1] By September 1, 2024, 14 states enacted total abortion bans: Alabama, Arkansas, Idaho, Indiana, Kentucky, Louisiana, Mississippi, Missouri, North Dakota, Oklahoma, South Dakota, Tennessee, Texas, and West Virginia.[2] Another 6 states restricted abortion at 6 or 12 weeks' gestation. Recent research estimated a 2.3% relative increase in births after *Dobbs* in states enforcing total abortion bans in early 2023, rising interstate travel for abortion, increased telemedicine medication abortion, and greater availability of medication abortion pills.[3–7] National clinician-provided abortion counts have also increased, partly because of expanded access in states where abortion remains legal.[7]

To better understand the consequences of *Dobbs*, we estimated the personal and external cost in the first year of total abortion bans for people who would have obtained in-clinic abortions in the 14 states with bans at the time of this study. We modeled the share of individuals who would (1) travel to another state for care, (2) experience miscarriage or stillbirth, (3) carry pregnancy to term, or (4) access abortion care outside the clinic setting, including telehealth under shield laws, community networks, or online vendors (Figure 1). For each pathway, we estimated the likelihood of adverse outcomes and modeled excess costs associated with these outcomes in the first year after states enacted total bans (July 2022 to June 2023 for most states; see Methods).

METHODS

We estimated the first-year cost of total abortion bans in the 14 states enforced as of September 1, 2024.[2] To provide conservative estimates, we focused on states with total bans, although 6-week and other gestational limits have also reduced access.[5,7] Our cost-of-illness model captured personal costs (borne by individuals) and external costs (borne by health care payers, employers, taxpayers, and state and federal governments), from

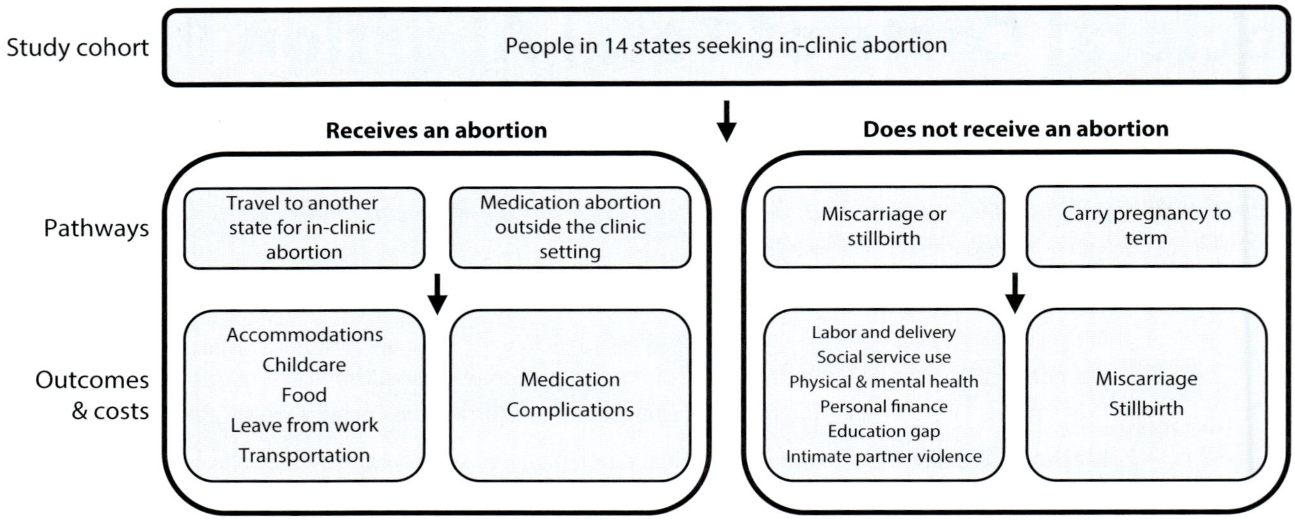

FIGURE 1— Conceptual Model of Alternative Pathways and Outcomes After a Total Abortion Ban, for People in 14 States With Bans Effective as of September 1, 2024: United States

Note. Medication abortion outside the clinic setting includes telehealth abortions conducted under shield law provision and self-managed abortions via online vendors or community networks.

conception through 1 year after pregnancy outcomes.

Literature Review

We conducted a literature review to identify impact estimates for outcomes across all pathways (Figure 1), compiled direct cost estimates, and inflation-adjusted pre-2022 figures to 2022 US dollars using the Personal Health Care price index.[8] We refined model assumptions and parameters through iterative consultation with our advisory panel (Appendix A, available as a supplement to the online version of this article at https://ajph.org), who evaluated our assumptions, methods, and findings. Full literature review methods appear in Appendix B (available as a supplement to the online version of this article at https://ajph.org).

Study Cohort

To construct our study cohort, we used published estimates from #WeCount of the average number of monthly in-clinic abortions in the 2 months preceding *Dobbs* (April and May 2022) as a baseline for the expected number of monthly in-clinic abortions in absence of a ban.[7] #WeCount accounted for selection bias among surveyed health centers, and at time of writing, represented the most recent available data.

We annualized each state's average monthly number of in-clinic abortions from the pre-*Dobbs* period to obtain our study cohort: the estimated number of people who would have received an in-clinic abortion in the year following implementation of a total abortion ban, had the ban not occurred. Although our model estimated costs over a 1-year period after the ban, the start date varied by state, depending on when each state's total ban went into effect. For example, bans became effective on June 24, 2022, in Alabama, Arkansas, Kentucky, Missouri, North Dakota, Oklahoma, and South Dakota; in July 2022 in Louisiana and Mississippi; in August 2022 in Idaho, Tennessee, and Texas; in September 2022 in West Virginia; and in June 2023 in Indiana. To avoid contamination of baseline data while reflecting abortion access trends, we used the 2 months preceding the *Dobbs* decision as the baseline period across all states, adjusted for seasonality.[9,10] We note some states had abortion restrictions in place before total ban enactment.[11]

Alternative Pathways Under a Total Abortion Ban

We modeled the share of our cohort that, under a total abortion ban, would follow 1 of 4 alternative pathways instead of receiving an in-clinic abortion in their home state (Figure 1). Appendix C (available as a supplement to the online version of this article at https://ajph.org) lists all sources used to model each pathway.

Travel out of state. We applied state-level estimates from literature on the impact of bans to model proportions of individuals by state who would travel to another state for an in-clinic abortion, after accounting for abortion outside the clinic setting.[3,5,7]

Medication abortion outside the clinic setting. We modeled the proportion of the cohort who would obtain abortion via shield law telehealth (where providers in states with legal abortion prescribe medication to patients in ban states) using recent estimated rates of telehealth abortion.[12] We used comparative rates of telehealth to self-managed medication abortion methods to estimate the proportion who would obtain abortion medication through online vendors or community networks.[3] Online vendors include e-commerce sites offering abortion pills, typically without health care provider involvement, whereas community networks (e.g., Las Libres, AccessMA) are volunteer groups that source medications internationally and provide peer support.[13]

Miscarriage or stillbirth. Our model assumed individuals who did not obtain an abortion through any pathway could not access abortion care. We applied national miscarriage and stillbirth rates to estimate the share of this group who would have had a miscarriage or stillbirth in each trimester.

Carrying pregnancy to term. Our model assumed that individuals who did not obtain an abortion and did not experience a miscarriage or stillbirth would carry their pregnancies to term.

Impact and Cost Estimates

We modeled costs associated with abortion bans for 4 pathways using estimates of the likelihood and cost of outcomes from literature, publicly available government data, and industry reports. When multiple estimates were available, we averaged the estimates, weighted by each source's sample size. We aggregated estimated costs across pathways and states to estimate the total cost associated with abortion bans in the first year after the *Dobbs* decision in ban states. We conducted analyses to explore the sensitivity of our analyses to variation in the likelihood and cost estimates.

Travel out of state. For people we estimated would travel out of state for abortion care, we modeled the incremental costs of travel to the nearest abortion clinic. We assumed travel by car, a 2-night hotel stay, and a travel companion for each person. Estimated costs included additional transportation, accommodations, childcare, time off work, and food. Transportation costs reflected increased driving distances after *Dobbs*.[5] Childcare and time-off-work costs captured extra time required beyond an in-state visit; food costs included the incremental expense of meals, likely more costly during travel. Since we assumed similar in-clinic abortion prices across states, we did not include procedure-related cost differences.

Abortion outside the clinic setting. For each type of abortion outside a clinic (telehealth, online vendors, or community networks), we included costs of abortion medication and potential treatment of complications. We estimated medication costs by averaging available price information for each of the 3 abortion types. We estimated complication costs using averages of major and minor complication rates from multiple studies, weighted based on each study's sample size. We applied corresponding treatment costs: emergency department visits for minor complications and hospital admissions for major complications. We subtracted costs associated with in-clinic abortion and expected complications, because individuals would forgo in-clinic care.

Miscarriage or stillbirth. To estimate additional costs from miscarriages and stillbirths, we multiplied per-person direct medical costs by the share of our study cohort who would have had a miscarriage or stillbirth after not obtaining an abortion. We presented conservative cost estimates because we did not include additional indirect costs (e.g., mental health services or productivity loss) because of a lack of relevant studies found in the literature. We subtracted the costs associated with in-clinic abortion and expected complications because individuals who experience a miscarriage or stillbirth would not receive an abortion.

Carrying pregnancy to term. To estimate the cost associated with carrying pregnancy to term after not obtaining an abortion, we included direct costs of labor, delivery, and expected costs of adverse outcomes. Outcomes included social service use, mental health, physical health, personal finance, reduced educational attainment, and intimate partner violence (Table 1). We used the baseline prevalence of each outcome to calculate the additional number of people who would experience each outcome after abortion denial.[11] We multiplied the incremental number of people experiencing each outcome by the cost per person and aggregated costs across all outcomes. For each person carrying their pregnancy to

TABLE 1— Estimated Cost of Abortion Bans by Pathway and Type of Cost: United States

Type of Cost	Cost in First Year After Enacting Ban, $ (% of Pathway Cost)	Average Cost Per Person, $[a]
Traveled to another state for in-clinic abortion	104.7 M	1 593
Leave from work	44.6 M (42.6)	679
Food for person and travel companion for 3 days and 2 nights	23.3 M (22.2)	354
Accommodations for 2 nights[b]	20.4 M (19.5)	310
Transportation by car	11.0 M (10.5)	167
Childcare	5.5 M (5.2)	83
Carried pregnancy to miscarriage or stillbirth	1.7 M	9 896
Miscarriage	2.2 M (80.2)	1 516
Stillbirth	0.5 M (19.8)	9 073
Forgone cost of in-clinic abortion procedure[c]	−1.0 M (−34.7)	−630
Forgone cost of in-clinic abortion complications	−0.1 M (−3.5)	−63
Carried pregnancy to term	233.2 M	25 632
Labor and delivery	165.9 M (69.3)	18 235
Social service use (SNAP, WIC, TANF, and Medicaid)[d]	32.4 M (13.5)	3 557
Personal finance (lost income and unemployment)	31.7 M (13.3)	3 487
Dropping out of college	4.3 M (1.8)	477
Mental health (anxiety, depression, tobacco use, suicidal ideation)	2.8 M (1.2)	308
Physical health (chronic pain, life-threatening complications, mortality, excluding labor and delivery)	2.1 M (0.9)	232
Intimate partner violence	29.7K (< 0.1)	3
Forgone cost of in-clinic abortion procedure	−5.5 M (−2.3)	−603
Forgone cost of in-clinic abortion complications	−0.6 M (−0.2)	−63
Decreased costs from post-*Dobbs* changes in abortion care	9.4 M	335
Medication abortion outside of clinic setting (telemedicine via shield law provision, community networks, online vendors)	6.2 M (74.9)	222
Complications from medication abortion outside of clinic setting	2.1 M (25.1)	74
Forgone cost of in-clinic abortion procedure	−5.9 M (−191.3)	−568
Forgone cost of in-clinic abortion complications	−1.8 M (−21.2)	−63

Note. K = thousand; M = million; SNAP = Supplemental Nutrition Assistance Program; TANF = Temporary Assistance for Needy Families; WIC = Special Supplemental Nutrition Program for Women, Infants, and Children. We estimated the first-year cost of total abortion bans in the 14 states enforced as of September 1, 2024.

[a]Average per-person costs account for estimated cost of each outcome and excess prevalence of people affected by each outcome. Average per-person costs may vary for the same type of cost across pathways to account for differing distribution of gestational duration within pathways. Percentage of pathway costs sum to 100% excluding forgone costs; percentages for forgone costs represent percentages of total pathway costs.

[b]Number of nights of accommodation varied by distance traveled, gestational duration, and other person-specific factors. We assumed 2 nights' accommodation for everyone to reflect time for travel and recommended recovery.

[c]We subtracted the costs associated with in-clinic abortion and expected complications because individuals would forgo in-clinic care.

[d]Increased rate of social service use for people who carried their pregnancy to term after abortion denial; does not include social service use for child.

term, we subtracted costs associated with in-clinic abortion and expected complications.

Appendices D through F (available as supplements to the online version of this article at https://ajph.org) provide a complete list of sources for baseline outcomes, impact estimates, and cost estimates. Appendices G through H (available as supplements to the online version of this article at https://ajph.org) provide additional methodological detail for our cost model and sensitivity analyses.

RESULTS

For our study cohort of 104 369 individuals, we estimated the cost of banning abortion in the first year after the abortion bans was $339.6 million, averaging $3254 per person. In addition to these costs, we estimated a decreased cost of $9.4 million attributable to changes in post-*Dobbs* abortion care delivery, such as telemedicine medication abortion under shield laws and modification of the Food and Drug Administration's Mifepristone Risk Evaluation and Mitigation Strategies program.[14] Figure 2 shows the distribution of the study cohort by pathway and associated costs.

Pathways

We estimated that 65 709 people (63.0% of the cohort) who would have obtained in-clinic abortion care would instead travel for abortion care in another state. We estimated that 28 033 people (26.9% of the cohort) would access abortion care outside the clinic, including 19 830 people (19.0% of the cohort, 70.7% of the pathway) who would use telehealth accessed under shield law provision, 6689 people (6.4% of the cohort, 23.9% of the pathway) who would access abortion care via community networks, and 1514 people (1.5% of the cohort, 5.4% of the pathway) who would purchase abortion medication through online vendors. We estimated that 1530 people (1.5% of the cohort) would have a miscarriage (1470 people; 1.4% of the cohort, 96.1% of the pathway) or stillbirth (60 people; 3.9% of the cohort, 19.8% of the pathway) after an inability to access abortion care. Finally, we estimated that 9097 people (8.7% of the cohort) would remain unable to access abortion care and carry their pregnancy to term.

Cost of Banning Abortion

Of the $339.6 million incremental cost of banning abortion in the first year after abortion bans, we estimated $104.7 million (30.8% of total costs) associated with travel to another state for in-clinic abortion care, $1.7 million (0.5% of total costs) associated with pregnancies ending in miscarriage or stillbirth, and $233.2 million (68.7% of total costs) associated with carrying pregnancy to term. We also estimated $9.4 million in decreased costs attributable to changes in post-*Dobbs* abortion care delivery. Table 1 details estimated costs by pathway.

The $104.7 million cost associated with travel primarily included the cost of leave from work ($44.6 million, 42.6% of cost associated with travel), followed by food costs ($23.3 million, 22.2% of cost associated with travel) and accommodations ($20.4 million, 19.5% of cost associated with travel). Remaining travel costs included transportation ($11.0 million, 10.5% of cost associated with travel) and childcare ($5.5 million, or 5.2% of cost associated with travel). The average excess cost per person traveling for an abortion totaled $1593, excluding the cost of an in-clinic abortion in another state.

The $1.7 million cost (0.5% of total cost) associated with people carrying pregnancy to miscarriage or stillbirth mostly consisted of costs associated with miscarriage ($2.2 million, 80.2% of the total pathway cost). Costs associated with stillbirth accounted for $0.5 million (19.8% of the total pathway cost). The $1.7 million cost included −$1.0 million accounting for forgone

AJPH May 2026, Vol. 116, No. 5

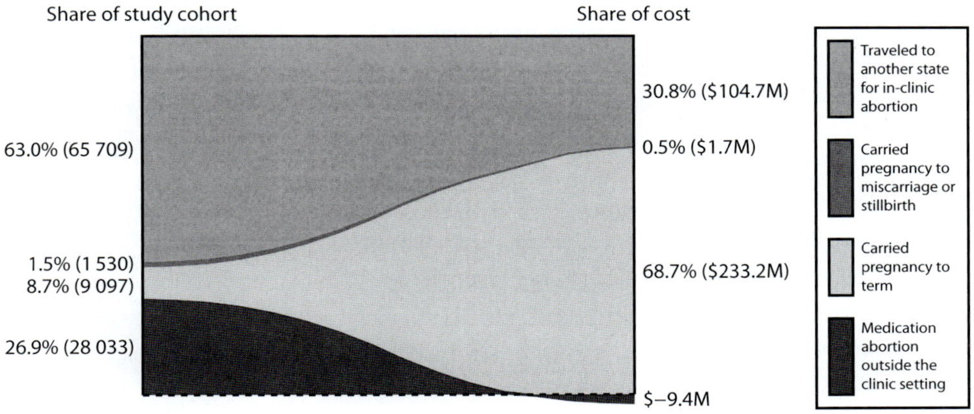

FIGURE 2— The Distribution of Alternatives to In-State, In-Clinic Abortion Among the Study Cohort, Compared With the Distribution of Estimated Costs Associated With Each Pathway: United States

Note. This figure compares the share of the study cohort in each pathway (left side of figure) with the share of costs that each pathway incurs (right side of figure). We estimated the first-year cost of total abortion bans in the 14 states enforced as of September 1, 2024. The numbers in parentheses represent the number of individuals in each pathway on the left and the total cost of each pathway on the right. We did not calculate the share of total cost for medication abortion outside the clinic setting as the pathway resulted in decreased costs because a medication abortion outside the clinic setting (approximately $220) costs less compared with an in-clinic procedure in the first trimester.

in-clinic abortion costs. The average per-person cost of a miscarriage was $1516; the average per-person cost of a stillbirth was $9073, excluding forgone costs (see Table 1).

The $233.2 million cost (68.7% of total cost) associated with carrying pregnancy to term instead of receiving an in-clinic abortion largely represented the cost of labor and delivery ($165.9 million, 71.1% of the total pathway cost). The average per-person cost of carrying pregnancy to term was $25 632 per person, of which $18 234 included estimated cost of labor and delivery. Other associated costs included increased social service use ($32.4 million, 13.9% of the total pathway cost) and lost income and unemployment ($31.7 million, 13.6% of the total pathway cost). Remaining costs of carrying a pregnancy to term remained comparatively small (Table 1). The $233.2 million cost included –$6.1 million accounting for forgone in-clinic abortion costs.

Decreased Costs From Changes in Abortion Care

We estimated that changes in post-*Dobbs* abortion care lowered costs by $9.4 million because of decreased costs of a medication abortion outside the clinic setting (approximately $220) compared with an in-clinic procedure in the first trimester (approximately $550 for medication abortion and $590 for procedural abortion). The increase in cost of complications from $1.8 million in-clinic to $2.1 million outside the clinic setting arose from differences in estimated complication rates (Table 1). Although the estimated minor complication rate remains lower outside the clinic setting (1.3 vs 4.9 per 100 people, costing $690 per person), the major complication rate is slightly higher outside the clinic setting, with markedly higher cost per person (0.58 vs 0.31 per 100 people, costing $11 172 per person).

Sensitivity Analysis

Across sensitivity analyses, we found the total cost (apart from decreased costs attributable to changes in post-*Dobbs* abortion care) could range from $278.9 million to $400.3 million, averaging $2673 to $3835 per person. The tornado diagram (Figure 3) summarizes our sensitivity analyses. Appendix H (available as a supplement to the online version of this article at https://ajph.org) contains additional methodology and inputs.

DISCUSSION

We estimated that in the year after enacting total abortion bans, 104 369 people in 14 states were unable to obtain an abortion in their home state, resulting in $339.6 million in combined private and external costs. These costs included medical expenses, travel, lodging, childcare, and lost income, and external costs borne by health care payers, employers, taxpayers, and state and federal governments.

Approximately one third of our estimated costs represented 63% of the study cohort traveling out of state for abortion care, at $1593 per person (excluding cost of abortion). These expenses, including transportation, accommodations, childcare, and time off work, disproportionately affect communities with less financial and social support.[15] Roughly half of US households with incomes less than $50 000 per year have no emergency savings, making these expenses especially burdensome.[16]

Interstate travel for abortion has increased nationwide, with more than 171 000 people traveling in 2023.[6] This surge may reflect, in part, rapid expansion of systems to help patients access abortion care in the months subsequent to our study period. Simultaneously, several states have enacted legislation restricting abortion-related travel and have pursued litigation against providers and abortion funds that facilitate interstate travel.[17] Although clinics, abortion funds, and logistical support organizations continue to assist patients as resources permit, donations have decreased since their post-*Dobbs* peak. These organizations were not intended to bear the unprecedented burden of interstate travel for abortion, and declining resources shift more of the financial burden back to patients.

Pregnancies ending in miscarriage or stillbirth accounted for $1.7 million, or 0.5% of total costs. This represents a conservative estimate because of limited data on to what extent costs differ for those unable to obtain an abortion.

About two thirds of our total costs accounted for 8.7% of the cohort who carried pregnancies to term. The average per-person cost was $25 632, including $18 234 in health care costs for labor, delivery, and treatment of physical and mental health complications in the year after abortion bans. These costs align with other findings that pregnant women of reproductive age who give birth incur significantly higher health costs than those who do not give birth.[18] Although private insurance or Medicaid may cover a portion of health care costs, giving birth remains unaffordable for many; nearly one third of households cannot afford typical employer-based deductibles.[19]

In addition to health care costs, an average of $7524 per person reflects lost income, unemployment, and increased reliance on social services, disproportionately affecting those already struggling to afford health care.

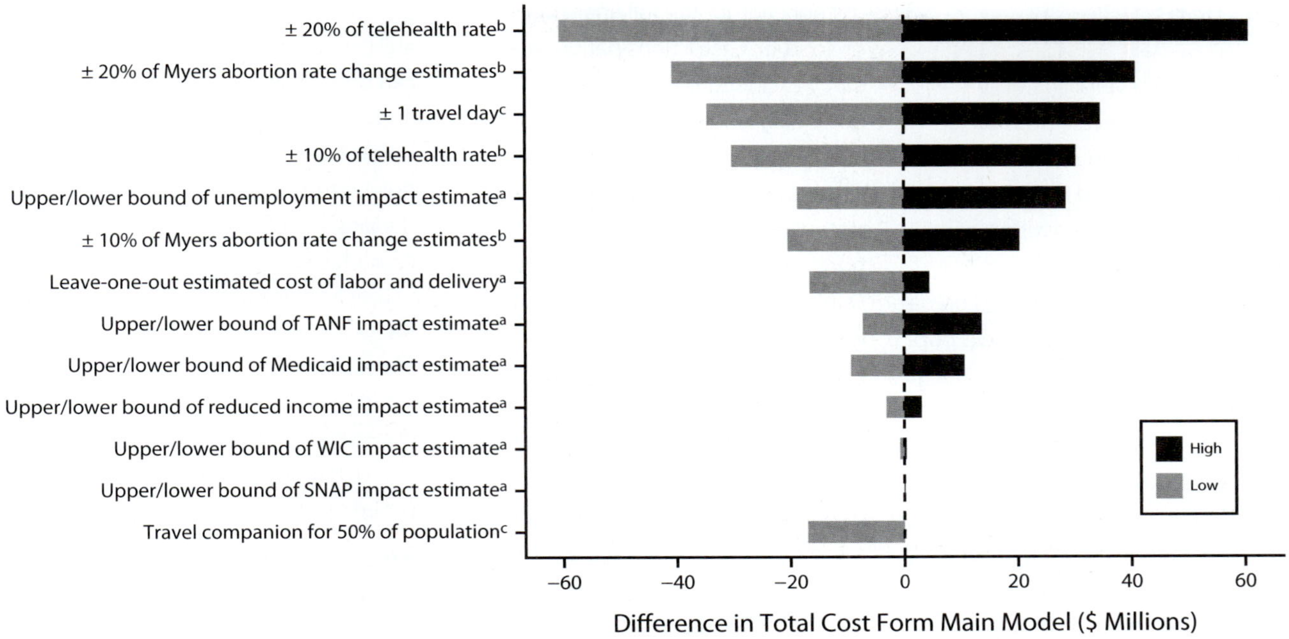

FIGURE 3— Tornado Diagram From Sensitivity Analysis of the Total Cost of Banning Abortion in the First Year After Enacting Bans Among 104 369 Individuals Across 14 US States

Note. SNAP = Supplemental Nutrition Assistance Program; TANF = Temporary Assistance for Needy Families; WIC = Special Supplemental Nutrition Program for Women, Infants, and Children. We estimated the first-year cost of total abortion bans in the 14 states enforced as of September 1, 2024. This diagram shows the results of our sensitivity analysis. Each row represents 1 model parameter that we modified. For model parameters based on estimates from a single study without accompanying confidence intervals, we varied the parameter by 10% and 20%; for model parameters based on estimates from a single study with accompanying confidence intervals, we used the upper and lower interval bounds; for model parameters based on estimates from multiple studies, we show the high and low total costs based on averaging the study estimates using a leave-one-out approach. As an example of how to interpret this graph, increasing the telehealth rate by 20% was associated with close to $60 million lower total cost compared with the main model (row 1, light gray), whereas decreasing the telehealth rate by 20% was associated with close to $60 million higher cost (row 1, dark gray).
[a]Impact estimate parameters.
[b]Rate parameter estimates for out-of-state travel and health.
[c]Parameters for travel time and companion.

States with abortion bans have less affordable health care; lower scores on measures of health care access, quality, and outcomes; and fewer maternity care providers relative to need, and many have not expanded Medicaid.[15,20] These figures represent conservative estimates of direct costs and do not capture the cost of raising a child in the first year. Abortion bans are therefore likely to deepen existing economic inequities, as states with restrictive policies often have structural conditions correlated with poorer economic outcomes, including low wages, limited public services, and the absence of paid leave or parental supports; access to abortion is closely linked to economic security, independence, and mobility, and the economic burden of abortion bans falls disproportionately on people already experiencing systematic disempowerment.[15]

Responding to rising demand in fewer states, telehealth abortion expanded rapidly after *Dobbs*. Evidence finds that telehealth abortion is effective and safe, reduces barriers to access, and helps address surges in demand in states where abortion is legal.[21,22] In addition, reliance on community networks and online vendors grew.[3] We estimated modest cost savings, averaging $335 per person, for the 26.9% of our study cohort accessing abortion outside the clinic setting, primarily because of the lower cost of telehealth and community-sourced medications.

However, people accessing abortion through shield law telehealth or other nonclinical routes face increasing risk of prosecution in states with abortion bans, which could lead to increased costs to individuals, friends and family that may assist them, and society.[23,24] Some states have also filed lawsuits against shield law providers, potentially deterring telehealth provision.[25] Furthermore, it remains unclear how much of the lower service cost is absorbed by telehealth providers, many of whom operate on a sliding-scale basis for patients unable to pay full price.[26,27]

Limitations

Our model had several limitations. First, we did not include every possible cost or outcome. We conducted a systematic literature review and included only direct costs and outcomes with recent, methodologically sound estimates. Costs and estimates were based on national averages and do not reflect population differences in states with bans or regional variation in resources or travel costs. Because state-specific data on shield law telemedicine was unavailable, we applied national rates.[7] Although we reported personal and external costs in aggregate, a detailed analysis of how these costs are distributed among different parties was beyond the scope of our study.

Our model also incorporated estimates from the Turnaway Study, the most comprehensive longitudinal data set on abortion seekers in the United States. Although the study included people seeking abortion at various gestations and supports similar impacts across gestational ages, its findings apply most directly to those near legal or facility gestational age limits and may not fully generalize to people who would have sought in-clinic abortion in states with full bans.[28]

Second, the rapidly evolving abortion policy landscape may affect generalizability. The #WeCount data provided the most recent data and accounted for selection bias among participating health centers but lacked data for periods prior to 2 months preceding *Dobbs*; although we accounted for seasonality, we could not account for other patterns in the months leading up to the *Dobbs* decision or reactions to the leaked draft opinion shared by *Politico* on May 2, 2022.[3] In addition, our study focused on 14 states with total post-*Dobbs* abortion bans; we did not capture the full financial burden of abortion restrictions nationwide. Our study excluded states with 6-week bans, potentially underestimating costs in states where neighboring states have since enacted bans, increasing travel distances. Increases in abortion rates in nonban states, likely reflecting post-*Dobbs* policy and services innovations, were beyond the scope of this study.[29]

Third, our model did not capture longer-term costs. Research links access to abortion to positive longer-term economic outcomes beyond the scope of our study, including lower rates of adolescent birth and increased educational attainment and labor force participation.[30,31] Research also supports negative longer-term economic outcomes of abortion bans.[32] We also did not capture the costs of raising a child during the first year or beyond, including child social services, which reflect broader public investments in family well-being.

Although our study estimated the cost of miscarriage and stillbirth for people unable to obtain an abortion, it did not capture heightened risks and costs for those not seeking abortion, such as complications or mortality from delayed or denied care, increased legal scrutiny, and mental health impacts. At least 210 pregnant people faced criminal charges in the year after *Dobbs*.[24]

Finally, we did not account for the psychological harm faced by those who want an abortion but cannot access one in their home state.[33]

Public Health Implications

Our study adds to a growing body of literature supporting that abortion bans carry significant costs for individuals, families, and society.[15,34,35] We provide evidence that restoring and protecting abortion access would improve economic outcomes, while expanding the availability of telehealth for abortion care can offer economic efficiencies. Our findings focused on the short-term economic harms of abortion bans and did not capture long-term consequences of denying people the ability to plan their reproductive and economic futures.

These findings provide important takeaways for policymakers in the United States. As states navigate the post-*Dobbs* landscape, this study provides critical evidence demonstrating the preventable and significant economic burdens imposed by abortion bans. AJPH

ABOUT THE AUTHORS

Jennifer E. Starling, Emma Pendl-Robinson, Sammie Chavez, and Kara Zivin are with Mathematica, Princeton, NJ. Divya Vohra and Isabel S. Platt were with Mathematica at the time of the study.

CORRESPONDENCE

Correspondence should be sent to Kara Zivin, 600 Alexander Park, Suite 100, Princeton, NJ 08543-2393 (e-mail: kzivin@mathematica-mpr.com). Reprints can be ordered at https://www.ajph.org by clicking the "Reprints" link.

PUBLICATION INFORMATION

Full Citation: Platt IS, Starling JE, Pendl-Robinson E, Chavez S, Vohra D, Zivin K. Societal costs of total abortion bans in 14 US states after *Dobbs*. *Am J Public Health*. 2026;116(5):683–691.

Acceptance Date: December 15, 2025.

DOI: https://doi.org/10.2105/AJPH.2025.308411

ORCID iDs:

Isabel S. Platt https://orcid.org/0000-0002-5229-0498

Jennifer E. Starling https://orcid.org/0000-0003-4765-360X

Emma Pendl-Robinson https://orcid.org/0000-0002-2318-9614

Sammie Chavez https://orcid.org/0009-0005-0251-3808

Divya Vohra https://orcid.org/0000-0001-9218-9397

Kara Zivin https://orcid.org/0000-0001-8246-6864

CONTRIBUTORS

I. S. Platt contributed to the design on the work, literature review, and writing. J. E. Starling contributed to design of the work, model development, and writing. E. Pendl-Robinson contributed to the design of the work, literature review, model development, and writing. S. Chavez contributed to the literature review and project management. D. Vohra and K. Zivin supervised the study and provided revisions to the article.

ACKNOWLEDGMENTS

This work was supported by The Commonwealth Fund (contracts 22-23171 and 23-23730).

The authors would like to thank the advisory panel (listed in Appendix A, available as a supplement to the online version of this article at https://ajph.org) for contributing to the model design and messaging of results. The authors would also like to thank Dana Johnson, So O'Neil, and Julia Strasser for their critical review of the article. Finally, we thank all the researchers and practitioners for conducting and publishing the studies used in our review.

CONFLICTS OF INTEREST

The authors have no conflicts of interest.

HUMAN PARTICIPATION PROTECTION

Data were retrieved from publicly available secondary data sources, so institutional review was not sought.

REFERENCES

1. Alito S. *Dobbs v. Jackson Women's Health Organization*. US Supreme Court. 2022. Available at: https://www.oyez.org/cases/2021/19-1392. Accessed September 26, 2024.
2. KFF. Abortion in the United States Dashboard. September 9, 2024. Available at: https://www.kff.org/womens-health-policy/dashboard/abortion-in-the-u-s-dashboard. Accessed September 26, 2024.
3. Aiken ARA, Wells ES, Gomperts R, Scott JG. Provision of medications for self-managed abortion before and after the *Dobbs v Jackson Women's Health Organization* decision. *JAMA*. 2024;331(18):1558–1564. https://doi.org/10.1001/jama.2024.4266
4. Dench D, Pineda-Torres M, Myers C. The effects of post-*Dobbs* abortion bans on fertility. *J Public Econ*. 2024;234:105124. https://doi.org/10.1016/j.jpubeco.2024.105124
5. Myers C. Forecasts for a post-Roe America: the effects of increased travel distance on abortions and births. *J Policy Anal Manage*. 2024;43(1):39–62. https://doi.org/10.1002/pam.22524
6. Guttmacher Institute. Monthly Abortion Provision Study. June 21, 2024. Available at: https://www.guttmacher.org/monthly-abortion-provision-study. Accessed September 27, 2024.
7. #WeCount Report: April 2022 to March 2024. Denver, CO: Society of Family Planning; 2024.
8. Dunn A, Grosse SD, Zuvekas SH. Adjusting health expenditures for inflation: a review of measures for health services research in the United States. *Health Serv Res*. 2018;53(1):175–196. https://doi.org/10.1111/1475-6773.12612
9. Parnell AM, Rodgers JL. Seasonality of induced abortion in North Carolina. *J Biosoc Sci*. 1998;30(3):321–332. https://doi.org/10.1017/s0021932098003216
10. Darrow LA, Strickland MJ, Klein M, et al. Seasonality of birth and implications for temporal studies of preterm birth. *Epidemiology*. 2009;20(5):699–706. https://doi.org/10.1097/EDE.0b013e3181a66e96
11. Luca DL, Margiotta C, Staatz C, Garlow E, Christensen A, Zivin K. Financial toll of untreated perinatal mood and anxiety disorders among 2017 births in the United States. *Am J Public Health*. 2020;110(6):888–896. https://doi.org/10.2105/AJPH.2020.305619
12. Center for Reproductive Rights. Interstate Shield Laws. June 26, 2024. Available at: https://reproductiverights.org/interstate-shield-laws. Accessed September 25, 2024.
13. Plan C. How to get an abortion pill by mail in 2–5 days. July 17, 2024. Available at: https://www.plancpills.org/abortion-pills/how-to-get-abortion-pill. Accessed September 25, 2024.
14. US Food and Drug Administration. Information about mifepristone for medical termination of pregnancy through ten weeks gestation. March 24, 2023. Available at: https://www.fda.gov/drugs/postmarket-drug-safety-information-patients-and-providers/information-about-mifepristone-medical-termination-pregnancy-through-ten-weeks-gestation. Accessed October 9, 2024.
15. Banerjee A. The economics of abortion bans: abortion bans, low wages, and public underinvestment are interconnected economic policy tools to disempower and control workers. Economic Policy Institute. 2023. Available at: https://www.epi.org/publication/economics-of-abortion-bans. Accessed October 9, 2024.
16. Middlewood B, Knoll M, Davies M, Guillory G. Emergency savings and financial security insights from the Making Ends: Meet Survey and Consumer Credit Panel. Consumer Financial Protection Bureau; Emergency Savings and Financial Security Insights from the Making Ends: Meet Survey and Consumer Credit Panel. Available at: https://www.consumerfinance.gov/data-research/research-reports/emergency-savings-financial-security-insights-from-making-ends-meet-survey-and-consumer-credit-panel. Accessed June 30, 2025.
17. Cohen IG, Adashi EY, Ziegler M. The new threat to medical travel for abortion. *Am J Med*. 2024;137(4):298–299. https://doi.org/10.1016/j.amjmed.2023.12.007
18. Rae M, Cox C, Dingel H. Health costs associated with pregnancy, childbirth, and postpartum care. Peterson–KFF Health System Tracker. 2022. Available at: https://www.healthsystemtracker.org/brief/health-costs-associated-with-pregnancy-childbirth-and-postpartum-care. Accessed September 14, 2023.
19. Young G, Rae M, Claxton G, Wager E, Amin K. How many people have enough money to afford private insurance cost sharing? Peterson–KFF Health System Tracker. March 10, 2022. Available at: https://www.healthsystemtracker.org/brief/many-households-do-not-have-enough-money-to-pay-cost-sharing-in-typical-private-health-plans. Accessed December 17, 2024.
20. Collins S, Radley D, Roy S, Zephyrin L, Shah A. 2024 state scorecard on women's health and reproductive care. Commonwealth Fund. 2024. Available at: https://www.commonwealthfund.org/publications/scorecard/2024/jul/2024-state-scorecard-womens-health-and-reproductive-care. Accessed October 9, 2024.
21. Upadhyay UD, Koenig LR, Meckstroth K, Ko J, Valladares ES, Biggs MA. Effectiveness and safety of telehealth medication abortion in the USA. *Nat Med*. 2024;30(4):1191–1198. https://doi.org/10.1038/s41591-024-02834-w
22. Aiken A, Lohr P, Lord J, Ghosh N, Starling J. Effectiveness, safety and acceptability of no-test medical abortion (termination of pregnancy) provided via telemedicine: a national cohort study. *BJOG*. 2021;128(9):1464–1474. https://doi.org/10.1111/1471-0528.16668
23. Dellinger J, Pell S. Bodies of evidence: the criminalization of abortion and surveillance of women in a post-*Dobbs* world. *SSRN Journal*. April 4, 2024:1–108. https://doi.org/10.2139/ssrn.4599445
24. Bach W, Wasilczuk M. Pregnancy as a crime: a preliminary report on the first year after *Dobbs*. Pregnancy Justice. 2024. Available at: https://www.pregnancyjusticeus.org/resources/pregnancy-as-a-crime-a-preliminary-report-on-the-first-year-after-dobbs. Accessed October 9, 2024.
25. Belluck P, Cochrane E. New York doctor indicted in Louisiana for sending abortion pills there. *New York Times*. January 31, 2025. Available at: https://www.nytimes.com/2025/01/31/health/abortion-louisiana-new-york-prosecution-shield-law.html. Accessed February 6, 2025.
26. Chaiyachati KH, Snider CK, Mitra N, et al. Economics of a health system's direct-to-consumer telemedicine for its employees. *Am J Manag Care*. 2023;29(6):284–290. https://doi.org/10.37765/ajmc.2023.89369
27. Ashwood JS, Mehrotra A, Cowling D, Uscher-Pines L. Direct-to-consumer telehealth may increase access to care but does not decrease spending. *Health Aff (Millwood)*. 2017;36(3):485–491. https://doi.org/10.1377/hlthaff.2016.1130
28. Biggs A, Foster DG, Gould H, et al. Commentary: The Turnaway Study: a case of self-correction in science upended by political motivation and unvetted findings. *Front Psychol*. 2022;13:1003116. https://doi.org/10.3389/fpsyg.2022.1003116
29. Ramaswamy A, Weigel G, Sobel L, Salganicoff A. Medication abortion and telemedicine: innovations and barriers during the COVID-19 emergency. KFF. June 16, 2021. Available at: https://www.kff.org/policy-watch/medication-abortion-telemedicine-innovations-and-barriers-during-the-covid-19-emergency. Accessed July 2, 2025.
30. Myers CK. The power of abortion policy: reexamining the effects of young women's access to reproductive control. *J Polit Econ*. 2017;125(6):2178–2224. https://doi.org/10.1086/694293
31. Angrist JD, Evans WN. Children and their parents' labor supply: evidence from exogenous variation in family size. *Am Econ Rev*. 1998;88(3):450–477.
32. Miller S, Wherry LR, Foster DG. The economic consequences of being denied an abortion. *Am Econ J Econ Policy*. 2023;15(1):394–437. https://doi.org/10.1257/pol.20210159
33. Kimport K, Rasidjan MP. Exploring the emotional costs of abortion travel in the United States due to legal restriction. *Contraception*. 2023;120:109956. https://doi.org/10.1016/j.contraception.2023.109956
34. Clark C, Jaimes MS, Rogers E. Updated analysis of the cost of abortion restrictions to states. Institute for Women's Policy Research. 2024. Available at: https://iwpr.org/2024-analysis-costs-of-reproductive-health-restrictions. Accessed October 9, 2024.
35. Economists Amicus Brief in *Dobbs v. Jackson Women's Health*. 2021. Available at: https://reproductiverights.org/wp-content/uploads/2021/09/Economists-Amicus-Brief.pdf. Accessed February 1, 2025.

Health Care Use and Health Care–Amenable Mortality Among US Adults With and Without a Bachelor's Degree, 1996–2023

Adam Gaffney, MD, MPH, Steffie Woolhandler, MD, MPH, Samuel L. Dickman, MD, Elizabeth Schrier, MD, Danny McCormick, MD, MPH, and David U. Himmelstein, MD

AJPH May 2026, Vol. 116, No. 5

Objectives. To describe health care–related educational divides in 2 dimensions—outpatient care utilization and medically preventable deaths—over the past 25 years.

Methods. We examined education-based disparities in ambulatory care utilization by analyzing data on 476 277 respondents aged 25 years or older to the 1996–2022 US Medical Expenditure Panel Survey, and in deaths potentially preventable by medical care (defined by *International Classification of Diseases, 10th Revision*, code) from 26 092 720 death certificates of individuals aged 25 to 74 years in the United States from 2001 to 2023.

Results. In 1996, the share of adults with zero provider visits was higher among those without (26.4%; 95% confidence interval [CI] = 25.3, 27.5) than with (20.2%; 95% CI = 18.5, 22.0) a bachelor's degree, a gap that widened to a nearly 2-fold difference by 2022; the gap in the proportion with no doctor visit also widened. Disparities in health care use were larger after adjustment for health factors. Separately, we observed large and growing education-based gaps in age-adjusted health care–amenable mortality.

Conclusions. Education-based disparities in ambulatory health care utilization have grown since 1996, as have medically preventable deaths.

Public Health Implications. Improved health care access for less-educated Americans might help address widening disparities in ambulatory health care use and, potentially, health outcomes. (*Am J Public Health*. 2026;116(5):692–701. https://doi.org/10.2105/AJPH.2025.308373)

In the decade before COVID-19, US life expectancy plateaued even as it continued to rise in other nations, a divergence in part driven by rising mortality among young adult and middle-aged Americans.[1,2] This disturbing development led to calls for a research "moonshot" to identify the causes of these trends.[2]

Previous research suggests that these trends may be driven by a growing socioeconomic divide in US health. The life expectancy gap by income has been widening[3]; multiple studies, moreover, have found that adverse life expectancy trends in the United States are explained by a growing divergence in health between more- and less-educated adults.[4–8] This widening gap—highlighted prominently by Case and Deaton[6,7]—has multiple drivers. Case and Deaton's 2015 analysis[6] emphasized "deaths of despair"—mortality from suicide, drug overdoses, and alcoholism—particularly among midlife non-Hispanic White Americans experiencing downward economic mobility. Subsequently, they[7,8] and others[9] found a similar education-based divide among Black persons and for a range of conditions other than deaths of despair, including cardiovascular disease. While education is only 1 metric of socioeconomic position (alongside income, wealth, and occupation), its stability over the life-course,[10] applicability to individuals not in the workforce,[10] and correlation with early life advantage and parental wealth[11] provide some methodologic advantages as an indicator of social inequality in health and medical care.

Before the modern era, health care had little impact on longevity: life expectancy gains were driven primarily by economic development and public health innovations.[12] However, over the past century, medical care has played an increasing role in extending longevity,[13] particularly through management of cardiovascular disease[13–15] and the provision of primary care.[16,17] Numerous studies have identified disparities in health care utilization by race, ethnicity, and socioeconomic status that are associated with disparities in health outcomes,[18] suggesting that widening disparities in health care use might contribute to the widening education-based gap in longevity.

The present study describes trends in health care–related educational divides along 2 dimensions using 2 separate and unlinked data sets over the past 25 years. First, for our primary analysis, we examined whether the education-based divide in the use (particularly no use) of outpatient care—the setting where most disease is diagnosed, prevented, and treated—has widened over time. Second, we separately examined trends in education-based disparities in medically preventable death[19,20] over a similar period.

METHODS

Our primary analyses used data from the 1996–2022 Medical Expenditure Panel Survey (MEPS), a nationally representative health care survey that collects data on health care utilization and expenditures among the noninstitutionalized US population.[21] We obtained data from IPUMS[22] on 859 723 individual-year–level records that we merged with office-based (n = 4 077 725) and outpatient (n = 412 441) event files providing data on physician visits by specialty. We restricted our sample to 515 503 individuals aged 25 years or older with nonzero sampling weights.

For our secondary analysis, we separately analyzed individual-level death certificate microdata on all (61 971 692) decedents in the United States from 2001 to 2023, obtained from the National Center for Health Statistics National Vital Statistics System via the National Bureau of Economic Research (2001–2021)[23] or the Centers for Disease Control and Prevention (2022–2023). We excluded 125 049 (0.2%) deaths among foreign residents. To estimate population denominators, we analyzed 63 702 892 individual-level records from corresponding years of the American Community Survey (ACS).[24] We restricted our sample to adults aged 25 to 74 years in each data set, leaving 26 092 720 death records and 39 485 434 ACS records.

Exposure

For both sets of analyses, the exposure was educational attainment, a proxy of social class[10] that we dichotomized as a 4-year or bachelor's college degree (hereinafter "BA") versus no such a degree ("no BA"), following previous studies.[8] We constructed this indicator for each data set as follows.

For our primary analyses examining MEPS data on health care utilization, our education indicator relied on the IPUMS-constructed detailed education variable (*educ*),[25] with BA defined as a "bachelor's degree (BA, AB, BS, BBA)" or a more advanced degree, and no BA as less educational attainment. We excluded 39 226 (7.6%) with "other degree," "no degree, years of education unknown," or "unknown," or missing data.

For our secondary analyses examining mortality data, we first aligned the education variable on death certificates, which changed during the study period. The 1989 version of the variable categorized education by years of schooling, while the 2003 version provides degree attainment; states implemented the 2003 version at different times following its introduction; by 2018, all states had completed the transition. We (following previous studies[7]) defined a BA as 4 or more years of college for records reporting the 1989 variable, and as a bachelor's, master's, doctorate, or professional degree for records reporting the 2003 variable. Some states did not report education early in our study period; overall, education was missing for 4% (n = 962 932) of decedents aged 25 to 74 years. For those individuals, we imputed education by first restricting our sample to "health care–amenable deaths," as described subsequently, and then, similar to a previously described approach,[7,8] assigning decedents with missing education data a BA (or no BA) in the same proportion as decedents with known BA status of the same year, age category, and sex.

The ACS (used to construct population denominators) assessed education consistently; as described previously, we defined a BA as having a bachelor's, master's, doctorate, or professional degree, excluding 1 individual with missing education data. We then used person-level weights to estimate the national population by year, age category, and education.

Outcomes

Our primary (MEPS-based) outcomes were 3 metrics of outpatient care use: provider visits, doctor visits, and primary-care physician (PCP) visits, all calculated by summing visits occurring in hospital outpatient departments and in office-based practices. We defined "provider visits" as visits to any medical provider (physicians, nurse practitioners, nurses, physician assistants, and other allied practitioners such as optometrists and physical therapists). Physician visits included visits to physicians of any specialty. We defined PCP visits (available since 2002) as visits to physicians of the following specialties: family practice, general practice, geriatrics, internal medicine, or pediatrics.

The outcome of our secondary (death certificate–based) analysis was "health care–amenable" mortality, defined according to the "underlying cause of death" reported on death certificates, using *International Classification of Diseases, 10th Revision*, codes included in the joint Organization for Economic Co-operation and Development (OECD)/Eurostat "avoidable mortality" lists.[26] That list subcategorizes "avoidable" deaths into "preventable deaths" (i.e., deaths "mainly avoid[able] through effective public health and primary prevention") and "treatable (or amenable)" causes of death (i.e., deaths "mainly avoid[able] through timely and effective health care interventions, including secondary prevention and treatment").[26] We only examined the latter category, which we term "health care–amenable deaths." Only deaths before age 75 are classified as avoidable in this schema. For deaths from causes designated as partially treatable or amenable, we considered 50% treatable or amenable following the OECD/Eurostat approach.[26] For this repeated cross-sectional analysis, we calculated crude health care–amenable death rates per 100 000 by year and age category using ACS population denominators, and the annual overall (age 25–74) age-adjusted health care–amenable mortality rate per 100 000, as described subsequently.

Analyses

We examined characteristics of our MEPS sample, overall and in the 2 earliest and 2 final years. We then examined 1996–2022 trends by education in the proportion with zero visits during each calendar year and mean number of visits per person per year. We assessed whether trends for each outcome differed by education by constructing linear (or logistic) multivariable regression models assessing the interaction of (continuous) calendar-year × BA status (along with main effects), and indicators for age (continuous) and gender.

We then examined education-based differences in health care use in recent years, using pooled 2018–2022 data (n = 83 661). We first examined differences in each outcome by individual year of age. For 2022, we then estimated the number of persons (by education status) with 1 or more chronic diseases who went without a single visit that year. We then performed 3 sets of multiple regression models to assess whether differences in age and sex and in health status explain education-based disparities in the use of care over 2018 to 2022. The first set of models was unadjusted; the second set adjusted only for age (25–34, 35–44, 45–54, 55–64, 65–74, ≥ 75 years) and sex (male/female); and the third "health needs" models additionally adjusted for the number of chronic diseases (hypertension, diabetes, stroke, cancer history, chronic lung disease, and heart disease), presence of a physical limitation (defined as any instrumental activity of daily living, activity of daily living, functional, or activity limitation), and 2 measures of acute health problems (having ≥ 1 emergency department visit or ≥ 1 night in a hospital in the calendar year). We used linear regressions for analyses of visit counts[27] and Poisson regressions for binary outcomes.[28] Multivariable analyses excluded 562 (0.7%) individuals with missing data for a health status covariate.

For sensitivity analyses, we repeated these regressions using zero-inflated Poisson regressions; we also repeated these analyses restricted to those with 1 or more chronic diseases and stratified by pre- (2018–2019) and post- (2020–2022) pandemic years.

Finally, for our separate (mortality) analyses, we examined time trends in treatable mortality per 100 000 by age group (25–34, 35–44, 45–54, 55–64, 65–74 years), and age-standardized for the overall population aged 25 to 74 years using direct standardization to the Census Bureau's Year 2000 reference population and these same 10-year age categories.

We used Stata/SE version 18 (StataCorp LP, College Station, TX), and (for MEPS analyses) population weights and complex survey procedures.

RESULTS

We first present results of our MEPS-based analyses examining health care use, followed by our death certificate analyses examining health care–amenable mortality.

Health Care Use

Our MEPS population was composed of 476 277 adults aged 25 years or older: 130 824 with and 345 453 without BAs. Appendix Table A (available as a supplement to the online version of this article at https://ajph.org) provides their characteristics. Compared with those with BAs, those with no BA were older (mean age 51.2 vs 48.3 years), had lower incomes, and worse health according to most indicators; more were Black, Hispanic, or American Indian, while fewer were White. Over time, the average age of both groups rose; educational disparities in income and physical limitations persisted, and the share of those with a BA who were female increased, as did the share without a BA who were Hispanic (Appendix Table B).

Figure 1 displays trends in total provider and doctor visits among those with and without a BA, including *P* values for the calendar-year*BA interaction terms evaluating differences in linear time trends between the 2 groups. In 1996, the proportion of adults with no visits to any medical provider was higher among those without (26.4%; 95% confidence interval [CI] = 25.3, 27.5) than with (20.2%; 95% CI = 18.5, 22.0) BAs, a gap that widened over time (*P* for interaction <.01) to a nearly 2-fold difference: in 2022, 28.6% (95% CI = 26.9, 30.3) of those with no BA had zero provider visits versus 15.6% (95% CI = 14.3, 17.0) of those with BAs.

In 1996, persons without a BA had only slightly lower mean numbers of provider visits than those with a BA, at 6.3 per year (95% CI = 5.9, 6.7) versus 6.8 per year (95% CI = 6.3, 7.3), respectively. Mean provider visits subsequently rose more steeply among the

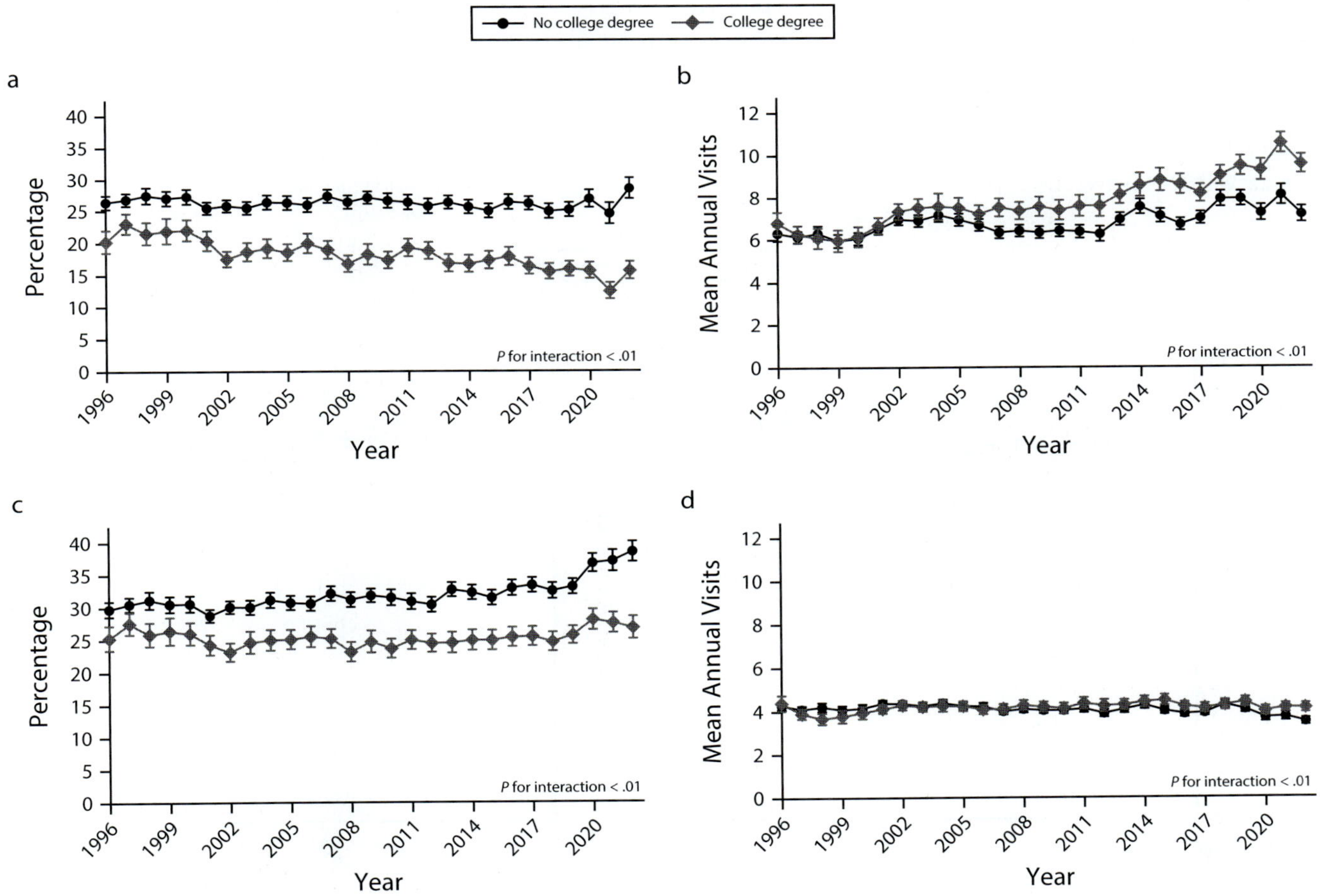

FIGURE 1— Metrics of Provider and Doctor Use by US Adults With and Without a BA, and by (a) Zero Provider Visits, (b) Provider Visits, (c) Zero Doctor Visits, (d) Doctor Visits: 1996–2022

Note. BA = bachelor's degree or greater. The sample size was n = 476 277. Visits are summed across outpatient and office-based practices. "Provider visits" were defined as visits to any medical provider (e.g., physicians, nurse practitioners, nurses, physician assistants, and other allied practitioners such as optometrists and physical therapists). Doctor visits included visits to physicians of any specialty. *P* value represents the significance of a linear (continuous) year × education group interaction term that was regressed onto each outcome along with main effects, a continuous age indicator, and a sex indicator. We used linear regressions for visit number and logistic regressions for the binary "zero visit" outcomes.

college educated (*P* for interaction <.01), to 9.6 per year (95% CI = 9.1, 10.0) in 2022 for those with BAs versus 7.2 per year (95% CI = 6.8, 7.6) for those with no BA.

In 1996, the share of those with no BA having zero doctor visits was 29.8% (95% CI = 28.6, 31.0) versus 25.3% (95% CI = 23.5, 27.3) among those with BAs, a gap that widened sharply thereafter (*P* for interaction <.01), with the divergence becoming more marked during COVID-19. In 2019, 33.1% of those without a BA had no doctor visit, rising to 38.5% in 2022. In contrast, among those with a BA, the share with no doctor visit rose little, from 25.7% in 2019 to 26.8% in 2022. Mean doctor visits were similar or slightly higher among those without versus with BAs between 1996 and 2007 but subsequently became lower (*P* for interaction <.01).

Figure 2 displays PCP visit trends. The share without PCP visits was similar in 2002 for those without and with BAs (44.2% [95% CI = 43.2, 45.2] and 42.7% [95% CI = 41.1, 44.3], respectively) and subsequently rose for both groups albeit more steeply among those with no BA (*P* for interaction <.01). By 2022, 54.5% of those with no BA had no PCP visits versus 46.4% of those with BAs.

In 2002, the PCP-visit rate was higher among those with no BA (1.8 per year; 95% CI = 1.7, 1.9) versus those with BAs (1.5 per year; 95% CI = 1.4, 1.5). Mean PCP visits fell over time for both groups, although more steeply among those with no BA (*P* for interaction <.01); by 2022, their mean PCP visits were similar.

Appendix Figures A and B display utilization of care at each year of age by education using pooled 2018–2022 data. Notably, education-based disparities in the proportion with zero provider, doctor, or PCP visits were largest among young and middle-aged adults and narrower among older adults.

In the subset of persons with a chronic disease in 2022, 15.6% of those without BAs had zero provider visits, 24.0% had zero doctor visits, and 40.7% had zero PCP visits; of adults with BAs, 8.3%, 15.9%, and 35.2% went without each type of visit, respectively (data not shown).

Table 1 provides regression results for our contemporary (pooled 2018–2022) sample: unadjusted, adjusted for age and sex, and additionally adjusted for health indicators ("Health Needs"

AJPH May 2026, Vol. 116, No. 5

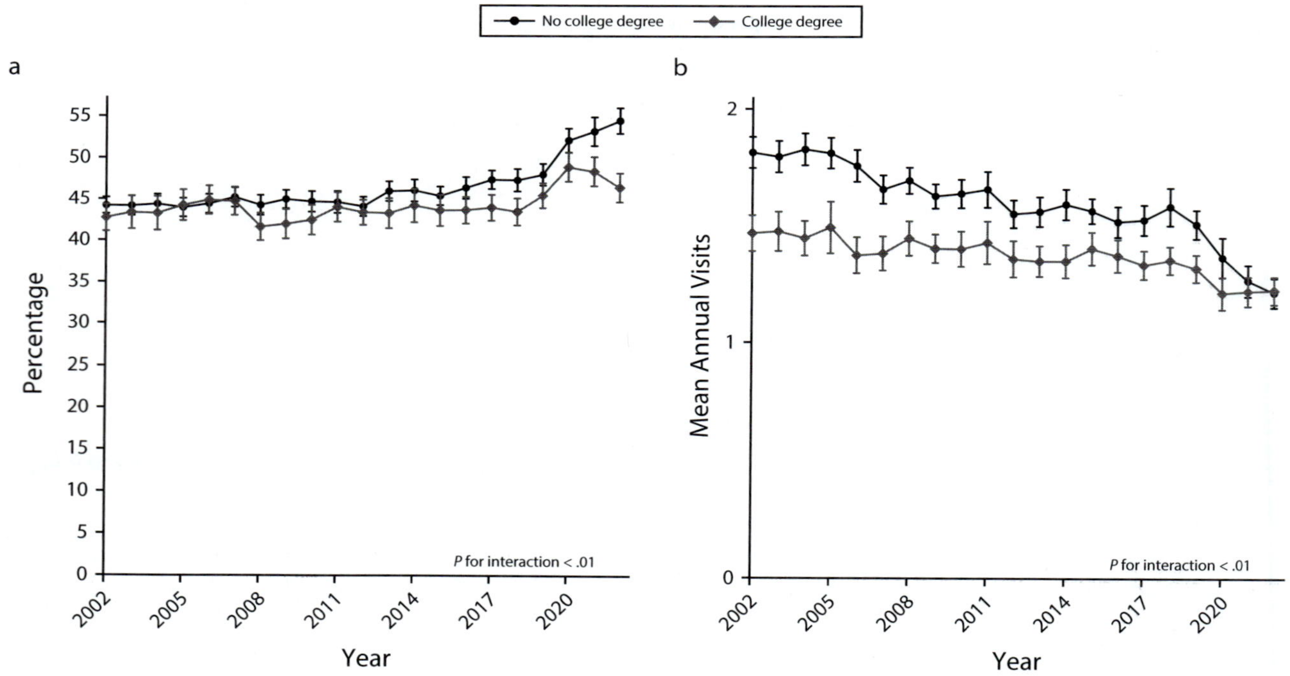

FIGURE 2— Primary Care Physician Use by US Adults With and Without a BA and by a) Zero Primary Care Visits, (b) Primary Care Visits: 2002–2022

Note. BA = bachelor's degree or greater. The sample size was n = 387 413. Primary care physician visits included visits to family practice, general practice, geriatrics, internal medicine, or pediatric physicians. *P* value represents the significance of a linear (continuous) year × education group interaction term that was regressed onto each outcome along with main effects, a continuous age indicator, and a sex indicator. We used linear regressions for visit number and logistic regressions for the binary "zero visit" outcomes.

TABLE 1— Unadjusted and Adjusted Differences in Provider and Physician Use Among US Adults Without a BA Versus With a BA: 2018–2022

	Unadjusted, b (95% CI)	Age and Sex-Adjusted,[a] b (95% CI)	Health Needs-Adjusted,[b] b (95% CI)
Number of visits (absolute difference)			
Provider visit	−1.92 (−2.31, −1.52)	−2.29 (−2.68, −1.90)	−3.65 (−4.01, −3.29)
Doctor visit	−0.32 (−0.48, −0.16)	−0.59 (−0.74, −0.43)	−1.25 (−1.38, −1.11)
PCP visit	0.13 (0.07, 0.18)	0.04 (−0.01, 0.09)	−0.14 (−0.18, −0.10)
Likelihood of zero visit (rate ratio)			
Provider visit	1.73 (1.64, 1.83)	1.81 (1.72, 1.91)	2.03 (1.92, 2.13)
Doctor visit	1.34 (1.28, 1.39)	1.40 (1.35, 1.45)	1.54 (1.49, 1.60)
PCP visit	1.09 (1.07, 1.13)	1.14 (1.11, 1.17)	1.21 (1.18, 1.24)

Note. BA = bachelor's degree or greater; PCP = primary care physician. The sample size was n = 83 661. Coefficients represent the absolute difference in the number of visits from linear regression models or in the relative likelihood of zero visits from Poisson regression models among those without a BA compared with those with a BA (the reference group). "Provider visits" were defined as visits to any medical provider (e.g., physicians, nurse practitioners, nurses, physician assistants, and other allied practitioners such as optometrists and physical therapists). Doctor visits included visits to physicians of any specialty. PCP visit includes visits to family practice, general practice, geriatrics, internal medicine, or pediatric physicians.

[a]Adjusted for age (25–34, 35–44, 45–54, 55–64, 65–74, and ≥75 years) and sex (male or female).

[b]Adjusted for age (25–34, 35–44, 45–54, 55–64, 65–74, and ≥75 years), sex (male or female), number of chronic diseases (hypertension, diabetes, stroke, cancer history, chronic lung disease, and heart disease), ≥1 emergency department visit indicator, ≥1 hospital night indicator, and physical limitation indicator. The sample size was n = 83 099 after exclusion of n = 562 with missing data for physical limitation or number of chronic diseases indicators.

model). Without adjustment, those without (vs with) BAs had 1.92 fewer provider visits (95% CI = -2.31, −1.52), 0.32 fewer doctor visits (95% CI = −0.48, −0.16), and slightly more PCP visits (0.13; 95% CI = 0.07, 0.18). Disparities emerged or widened with adjustment for age and sex, and further with adjustment for health factors. In the fully adjusted model, those without (vs with) BAs had 3.65 fewer provider visits (95% CI = −4.01, −3.29), 1.25 fewer doctor visits (95% CI = −1.38, −1.11), and 0.14 fewer PCP visits annually (95% CI = −0.18, −0.10). Moreover, they were twice as likely to go without any provider visits (rate ratio = 2.03; 95% CI = 1.92, 2.13), 54% more likely to have no doctor visits (95% CI = 1.49, 1.60), and 21% more likely to have no PCP visits (95% CI = 1.18, 1.24).

Results were consistent among those with a chronic disease (Appendix Table C), and before (2018–2019) and after (2020–2022) the COVID-19 pandemic onset (Appendix Table D). Zero-inflated Poisson models (Appendix Table E) produced consistent results for zero care use for all 3 visit types. However, among noncertain zeroes, persons without a BA also received fewer provider visits but more PCP visits; they received more doctor visits without adjustment but fewer with adjustment. In other words, while individuals without a BA were more likely to not see a PCP at all versus those with a BA, they saw PCPs more frequently contingent on having 1 or more visits.

Health Care–Amenable Mortality

Figure 3 provides trends in age-adjusted and age-specific health care–amenable mortality for persons without versus with BAs. In 2001, the age-adjusted health care–amenable mortality for persons aged 25 to 74 years was 71% higher among those without versus with BAs (175.3 vs 102.7 per 100 000). Over the subsequent decade, such mortality fell for both groups, to 140.0 versus 68.1 per 100 000 in 2012, respectively. However, the gap widened over the following decade, as mortality continued to decline (slowly) for those with BAs to 63.8 per 100 000 in 2019, before rising to 66.0 per 100 000 in 2020 during the pandemic. In contrast, among those with no BA, health care–amenable mortality began rising after 2012, reaching 145.4 per 100 000 in 2019 (128% higher than those with BAs), and 161.6 per 100 000 in 2021. The health care–amenable mortality rate fell after 2021 for both education groups as the pandemic receded. However, in 2023, age-adjusted treatable mortality remained higher among non–college-educated (150.8 per 100 000) compared with every prepandemic year since 2009, whereas among college-educated (61.9 per 100 000) individuals the rate in 2023 was lower than any previous year in our series.

The rise in health care–amenable mortality among those with no BA was

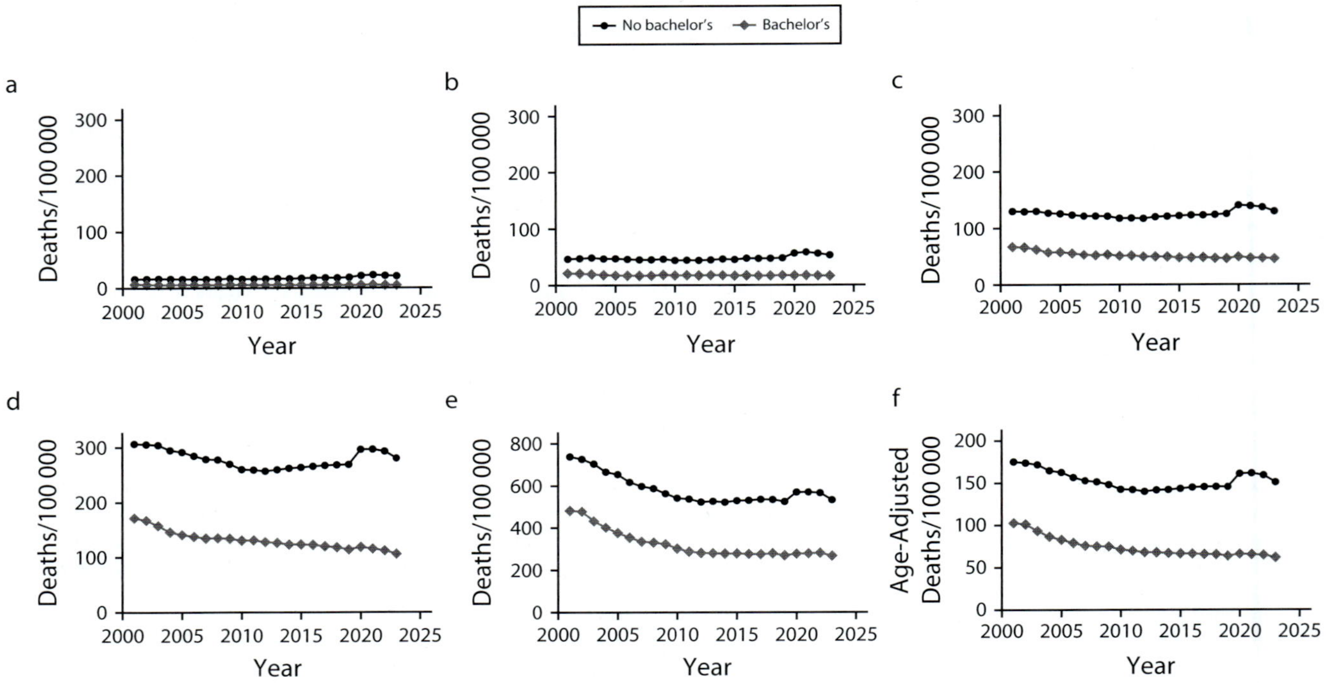

FIGURE 3— Age-Adjusted Health Care–Amenable Mortality by Education and Age Among US Adults Aged (a) 25–34 Years, (b) 35–44 Years, (c) 45–54 Years, (d) 55–64 Years, (e) 65–74 Years, and (f) Overall: 2001–2023

Note. Health care–amenable mortality defined by *International Classification of Diseases, 10th Revision*, code of the underlying cause of death per Organization for Economic Co-operation and Development (OECD)/Eurostat "treatable mortality" list (January 2022 version).[26] Overall mortality is age-adjusted rate per 100 000 using direct standardization to the US Census Bureau Year 2000 reference population and 10-year age categories (25–34, 35–44, 45–54, 55–64, and 65–74 years). For direct age-standardization of mortality rates, we used Stata's DSTDIZE command (version 18; StataCorp LP, College Station, TX). Analysis was based on analysis of death certificate data on 26 092 720 decedents aged 25 to 74 years. Education status was classified (and imputed where missing) as described in the article.
[a]The y-axes of these graphs are shown on different scales than the other graphs.

seen in all but the oldest (65–74 years) age group but was particularly steep among adults aged 25 to 34 years, who experienced a 32% increase between 2010 (15.8 per 100 000) and 2023 (20.8 per 100 000).

DISCUSSION

Education-based disparities in outpatient health care use are widening. At the turn of the millennium, Americans without BAs had similar rates of provider and doctor visits (and more PCP visits) compared with those with BAs—although they more often went without any visits. Today, adults without BAs make fewer visits to providers and physicians overall (although not to PCPs) and are even more likely to go without any such ambulatory care.

The education-based divide in health care–amenable mortality has simultaneously widened: in 2023, despite the waning of the COVID-19 pandemic, treatable mortality among less-educated adults was the highest in almost 15 (nonpandemic) years. Although the increasing disparities in health care use and health care–amenable mortality are both indicative of growing social inequalities in health care, our study could not assess whether these trends are linked.

Our analysis additionally highlights the declining provision of primary care[29–31] and identifies a recent rise in the share of Americans who receive no primary care, driven by falling use among less-educated Americans. In recent years, about half of adults, regardless of education, had no encounter with a primary care doctor. Annual primary care visits may not be necessary for some young, healthy individuals. Yet absent any visit, delivery of the burgeoning number of recommended preventive services and counseling, or ascertainment (and treatment) of asymptomatic conditions (e.g. hypertension) seems unlikely to occur.

The care gaps we observed—particularly the large number of less-educated Americans who receive no outpatient care—could plausibly contribute to growing gaps in health care–amenable mortality,[7,8] although our study was not designed to address such a linkage. The concept of preventable mortality as a measure of good medical care has been developed over decades[19,20]; today, the OECD tracks this metric across member states. A recent study by Papanicolas et al. examined overall "avoidable" (treatable plus preventable) mortality in the United States (through 2021), finding an increase that was mostly (but not entirely) driven by preventable deaths.[32] We expand upon their findings by examining treatable mortality by social class and finding a growing divergence that extends to the postpandemic period (i.e., through 2023).

However, both the study by Papanicolas et al. and our study lack clinical data to assess the extent to which any individual death might have been prevented with better or earlier care. Moreover, "treatable" deaths often have multiple contributing causes, including behaviors such as tobacco use. Certifiers can also err in ascertaining the cause(s) of death: the rise in health care–amenable mortality we observed during the COVID-19 pandemic may reflect deferred care, but also undiagnosed COVID-19.[33]

The increasing education-based disparities we observed in health care use and health care–amenable mortality are each concerning on their own terms; as noted, however, the design of our study did not permit us to determine whether, or to what extent, the former caused the latter, and we make no assertions about a causal relationship. Future research could further explore the relationship between social position, health care access or use (whether mediating, or interacting with, social position[34]), and health. In addition, we do not view lower educational attainment as a direct causal exposure but, rather, as a surrogate for lower socioeconomic status associated with numerous forms of disadvantage (e.g., adverse early life exposures, low lifetime earnings, and inferior health insurance coverage).

We also did not assess the cause of lower health care utilization among less-educated individuals, although our "health-adjusted" models indicate that they are not attributable to lesser health needs as reflected by age, chronic disease prevalence, or physical limitations. Lack of insurance, cost barriers like copayments and deductibles, geographic inaccessibility of providers, inability to navigate the complexities of securing appointments, and low health literacy, among other factors, might contribute.

Our study has additional limitations. Use of large data sets can increase the likelihood of finding statistically, but not clinically, significant differences. We assessed PCP visits, but not primary care visits provided by nonphysician professionals, although visits to these professionals were included in our provider visit outcomes. We examined "visits"—which are only 1 type of outpatient service—although visits reasonably assess the allocation of professionals' time, which underlies counseling, diagnosis, and treatment. We could not assess whether differences in average visits reflect only underuse among the less-educated or some overuse among the college-educated. However, overuse is unlikely to explain higher rates of zero use among those lacking a BA, including those with a serious chronic disease who almost always will require at least 1 annual provider visit.

Utilization, including the specialty of consulted physicians, is self-reported by MEPS respondents. Funeral directors, who usually record decedents' education on death certificates, may also err; however, previous analyses, including Case and Deaton's,[7,8] also relied on those data, and longitudinal survey-based studies[35] using self-reported education have also found social divides in all-cause mortality. Our death certificate analysis examined underlying (but not all contributing) causes of death; particularly in older individuals, the confluence of many acute and chronic processes often leads to death. Finally, we did not assess the impacts of compositional changes caused by the falling proportion of individuals without BA degrees, which might contribute to growing disadvantage of this group and higher relative mortality; such compositional change would not lessen the salience of the social disparities we observed, however.

In conclusion, the utilization of ambulatory health care has become more inequitable across the lines of social class in 21st century America. Meanwhile, the provision of primary care is falling among all adults. Most recently, declines in health care–amenable mortality have slowed for the better-educated and reversed for the less-educated. Reforms to achieve a more equitable distribution of care—such as universal coverage and the lowering of cost barriers, greater geographic equity in provider supply, and a reinvigoration of primary care—could potentially help (in part) to reverse the disturbing trends in health care equity we observed; whether this would mitigate educational divides in population health, which reflects diverse drivers, is less certain. AJPH

ABOUT THE AUTHORS

Adam Gaffney and Danny McCormick are with Harvard Medical School and the Department of Medicine at the Cambridge Health Alliance, Cambridge, MA. Steffie Woolhandler and David U. Himmelstein are with the City University of New York Hunter College, New York, NY. Samuel L. Dickman is with Planned Parenthood Montana,

Billings. Elizabeth Schrier is with the Department of Medicine at the University of California San Francisco.

CORRESPONDENCE

Correspondence should be sent to Adam Gaffney, 1493 Cambridge St, Cambridge, MA 02139 (e-mail: agaffney@challiance.org). Reprints can be ordered at https://www.ajph.org by clicking the "Reprints" link.

PUBLICATION INFORMATION

Full Citation: Gaffney A, Woolhandler S, Dickman SL, Schrier E, McCormick D, Himmelstein DU. Health care use and health care–amenable mortality among US adults with and without a bachelor's degree, 1996–2023. *Am J Public Health*. 2026;116(5):692–701.

Acceptance Date: November 20, 2025.

DOI: https://doi.org/10.2105/AJPH.2025.308373

ORCID iDs:

Samuel L. Dickman https://orcid.org/0000-0003-3126-786X

Elizabeth Schrier https://orcid.org/0000-0001-5118-6085

CONTRIBUTORS

All authors made substantial contributions to the conceptualization and design of the study, the interpretation of data, and critical revision of the article. A. Gaffney conducted the analyses and wrote the original draft. All authors approved the final version of the article.

CONFLICTS OF INTEREST

A. Gaffney is a former president of Physicians for a National Health Program, a nonprofit organization that favors coverage expansion through a single-payer program. A. Gaffney's spouse is a former employee of Treatment Action Group, a nonprofit research and policy think tank focused on HIV, tuberculosis, and hepatitis C treatment, and is a current employee at the nonprofit organization Health Care for All Massachusetts. The authors report no conflicts of interest.

HUMAN PARTICIPANT PROTECTION

This study used only publicly available, de-identified data and, hence, is not considered human participant research by the authors' institutional review boards consistent with the Common Rule; review was hence not required or sought.

REFERENCES

1. Woolf SH, Schoomaker H. Life expectancy and mortality rates in the United States, 1959–2017. *JAMA*. 2019;322(20):1996–2016. https://doi.org/10.1001/jama.2019.16932
2. Woolf SH. Increasing mortality rates in the US, but not from COVID-19. *JAMA*. 2024;332(12): 959–960. https://doi.org/10.1001/jama.2024.13626
3. Chetty R, Stepner M, Abraham S, et al. The association between income and life expectancy in the United States, 2001–2014. *JAMA*. 2016;315(16): 1750–1766. https://doi.org/10.1001/jama.2016.4226
4. Meara E, Richards S, Cutler D. The gap gets bigger: changes in mortality and life expectancy by education, 1981 – 2000. *Health Aff (Millwood)*. 2008;27(2):350–360. https://doi.org/10.1377/hlthaff.27.2.350
5. Olshansky SJ, Antonucci T, Berkman L, et al. Differences in life expectancy due to race and educational differences are widening, and many may not catch up. *Health Aff (Millwood)*. 2012;31(8): 1803–1813. https://doi.org/10.1377/hlthaff.2011.0746
6. Case A, Deaton A. Rising morbidity and mortality in midlife among White non-Hispanic Americans in the 21st century. *Proc Natl Acad Sci U S A*. 2015;112(49):15078–15083. https://doi.org/10.1073/pnas.1518393112
7. Case A, Deaton A. Life expectancy in adulthood is falling for those without a BA degree, but as educational gaps have widened, racial gaps have narrowed. *Proc Natl Acad Sci U S A*. 2021;118(11): e2024777118. https://doi.org/10.1073/pnas.2024777118
8. Case A, Deaton A. Accounting for the widening mortality gap between American adults with and without a BA. *Brookings Pap Econ Act*. 2023; 2023(2):1–78. https://doi.org/10.1353/eca.2023.a935412
9. Geronimus AT, Bound J, Waidmann TA, Rodriguez JM, Timpe B. Weathering, drugs, and whack-a-mole: fundamental and proximate causes of widening educational inequity in US life expectancy by sex and race, 1990–2015. *J Health Soc Behav*. 2019;60(2):222–239. https://doi.org/10.1177/0022146519849932
10. Krieger N, Williams DR, Moss NE. Measuring social class in US public health research: concepts, methodologies, and guidelines. *Annu Rev Public Health*. 1997;18(1):341–378. https://doi.org/10.1146/annurev.publhealth.18.1.341
11. Pfeffer FT. Growing wealth gaps in education. *Demography*. 2018;55(3):1033–1068. https://doi.org/10.1007/s13524-018-0666-7
12. McKeown T. *The Modern Rise of Population*. London, England: Edward Arnold; 1976:168.
13. Mackenbach JP. The contribution of medical care to mortality decline: McKeown revisited. *J Clin Epidemiol*. 1996;49(11):1207–1213. https://doi.org/10.1016/s0895-4356(96)00200-4
14. Bunker JP, Frazier HS, Mosteller F. Improving health: measuring effects of medical care. *Milbank Q*. 1994;72(2):225–258. https://doi.org/10.2307/3350295
15. Cutler DM, Rosen AB, Vijan S. The value of medical spending in the United States, 1960–2000. *N Engl J Med*. 2006;355(9):920–927. https://doi.org/10.1056/NEJMsa054744
16. Basu S, Berkowitz SA, Phillips RL, Bitton A, Landon BE, Phillips RS. Association of primary care physician supply with population mortality in the United States, 2005–2015. *JAMA Intern Med*. 2019;179(4):506–514. https://doi.org/10.1001/jamainternmed.2018.7624
17. Starfield B, Shi L, Macinko J. Contribution of primary care to health systems and health. *Milbank Q*. 2005;83(3):457–502. https://doi.org/10.1111/j.1468-0009.2005.00409.x
18. *Unequal Treatment: Confronting Racial and Ethnic Disparities in Health Care* (with CD). Washington, DC: National Academies Press; 2003 Available at: http://www.nap.edu/catalog/12875. Accessed September 11, 2024.
19. Rutstein DD, Berenberg W, Chalmers TC, Child CG, Fishman AP, Perrin EB. Measuring the quality of medical care. *N Engl J Med*. 1976; 294(11):582–588. https://doi.org/10.1056/NEJM197603112941104
20. Nolte E, McKee CM. In amenable mortality—deaths avoidable through health care—progress in the US lags that of three European countries. *Health Aff (Millwood)*. 2012;31(9):2114–2122. https://doi.org/10.1377/hlthaff.2011.0851
21. Agency for Healthcare Research and Quality. Medical Expenditure Panel Survey data overview. Available at: https://meps.ahrq.gov/mepsweb/data_stats/data_overview.jsp. Accessed August 18, 2024.
22. Blewett LA, Rivera Drew JA, Backman D, et al. IPUMS Health Surveys: Medical Expenditure Panel Survey, Version 2.3. Minneapolis, MN: IPUMS; 2023. https://doi.org/10.18128/D071.V2.3
23. National Bureau of Economic Research. Mortality Data - Vital Statistics NCHS Multiple Cause of Death Data. 2023. Available at: https://www.nber.org/research/data/mortality-data-vital-statistics-nchs-multiple-cause-death-data. Accessed August 18, 2024.
24. Ruggles S, Flood S, Sobek M, et al. IPUMS USA: Version 15.0. Minneapolis, MN: IPUMS; 2024. https://doi.org/10.18128/D010.V15.0
25. IPUMS Medical Expenditure Panel Survey. EDUC. Available at: https://meps.ipums.org/meps-action/variables/EDUC#comparability_section. Accessed August 15, 2024.
26. OECD/Eurostat. Avoidable mortality: OECD/Eurostat lists of preventable and treatable causes of death (January 2022 version). January 2022. Available at: https://www.oecd.org/content/dam/oecd/en/data/datasets/oecd-health-statistics/avoidable-mortality-2019-joint-oecd-eurostat-list-preventable-treatable-causes-of-death.pdf. Accessed August 16, 2024.
27. Lumley T, Diehr P, Emerson S, Chen L. The importance of the normality assumption in large public health data sets. *Annu Rev Public Health*. 2002;23:151–169. https://doi.org/10.1146/annurev.publhealth.23.100901.140546
28. Zou G. A modified Poisson regression approach to prospective studies with binary data. *Am J Epidemiol*. 2004;159(7):702–706. https://doi.org/10.1093/aje/kwh090
29. Johansen ME, Niforatos JD. Decreasing use of primary care: a repeated cross-sectional study of MEPS 2007–2017. *Ann Fam Med*. 2021;19(1): 41–43. https://doi.org/10.1370/afm.2631
30. Ganguli I, Shi Z, Orav EJ, Rao A, Ray KN, Mehrotra A. Declining use of primary care among commercially insured adults in the United States, 2008–2016. *Ann Intern Med*. 2020;172(4): 240–247. https://doi.org/10.7326/M19-1834
31. Gaffney A, Himmelstein DU, Dickman S, McCormick D, Cai C, Woolhandler S. Trends and disparities in the distribution of outpatient physicians' annual face time with patients, 1979–2018. *J Gen Intern Med*. 2023;38(2):434–441. https://doi.org/10.1007/s11606-022-07688-x

32. Papanicolas I, Niksch M, Figueroa JF. Avoidable mortality across US states and high-income countries. *JAMA Intern Med.* 2025;185(5):583–590. https://doi.org/10.1001/jamainternmed.2025.0155

33. Luck AN, Preston SH, Elo IT, Stokes AC. The unequal burden of the Covid-19 pandemic: capturing racial/ethnic disparities in US cause-specific mortality. *SSM Popul Health.* 2022;17:101012. https://doi.org/10.1016/j.ssmph.2021.101012

34. Diderichsen F, Hallqvist J, Whitehead M. Differential vulnerability and susceptibility: how to make use of recent development in our understanding of mediation and interaction to tackle health inequalities. *Int J Epidemiol.* 2019;48(1):268–274. https://doi.org/10.1093/ije/dyy167

35. Montez JK, Zajacova A, Hayward MD, Woolf SH, Chapman D, Beckfield J. Educational disparities in adult mortality across US states: how do they differ, and have they changed since the mid-1980s? *Demography.* 2019;56(2):621–644. https://doi.org/10.1007/s13524-018-0750-z

Economic Hardship; Coronavirus Aid, Relief, and Economic Security (CARES) Act Payments; and Self-Rated Health: A Longitudinal Analysis From the Health and Retirement Study, United States, 2020–2022

Samuel L. Swift, PhD, MPH, Brady P. Horn, PhD, Barbara N. Harding, PhD, Macaiah Shendo, BA, Tracie C. Collins, MD, MPH, MHCDS, and Adina Zeki Al Hazzouri, PhD, MSc

AJPH May 2026, Vol. 116, No. 5

Objectives. To determine the longitudinal relationships between economic hardship in 2020 and self-rated health (SRH) in 2022, and whether monetary stimulus payments offset negative health consequences of economic hardship among older adults living in the United States.

Methods. We used data from 7549 adults aged 50 years or older from all US states in the longitudinal Health and Retirement Study cohort. Using Poisson regression models, we evaluated the relationship between economic hardship in 2020 and "fair or poor" SRH in 2022, and whether receipt of stimulus payments modified this relationship, controlling for covariates.

Results. In stratified analysis, among persons who did not receive a stimulus payment, economic hardship was associated with higher risk of "fair or poor" SRH (risk ratio [RR] = 1.50; 95% confidence interval [CI] = 1.22, 1.85). Among persons who received a stimulus payment, the relationship between economic hardship and "fair or poor" SRH was nonsignificant (RR = 1.06; 95% CI = 0.96, 1.17).

Conclusions. Receipt of a stimulus payment may have offset the negative consequences of economic hardship on SRH among persons aged 50 years and older.

Public Health Implications. Monetary payments may be an effective health intervention for persons experiencing economic hardship. (*Am J Public Health*. 2026;116(5):702–710. https://doi.org/10.2105/AJPH.2025.308414)

Economic hardship during recessions is strongly associated with adverse health outcomes,[1–6] including self-rated health (SRH).[7,8] The economic recession caused by the disruption in labor markets during the 2020 COVID-19 pandemic provides a unique opportunity for studying the relationship between recessionary economic conditions and health within the United States.[9] Like other types of economic hardship, economic hardship during the COVID-19 pandemic has been shown to be associated with negative health outcomes.[2,5,6,10,11]

To alleviate the loss of income caused by the recession, in 2020, the US government (and governments in many other countries) provided direct economic stimulus relief payments to income-eligible citizens.[12] In the United States, this was done through the Coronavirus Aid, Relief, and Economic Security (CARES) Act, which provided direct monetary payments to income-eligible citizens between March 2020 and January 2021.[12] These payments ranged in value, but individuals were eligible for 1-time payments of up to $1200, while married couples filing jointly were eligible for up to $2400, with additional money available for persons with dependent children.[12] The use of such direct monetary payments during a recession is novel, and consequently understudied. However, there is a robust literature demonstrating social assistance programs like cash transfers may improve health for persons experiencing financial hardship.[13–15]

For the present analysis, we examined the relationship between economic hardship in 2020, CARES Act stimulus payments, and SRH. SRH has been shown to be a strong predictor of mortality,[16] depression,[17] and composite variables of physical health,[17] giving this measure strong predictive validity as a health outcome. Some literature has demonstrated that the CARES Act payments were helpful to counteract the negative health consequences of economic hardship during the pandemic, at least partially.[5,6,18] However, to our knowledge, no research has examined the longitudinal relationship between hardship, stimulus payments, and SRH. The objective of this analysis was to determine the longitudinal relationships between economic hardship in 2020, CARES Act stimulus payments, and SRH in 2022, among Health and Retirement Study (HRS) participants. We investigated 2 hypotheses: (1) that economic hardship experienced during 2020 is longitudinally associated with worse SRH in 2022 and (2) that receipt of a CARES Act stimulus payment modifies the relationship between economic hardship and SRH, offsetting the negative consequences of economic hardship on SRH.

METHODS

The HRS (University of Michigan, National Institute on Aging U01AG009740), which began in 1992, is an ongoing longitudinal cohort of adults living in the United States aged 50 years and older.[19] The study methods are described elsewhere.[20] In brief, the HRS uses "steady state" design, which means that every 6 years the HRS replenishes the cohort sample by recruiting a younger cohort of participants. Participants are recontacted every 2 years using telephone and mail-in interviews, and proxy interviews in which household members may answer questions for themselves and others within the household. In the 2020 wave (2020–2021), 15 171 participants responded to these interviews. A portion of the sample was then randomly selected to answer questions about experiences of the COVID-19 pandemic, which included our primary exposure.[21] Of those, approximately 75% answered questions on our outcome in 2020–2021 and again in a 2022–2023 follow-up interview, giving us an analytical sample of 7549 for unadjusted models examining the association between hardship and self-rated health. Figure 1 details subsequent restrictions that we made for different levels of our analysis.

Outcome

In both waves, participants reported their SRH using the following 5-point question: "Would you say your health is (1) excellent, (2) very good, (3) good, (4) fair, or (5) poor?" As is commonly done in studies using self-rated health as the outcome,[22] we dichotomized this variable into "fair or poor" SRH versus "excellent, very good, or good" SRH. To evaluate the longitudinal consequences of economic hardship during the pandemic, our study outcome was "fair or poor" SRH in 2022, controlled for continuous 2020 SRH status.

Exposures

The 2020 wave of the HRS study administered a special core module on the COVID-19 pandemic to a random subsample of participants. This module included questions on hardship during 2020 and whether participants received the CARES Act stimulus payment. Economic hardship was measured in the 2020 HRS using a question that asked, "Did you experience any of the following: (1) missed any regular payments on rent or mortgage, (2) missed any regular payments on credit cards or other debt, (3) missed any other regular payments such as utilities or insurance, (4) could not pay medical bills, (5) didn't have enough money to buy food, (6) had trouble buying food even though had enough money, or (7) no hardship, or (8) other material hardship?" For our main analysis, we categorized participants experiencing economic hardship as a "yes" answer to any of the choices (1–6) and not experiencing economic hardship as reporting "no hardship" (choice 7). We coded "other material hardship" as missing, given that category was unquantifiable in comparison with the other categories.

Stimulus payment was defined using the following question, asked only of the designated household financial respondent: "Because of the coronavirus crisis, many families will receive an economic impact payment of up to twelve hundred dollars for individuals, twenty-four hundred dollars for couples, and five hundred dollars for each interviewer dependent child." For participants

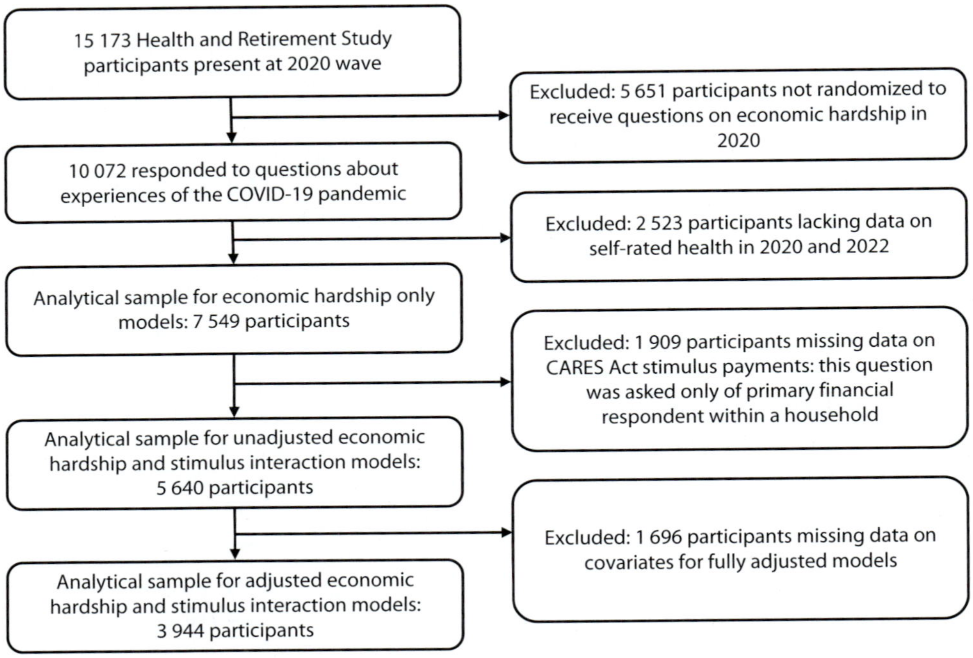

FIGURE 1— Study Flow Diagram and Analytical Samples, the Health and Retirement Study: United States, 2020–2022

Note. CARES = Coronavirus Aid, Relief, and Economic Security.

contacted later in 2020 and 2021, this question was slightly amended to reflect the timing of the payments and possible amounts.[21] Participants were able to select 1 of 3 answer choices: "Yes/yes both [persons in the household] received payment" (if there were more than 2 HRS respondents in the household), "Yes, but only one person in the household received the payment" (if there were more than 2 HRS respondents in the household and only 1 person received it), versus "no one received the payment." We operationalized receiving a CARES Act stimulus payment for our primary analysis as "anyone in the household received a payment" (yes, 1 or yes, both received it) versus "no one in the household received a payment." In all analysis, CARES Act payment was treated as an effect modifier to evaluate our hypothesis that CARES Act payment could offset the negative health outcomes of economic hardship in 2020.

Covariates

We included the following confounders in our models. We defined age in 2020 as self-reported in continuous years. To control for a more granular construct of baseline SRH, we adjusted all models for continuous 5-point scale 2020 self-rated health, which was collected as explained previously. We included level of education, operationalized as "high school education or less," "degree unknown or some college," and "2-year college or more." We defined self-reported race/ethnicity using the categories "non-Hispanic white/Caucasian," "non-Hispanic Black/African American," "non-Hispanic Other," and "Hispanic." We included self-reported "male" or "female" gender. We defined 2020 employment status using the categories "employed," "unemployed," "retired," and "laid off, either temporarily laid off or due to the pandemic." We defined 2020 marital status using the categories "married," "separated," "divorced," "single," or "widowed." We defined 2020 health insurance status using categories of "any health insurance" versus "no health insurance." Health insurance status was defined using self-reported and imputed data, using methods described elsewhere.[23] We defined nativity using the self-reported categories "US-born" versus "not US-born." We defined body mass index in continuous units (weight in kilograms divided by the square of height in meters) in 2020, using self-reported height and weight and the metric conversion formula weight in pounds divided by the square of height in inches multiplied by 703. We defined dichotomous physical activity as self-reported "vigorous" or "moderate" physical activity "more than once a week" versus "once per week or less." We defined 2020 smoking status using the self-reported categories "never smoker," "former smoker," and "current smoker." For our descriptive analysis, we provided data on 2020 household income, measured in dollars from all income sources, as well as 2020 household assets, measured as the sum total value of all household assets in dollars (which are derived from the HRS RAND data, described elsewhere).[23]

Statistical Analysis

First, we presented basic descriptive statistics of our study sample, stratified by hardship in 2020. In this descriptive analysis, we evaluated differences in covariates across strata of hardship using the *t* test for continuous variables and the χ^2 test for categorical variables. In our descriptive analysis, we also included measures of household income and household assets.

In our main analysis, we used Poisson models with robust standard errors to investigate the cumulative incidence risk ratio of "fair or poor" SRH among persons who experienced hardship and received CARES Act stimulus payments. Poisson models are appropriate for this scenario because "fair or poor" SRH is relatively common in our sample, and in this situation an odds ratio produced by logistic regression will overestimate the relative risk.[24]

We presented 4 models, adding additional confounders in stages to check for robustness of our associations across models. Model 1 examined the association between economic hardship and SRH, adjusted only for 2020 baseline SRH. In model 2, we additionally adjusted for receipt of a stimulus payment. In model 3, we additionally adjusted for age, level of education, self-reported race, self-reported sex or gender, employment status, marital status, health insurance status, and US-born (vs not).

In our final model (model 4) we additionally included covariates for 2020 body mass index, physical activity status, and smoking status. For model 4, we also included a variable to reflect the interaction between economic hardship and stimulus payment, with the following 4 levels: "had hardship and received payment," "had hardship and did not receive payment," "did not have hardship and received payment," and "no hardship and no payment" as the reference group. For model 4 we did not include the separate variables for stimulus and hardship.

We did not adjust these models for household income or household wealth, as these variables are highly colinear with economic hardship in 2020. Because of the sample subsetting, that the COVID-19 module was given to a random subsample of participants with different probabilities of selection than their survey weights reflect, and the potential for overinflating of variance, we did not use HRS study weights in our main analysis models, nor did we interpret our results as nationally representative. This approach is supported by recent recommendations for statistical survey weighted research.[25,26] We considered main effects in our models statistically significant at $P < .05$. Because of the potential for interaction terms being underpowered, we focused on consistency in the direction of the effect size for our interaction terms[27] and further investigated interactions at $P < .1$.

To investigate our hypothesis on the modifying role of stimulus payments in the relationship between hardship and SRH, we stratified our analysis by both CARES Act payments and hardship, examining the effect of hardship within strata of payment and payment within strata of hardship adjusting for all model 4 covariates.

Finally, we provide descriptive statistics on why persons who experienced an economic hardship did not receive CARES Act stimulus payments, assessed in HRS by asking "Do you expect to receive this payment, and if no, why not?"

Sensitivity Analysis

We conducted 8 sensitivity analyses. For these analyses, we repeated our main analysis with the covariates included in model 4. First, we accounted for income by adjusting for individual income, household income, household assets, and social security income, and we limited our sample to income-eligible CARES Act recipients in separate models (Table A, available as a supplement to the online version of this article at https://ajph.org). The income eligibility criteria for CARES Act stimulus payments was income of up to $75 000 for singles and married persons filing a separate return, up to $112 500 for heads of household, and up to $150 000 for married couples filing joint returns and surviving spouses.[12] We operationalized income eligibility according to marital status and income data from the RAND imputations.[23]

Second, we accounted for missing data in our analysis by first assuming that all persons who shared a household with persons who answered the stimulus question would have the same stimulus payment value as the person who answered the question, and by using multiple imputation on missing covariates in our main analysis using the mice package in R,[28] without robust standard errors, which are not available in the mice package. Third, we reran our main analysis using ordinal regression and a 5-level ordinal categorization of self-rated health, as well as logistic regression with our 2-level categorization (Table C, available as a supplement to the online version of this article at https://ajph.org). We also conducted 5 additional sensitivity analyses (not shown in the online supplement) as follows: (1) we conducted our main analysis using a 3-level categorization of stimulus payment (all persons in household got the payment, 1 out of 2 persons in the household got the payment, no one in the household got the payment); (2) we conducted our main analysis additionally adjusting for doctor-diagnosed heart disease and diabetes; (3) we conducted our main analysis examining a 3-level version of hardship, which allowed "trouble paying for food" to be its own category of hardship separate from the others and including "other material hardship" with all other hardships; (4) our main analysis examining continuous amount of stimulus payment; and (5) our main analysis conducted within a propensity score matched sample.

RESULTS

At baseline, 2332 persons experienced hardship in 2020, whereas 5217 persons did not. Those who experienced hardship were slightly more likely to have received a CARES Act stimulus payment, with 82.1% of those experiencing a hardship receiving a payment compared with 81.0% of those not experiencing a hardship. Other descriptive statistics stratified by experience of hardship can be found in Table 1.

In our main analysis (Table 2), we found that persons who experienced a hardship had a higher risk of "fair or poor" SRH, in our model unadjusted for stimulus payment and covariates. This relationship was consistent across models. Across models, the receipt of CARES Act stimulus payment was not associated with "fair or poor" SRH. In our final model, the interaction between hardship and payment was statistically significant for persons who had a hardship but did not receive a payment (risk ratio [RR] = 1.38; 95% confidence interval [CI] = 1.14, 1.69), and smaller but significant among those who had a hardship and received a payment (RR = 1.17; 95% CI = 1.00, 1.37), compared with those who did not have a hardship or receive a payment.

In our stratified analysis (Table 3), among persons who did not receive a stimulus payment, we found a strong relationship between economic hardship and "fair or poor" SRH (RR = 1.50; 95% CI = 1.22, 1.85). Among persons who received a stimulus payment, this relationship between economic hardship and "fair or poor" SRH was smaller and nonsignificant (RR = 1.06; 95% CI = 0.96, 1.17).

Table D (available as a supplement to the online version of this article at https://ajph.org) displays the reasons persons may have not received a stimulus check, among persons who reported hardship. The majority of the persons who experienced hardship were missing an answer to this question (45.9%); however, some reported income too high (11.8%), not being a US citizen (7.3%), and not paying taxes (4.2%) as reasons for not receiving payment.

Our 8 sensitivity analyses were consistent with our main analysis in direction and magnitude of association (Tables A–C, and supplementary analyses 1–5 not shown). The association attenuated slightly in our models limited to persons eligible for CARES Act payments (Table A) and with multiple imputation of covariates (Table B) but was robust to all other sensitivity analyses.

DISCUSSION

Our results provide consistent evidence that economic hardship during 2020 was associated with increased risk of self-rated health being "fair or poor" in 2022, adjusted for baseline self-rated health, stimulus payments, and other covariates. The results of our stratified analysis suggest that receipt of a CARES Act stimulus payment in 2020 may have offset the longitudinal consequences of economic hardship on SRH among persons aged 50 years or older in the HRS.

When we examined why people did not receive payment although they experienced hardship, the available data suggest that some participants' incomes were too high, some did not pay taxes, and others were not US citizens. This information helps us better understand this portion of the sample and the types of people that the policy did not reach.

Our results add important new information that complements existing similar studies that found that hardship in 2020 had negative health consequences,[2,5,6,10,11] as well as studies that found stimulus payments may have offset negative health consequences.[5,6,18,29] One meta-analysis found that across 49 studies, job loss during the pandemic was consistently associated with negative health outcomes, and that in 3 studies, stimulus payments mitigated the negative associations of these job losses.[6] Our study adds longitudinal evidence to previous cross-sectional analyses that also examined the interaction between

TABLE 1— Characteristics of Study Sample Stratified by Hardship, the Health and Retirement Study: United States, 2020

	Experienced Hardship in 2020 (n = 2332), No. (%) or Mean ±SD	Did Not Experience Hardship in 2020 (n = 5217), No. (%) or Mean ±SD	P[a]
Received CARES Act payment, anyone in HH (Ref = no one in HH received payment)	1 521 (82.1)	3 067 (81.0)	.31
2020 age, y	64.48 ±9.75	68.37 ±10.54	<.001
2020 self-rated health	2.81 ±1.02	3.24 ±0.97	<.001
2020 education level			
2 years of college or more	619 (26.5)	1 963 (37.6)	<.001
High school education or less	1 223 (52.4)	2 592 (49.7)	
Degree unknown or some college	490 (21.0)	662 (12.7)	
Race/ethnicity			<.001
Non-Hispanic White	902 (38.7)	3 109 (59.7)	
Non-Hispanic Black or African American	698 (29.9)	1 062 (20.4)	
Non-Hispanic other	148 (6.3)	243 (4.7)	
Hispanic	583 (25.0)	797 (15.3)	
Female gender (Ref = male)	1 529 (65.6)	3 035 (58.2)	<.001
2020 employment status			<.001
Employed	739 (31.9)	1 693 (32.6)	
Other	622 (26.8)	754 (14.5)	
Retired	742 (32.0)	2 525 (48.6)	
Unemployed	215 (9.3)	228 (4.4)	
2020 marital status			<.001
Married	1 024 (44.2)	2 897 (55.7)	
Separated or divorced	646 (27.9)	1 006 (19.3)	
Single	274 (11.8)	374 (7.2)	
Widowed	373 (16.1)	927 (17.8)	
Had health in insurance in 2020 (Ref = no health insurance)	1 919 (84.3)	4 568 (88.8)	<.001
Not born in the United States (Ref = born in United States)	562 (24.1)	800 (15.3)	<.001
2020 body mass index, kg/m^2	30.26 ±7.03	28.87 ±6.09	<.001
2020 physical activity "> weekly" (Ref = "once a week or less")	1 150 (49.5)	3 021 (58.1)	<.001
2020 smoking status			<.001
Never	953 (41.4)	2 533 (49.2)	
Former	910 (39.6)	2 121 (41.2)	
Current	437 (19.0)	498 (9.7)	
2020 total household income, US $	53 603.99 ±68 358.11	83 727.26 ±109 026.98	<.001
2020 total household assets, US $	303 995.18 ±929 193.28	651 696.61 ±1 259 364.82	<.001
Income eligible for CARES payment	1 885 (89.5)	3 936 (81.3)	<.001

Note. CARES = Coronavirus Aid, Relief, and Economic Security; HH = household.
[a]*P* values assessed with *t* test for continuous variables and χ^2 test for categorical variables.

hardship and stimulus. In the HRS, 1 cross-sectional study found that the stimulus mitigated depression among persons experiencing a hardship.[5] Another cross-sectional study in the US Household Pulse Survey found that stimulus payments had a stronger positive association with depression and anxiety among persons with low income or job loss.[18] Another cross-sectional study examined the relationships between stimulus payments and health outcomes; however, this study examined prevalent health outcomes and, therefore, did not

TABLE 2— Associations Between Economic Hardship in 2020, CARES Act Stimulus Payment in 2020, and "Fair or Poor" Self-Rated Health in the Health and Retirement Study in 2022: United States

	Main Effects and Interaction Terms for Persons Who Experienced Economic Hardships and Received CARES Act Stimulus Payments			
	Model 1, RR (95% CI)	Model 2, RR (95% CI)	Model 3, RR (95% CI)	Model 4, RR (95% CI)
Economic hardship during 2020 (Ref = no hardship)	1.17 (1.10, 1.24)	1.17 (1.09, 1.25)	1.16 (1.09, 1.25)	. . .
Anyone in household received payment (Ref = no payment)	. . .	0.93 (0.86, 1.01)	0.95 (0.88, 1.04)	. . .
Had hardship and received payment	. . .	. . .	. . .	1.17 (1.00, 1.37)
Had hardship and did not receive payment	. . .	. . .	. . .	1.38 (1.14, 1.69)
Did not have hardship and received payment	. . .	. . .	. . .	1.09 (0.94, 1.27)
Did not have hardship and did not receive payment	. . .	. . .	. . .	Ref

Note. CARES = Coronavirus Aid, Relief, and Economic Security; CI = confidence interval; RR = risk ratio. Model 1 adjusted for 2020 self-rated health alone. Model 2 is additionally adjusted for stimulus payment. Model 3 is additionally adjusted for age, level of education, self-reported race/ethnicity, self-reported sex or gender, employment status, marital status, US-born (vs not) and health insurance status. Model 4 additionally adjusted for body mass index in 2020, physical activity score in 2020, and smoking status in 2020, and includes a 4-level variable to reflect the interaction between hardship and payment.

evaluate the stimulus.[30] Finally, a small (n = 392) randomized controlled trial of a 2020 cash-transfer program in Canada found that among persons facing hardship, a cash payment of 1000 Canadian dollars was not associated with a subsequent improvement in self-rated health.[29]

Our study has limitations. First, the HRS only includes persons aged 50 years or older, which reduces generalizability. The observational study design increases the possibility that our results may be attributable to confounding by some unmeasured underlying difference between subpopulations; however, our results were robust to several sensitivity analyses. We believe that the similar numbers of persons who received the payment across strata of hardship may be attributable to the high-income threshold for stimulus eligibility, which raises questions about whether the payment was accurately targeted to assist persons experiencing hardship.

In addition, our measurements of hardship may not have fully captured all possible economic hardships, and categorizing all of these diverse hardships as 1 variable may have induced measurement error. However, using

TABLE 3— Association Between Economic Hardship and Receipt of a CARES Act Stimulus Payment in 2020 and "Fair or Poor" Self-Rated Health in 2022, Stratified Analysis, the Health and Retirement Study: United States

Stratification Variable and Strata	Model 1, RR (95% CI)
Stratified by payment receipt	
Effect of hardship among persons who did not receive stimulus (n = 4588)	1.50 (1.22, 1.85)
Effect of hardship among persons who received stimulus (n = 1052)	1.06 (0.96, 1.17)
Stratified by hardship	
Effect of stimulus among persons who experienced a hardship (n = 1852)	0.82 (0.71, 0.96)
Effect of stimulus among persons who did not experience hardship (n = 3788)	1.11 (0.95, 1.30)

Note. CARES = Coronavirus Aid, Relief, and Economic Security; CI = confidence interval; RR = risk ratio. All models are adjusted for 2020 self-rated health, age, level of education, self-reported race/ethnicity, self-reported sex or gender, employment status, marital status, US-born (vs not), health insurance status, body mass index in 2020, physical activity score in 2020, and smoking status in 2020.

the composite hardship variable captures a wider range of hardships than previous research that only looked at job loss in 2020,[6,18] and our analysis was robust to a sensitivity analysis using a 3-level construction of economic hardship.

Furthermore, SRH as an outcome is subjective and, therefore, may be at risk for some forms of response bias; however, SRH is associated with life satisfaction and may also capture a more holistic picture of how people view their own health.[31] SRH is a strong predictor of mortality[16] and other health outcomes,[17] demonstrating its validity as a health outcome for epidemiological research.

Another limitation is that while the HRS captured receipt of CARES Act payments, the question did not capture receipt of additional payments in 2021 from the American Rescue Plan Act, which provided additional economic stimulus payments to income-eligible US citizens.[32] As the eligibility criteria for both policies were the same,[12,32] it is likely that persons who received or did not receive payments were the same persons for both policies, so our results would likely be similar if we had this information.

Finally, a large number of participants were missing information because of only a subset of participants being randomized to receive hardship questions. Given the randomization, our analytic sample was less likely to be biased by this missingness.

Our study has notable strengths as well. By examining the relationship between economic hardship, CARES Act stimulus, and SRH longitudinally and controlling for baseline SRH, we ruled out demonstrated reverse causation[33] in the relationship between our exposures and SRH. Another notable strength is that by examining the interaction between the hardship and the stimulus, we provide evidence supporting the stimulus as an intervention, which is something that studies that only examined economic hardship are unable to do. Unlike economic hardship, which may be related to lifelong conditions, the stimulus presents an actionable intervention, strengthening the implications of our results. Our sample size was considerably large, which allowed for stratified analysis by receipt of a stimulus payment. Finally, although not always achieving the same statistical significance, our results were robust in magnitude and direction across our 8 sensitivity analyses. By demonstrating relatively consistent associations across models adjusted for different income-related constructs, different strategies for addressing missing data, and different statistical techniques, we further supported our results.

In conclusion, our results support the use of interventions like stimulus payments to offset the negative health-related consequences of hardship during an economic recession. These results may inform the use of similar interventions during future economic recessions. In addition, our results may inform broader conversations around the potential of sustained cash assistance programs like Universal Basic Income,[34] which may become important given changing global economic conditions.[35] We recommend future research on the associations between these types of payments and long-term health outcomes. Finally, we recommend that policies designed to address economic hardship also consider the potential positive outcomes of these policies on SRH and other health outcomes. AJPH

ABOUT THE AUTHORS

Samuel L. Swift, Barbara N. Harding, Macaiah Shendo, and Tracie C. Collins are with the College of Population Health, University of New Mexico, Albuquerque. Brady P. Horn is with the Department of Economics, and the Center on Alcohol, Substance Use, and Addictions, University of New Mexico, Albuquerque. Adina Zeki Al Hazzouri is with the Mailman School of Public Health, Columbia University, New York, NY.

CORRESPONDENCE

Correspondence should be sent to Samuel L. Swift, PhD, MPH, Assistant Professor, College of Population Health, University of New Mexico, 2300 Tucker Ave NE, Albuquerque, NM 87131 (e-mail: samswift@salud.unm.edu). Reprints can be ordered at https://www.ajph.org by clicking the "Reprints" link.

PUBLICATION INFORMATION

Full Citation: Swift SL, Horn BP, Harding BN, Shendo M, Collins TC, Zeki Al Hazzouri A. Economic hardship; Coronavirus Aid, Relief, and Economic Security (CARES) Act payments; and self-rated health: a longitudinal analysis from the Health and Retirement Study, United States, 2020–2022. *Am J Public Health*. 2026;116(5): 702–710.

Acceptance Date: December 26, 2025.

DOI: https://doi.org/10.2105/AJPH.2025.308414

ORCID iDs:

Samuel L. Swift https://orcid.org/0000-0001-5858-8247

Barbara N. Harding https://orcid.org/0000-0002-9460-9399

Macaiah Shendo https://orcid.org/0009-0008-8511-3886

CONTRIBUTORS

S. L. Swift originated the study design, performed analysis, and drafted the article. B. P. Horn provided technical guidance for analysis and provided a critical review of the article. B. N. Harding provided help drafting the article. M. Shendo assisted with coding in the analysis and provided a critical review of the article. T. C. Collins and A. Zeki Al Hazzouri provided a critical review of the article.

ACKNOWLEDGMENTS

The Health and Retirement Study is sponsored by the National Institute on Aging (grant NIA U01AG009740) and is conducted by the University of Michigan.

CONFLICTS OF INTEREST

The authors have no conflicts of interest to report for this research.

HUMAN PARTICIPANT PROTECTION

The Health and Retirement Study procedures are approved by the University of Michigan institutional review board and conform to the principles of the Declaration of Helsinki.

REFERENCES

1. Noelke C, Avendano M. Who suffers during recessions? Economic downturns, job loss, and cardiovascular disease in older Americans. *Am J Epidemiol.* 2015;182(10):873–882. https://doi.org/10.1093/aje/kwv094
2. Banks J, Karjalainen H, Propper C. Recessions and health: the long-term health consequences of responses to the coronavirus. *Fisc Stud.* 2020;41(2):337–344. https://doi.org/10.1111/1475-5890.12230
3. Swift SL, Elfassy T, Bailey Z, et al. Association of negative financial shocks during the Great Recession with depressive symptoms and substance use in the USA: the CARDIA study. *J Epidemiol Community Health.* 2020;74(12):995–1001. https://doi.org/10.1136/jech-2020-213917
4. Riumallo-Herl C, Basu S, Stuckler D, Courtin E, Avendano M. Job loss, wealth and depression during the Great Recession in the USA and Europe. *Int J Epidemiol.* 2014;43(5):1508–1517. https://doi.org/10.1093/ije/dyu048
5. Liu Y, Zhang Y, Chatterjee S. Financial hardship and depression experienced by pre-retirees during the COVID-19 pandemic: the mitigating role of stimulus payments. *Appl Econ Lett.* 2023;30(3):391–396. https://doi.org/10.1080/13504851.2021.1989364
6. McNamara CL, Kotzias V, Bambra C, Labonté R, Stuckler D. Have COVID-19 stimulus packages mitigated the negative health impacts of pandemic-related job losses? A systematic review of global evidence from the first year of the pandemic. *Int J Soc Determinants Health Health Serv.* 2023;53(3):311–322. https://doi.org/10.1177/27551938231176374
7. Mulia N, Ye Y, Karriker-Jaffe KJ, Li L, Kerr WC, Greenfield TK. The Great Recession, behavioral health, and self-rated health: an examination of racial/ethnic differences in the US. *Addict Behav.* 2021;118:106873. https://doi.org/10.1016/j.addbeh.2021.106873
8. Huijts T, Reeves A, McKee M, Stuckler D. The impacts of job loss and job recovery on self-rated health: testing the mediating role of financial strain and income. *Eur J Public Health.* 2015;25(5):801–806. https://doi.org/10.1093/eurpub/ckv108
9. Brenner MH. Will there be an epidemic of corollary illnesses linked to a COVID-19–related recession? *Am J Public Health.* 2020;110(7):974–975. https://doi.org/10.2105/AJPH.2020.305724
10. Witteveen D, Velthorst E. Economic hardship and mental health complaints during COVID-19. *Proc Natl Acad Sci U S A.* 2020;117(44):27277–27284. https://doi.org/10.1073/pnas.2009609117
11. Odani S, Shinozaki T, Shibuya K, Tabuchi T. Economic hardships and self-reported deterioration of physical and mental health under the COVID-19 pandemic: a cross-sectional study, 2020, Japan. *J Epidemiol.* 2022;32(4):195–203. https://doi.org/10.2188/jea.JE20210268
12. Murphy D. *Economic Impact Payments.* Washington, DC: Brookings Institution; 2021.
13. Courtin E, Kim S, Song S, Yu W, Muennig P. Can social policies improve health? A systematic review and meta-analysis of 38 randomized trials. *Milbank Q.* 2020;98(2):297–371. https://doi.org/10.1111/1468-0009.12451
14. Shahidi FV, Ramraj C, Sod-Erdene O, Hildebrand V, Siddiqi A. The impact of social assistance programs on population health: a systematic review of research in high-income countries. *BMC Public Health.* 2019;19(1):2. https://doi.org/10.1186/s12889-018-6337-1
15. Sun S, Huang J, Hudson DL, Sherraden M. Cash transfers and health. *Annu Rev Public Health.* 2021;42:363–380. https://doi.org/10.1146/annurev-publhealth-090419-102442
16. Schnittker J, Bacak V. The increasing predictive validity of self-rated health. *PLoS One.* 2014;9(1):e84933. https://doi.org/10.1371/journal.pone.0084933
17. Baćak V, Ólafsdóttir S. Gender and validity of self-rated health in nineteen European countries. *Scand J Public Health.* 2017;45(6):647–653. https://doi.org/10.1177/1403494817717405
18. Chu L, Teng L. Does stimulus check payment improve people's mental health in the COVID-19 pandemic? Evidence from US Household Pulse Survey. *J Ment Health Policy Econ.* 2022;25(4):133–142. https://doi.org/10.1016/j.enpol.2022.113011
19. Sonnega A, Faul JD, Ofstedal MB, Langa KM, Phillips JW, Weir DR. Cohort profile: the Health and Retirement Study (HRS). *Int J Epidemiol.* 2014;43(2):576–585. https://doi.org/10.1093/ije/dyu067
20. Juster FT, Suzman R. An overview of the Health and Retirement Study. *J Hum Resour.* 1995;30:S7–S56. https://doi.org/10.2307/146277
21. Health and Retirement Study. 2020 Core, Final, Version 1.0, Data Description and Usage. May 2023. Available at: https://hrsdata.isr.umich.edu/sites/default/files/documentation/data-descriptions/1686078541/h20dd.pdf. Accessed December 15, 2024.
22. Tucker-Seeley RD, Harley AE, Stoddard AM, Sorensen GG. Financial hardship and self-rated health among low-income housing residents. *Health Educ Behav.* 2013;40(4):442–448. https://doi.org/10.1177/1090198112463021
23. Chien S, Campbell N, Hayden O, et al. RAND HRS data documentation, version N. RAND Corporation. 2015. Available at: https://hrsonline.isr.umich.edu/modules/meta/rand/randhrso/randhrs_O.pdf. Accessed December 15, 2024.
24. Knol MJ, Le Cessie S, Algra A, Vandenbroucke JP, Groenwold RH. Overestimation of risk ratios by odds ratios in trials and cohort studies: alternatives to logistic regression. *CMAJ.* 2012;184(8):895–899. https://doi.org/10.1503/cmaj.101715
25. Bollen KA, Biemer PP, Karr AF, Tueller S, Berzofsky ME. Are survey weights needed? A review of diagnostic tests in regression analysis. *Annu Rev Stat Appl.* 2016;3(1):375–392. https://doi.org/10.1146/annurev-statistics-011516-012958
26. Solon G, Haider SJ, Wooldridge JM. What are we weighting for? *J Human Resources.* 2015;50(2):301–316. https://doi.org/10.3368/jhr.50.2.301
27. Matthews JNS, Altman DG. Statistics notes: interaction 2: compare effect sizes not *P* values. *BMJ.* 1996;313(7060):808. https://doi.org/10.1136/bmj.313.7060.808
28. Van Buuren S, Groothuis-Oudshoorn K. mice: Multivariate imputation by chained equations in R. *J Stat Soft.* 2011;45(3):1–67. https://doi.org/10.18637/jss.v045.i03
29. Persaud N, Thorpe KE, Bedard M, DISTANSE COVID-19 Study Team, et al. Cash transfer during the COVID-19 pandemic: a multicentre, randomised controlled trial. *Fam Med Community Health.* 2021;9(4):e001452. https://doi.org/10.1136/fmch-2021-001452
30. Tsai J, Huang M, Montgomery AE, Elbogen EB. Receipt, spending, and clinical correlates of the economic impact payment among middle- and low-income US adults. *Psychiatr Serv.* 2021;72(12):1377–1384. https://doi.org/10.1176/appi.ps.202100001
31. Siahpush M, Spittal M, Singh GK. Happiness and life satisfaction prospectively predict self-rated health, physical health, and the presence of limiting, long-term health conditions. *Am J Health Promot.* 2008;23(1):18–26. https://doi.org/10.4278/ajhp.061023137
32. US Department of Treasury. Economic Impact Payments. 2025. Available at: https://home.treasury.gov/policy-issues/coronavirus/assistance-for-american-families-and-workers/economic-impact-payments. Accessed December 15, 2024.
33. Bierman A, Upenieks L, Glavin P, Schieman S. Accumulation of economic hardship and health during the COVID-19 pandemic: social causation or selection? *Soc Sci Med.* 2021;275:113774. https://doi.org/10.1016/j.socscimed.2021.113774
34. Johnson AF, Roberto KJ. The COVID-19 pandemic: time for a universal basic income? *Public Adm Dev.* 2020;40(4):232–235. https://doi.org/10.1002/pad.1891
35. Virgilio GPM, Saavedra Hoyos F, Bao Ratzemberg CB. The impact of artificial intelligence on unemployment: a review. *IJSE.* 2024;51(12):1680–1695. https://doi.org/10.1108/IJSE-05-2023-0338

Psychosocial Risk and Resilience as Moderators of the Association Between Neighborhood Disadvantage and Incident Cardiovascular Disease Across Ethnoracial Groups: Multi-Ethnic Study of Atherosclerosis, United States, 2000–2019

Hannah Pleasants, BA, James R. Pike, MS, Priya Palta, PhD, Alain G. Bertoni, MD, PhD, Timothy M. Hughes, PhD, Qian Xiao, PhD, Jana A. Hirsch, PhD, MES, and Ganga S. Bey, PhD, MPH

AJPH May 2026, Vol. 116, No. 5

Objectives. To determine whether optimism and anger modify the association between neighborhood disadvantage and incident cardiovascular disease (CVD) and whether these relationships vary by ethnoracial group.

Methods. We drew data from 4326 participants in the Multi-Ethnic Study of Atherosclerosis (MESA: 2000–2019), a cohort of US adults aged 45 to 84 years without baseline CVD. We measured neighborhood disadvantage using the Area Deprivation Index. We assessed optimism and anger (reaction and temperament) by self-report. We used multilevel Cox proportional hazards models to estimate hazard ratios for incident CVD over 19 years of follow-up, adjusting for demographic, behavioral, and clinical factors.

Results. A total of 879 incident CVD events occurred. Greater neighborhood disadvantage was associated with higher CVD risk. Tract-level optimism attenuated this association, whereas tract-level anger amplified it. Effects of optimism were stronger among Black participants, whereas anger more strongly exacerbated risk among Hispanic participants.

Conclusions. Psychosocial resilience and risk factors modify the impact of neighborhood disadvantage on CVD, with important ethnoracial differences.

Public Health Implications. Structural and community-partnered strategies are needed to address ethnoracial differences in how psychosocial factors modify the cardiovascular effects of neighborhood disadvantage. (*Am J Public Health*. 2026;116(5):711–721. https://doi.org/10.2105/AJPH.2025.308407)

Cardiovascular disease (CVD) remains a leading cause of death in the United States, with marked disparities in incidence across neighborhoods. Individuals living in disadvantaged neighborhoods face elevated CVD risk regardless of individual socioeconomic status, yet those exposed to similar neighborhood stressors may exhibit different levels of resilience or vulnerability.[1,2] Modifiable psychosocial factors such as dispositional optimism and anger shape an individual's resilience or susceptibility to the harmful effects of chronic stress on cardiovascular health.[3,4] These factors influence how individuals perceive and experience stress related to living in disadvantaged neighborhoods, ultimately modulating physiological pathways linked to CVD risk.[5,6]

Structural factors, including long-standing discriminatory policies, have concentrated marginalized ethnoracial communities in disadvantaged neighborhoods, exacerbating CVD risk among ethnically and racially minoritized groups.[7] However, our previous work reveals that psychosocial resilience, particularly through dispositional optimism, plays a protective role by reducing the risk of incident heart failure among Black individuals.[8] Similarly, in a study of a diverse Hispanic/Latina/o ("Hispanic" from here on) population, higher levels of optimism were associated with better cardiovascular health outcomes, further suggesting that psychosocial factors can positively influence health even in the context of adversity.[9] Conversely, we found that psychosocial risk amplifies the impact of perceived neighborhood problems on incident heart failure by accelerating biological aging among Black persons.[10]

Despite growing evidence on the interplay between social environment, individual psychosocial factors, and CVD risk, to our knowledge, no study has explored how these factors interact across different ethnoracial groups. Comparing socially defined groups solely by the extent of disadvantage they experience overlooks key sociocultural differences in psychosocial factors that influence how social stressors affect health within and across populations. Understanding how psychosocial risk and resilience shape the association between neighborhood disadvantage and CVD across ethnoracial groups is key to developing interventions that consider sociocultural and psychosocial determinants of health. We evaluated whether psychosocial risk and resilience—operationalized as anger and optimism, respectively—modify the association between neighborhood disadvantage and incident CVD and whether these associations differ across ethnoracial groups. We hypothesized that optimism would attenuate and anger would amplify the association between neighborhood disadvantage and CVD with variation in these associations across racial and ethnic groups.

METHODS

The Multi-Ethnic Study of Atherosclerosis (MESA) is a prospective cohort study initiated in 2000 that investigates risk factors for subclinical CVD and its progression to clinical CVD events.[11]

Study Population

The cohort enrolled 6814 CVD-free participants aged 45 to 84 years from 6 US communities (New York, NY; Chicago, IL; Los Angeles, CA; Twin Cities, MN; Baltimore, MD; Winston-Salem, NC). For this investigation of neighborhood-level factors associated with incident CVD from 2000 to 2019, we excluded participants from the analytic sample (Figure 1) if their 9-digit zip code was unknown (n = 651), if they resided in a census tract with less than 5 participants (n = 1835), or if they had an incident CVD event before baseline (n = 2).

Measures

We measured neighborhood disadvantage using the National Area Deprivation Index (ADI),[12] which is derived from 5-year data from the 2000 American Community Survey. The ADI, a widely used metric of neighborhood deprivation, includes 17 indicators of income, education, employment, and housing quality at the census block group level.[12] Rankings range from 1 (least deprived) to 100 (most deprived) and are standardized to the census tract level.

Optimism was assessed at the second MESA examination (exam 2; 2002–2004) with the Life Orientation Test-Revised (LOT-R), a validated 6-item scale[13] in which higher scores represent higher levels of self-reported optimism. At the baseline examination (exam 1; 2000–2002), trait anger was assessed using the 10-item Spielberger Trait Anger Scale,[14] in which higher scores correspond to an angrier disposition. We separately assessed the 2 predefined subscales of the Spielberger Trait Anger Scale: anger temperament and anger reaction.[14] Higher scores on the anger temperament subscale correspond to a tendency to experience intense, unprovoked anger across various situations, and higher scores on the anger reaction subscale correspond to a tendency to anger in response to perceived criticism, injustice, or frustration. An examination of the distribution of responses revealed sizable skew (> 1) and kurtosis (> 6) across LOT-R and Spielberger Trait Anger Scale items. Consequently, we treated all items as categorical indicators in a multilevel confirmatory factor analysis[15] model that computed 2 factor scores for each moderator: 1 at the neighborhood level (census tract) and 1 representing subject-specific deviation from that mean.

Participants were contacted every 9 to 12 months to report hospital admissions, outpatient CVD diagnoses, and deaths. Diagnoses included myocardial

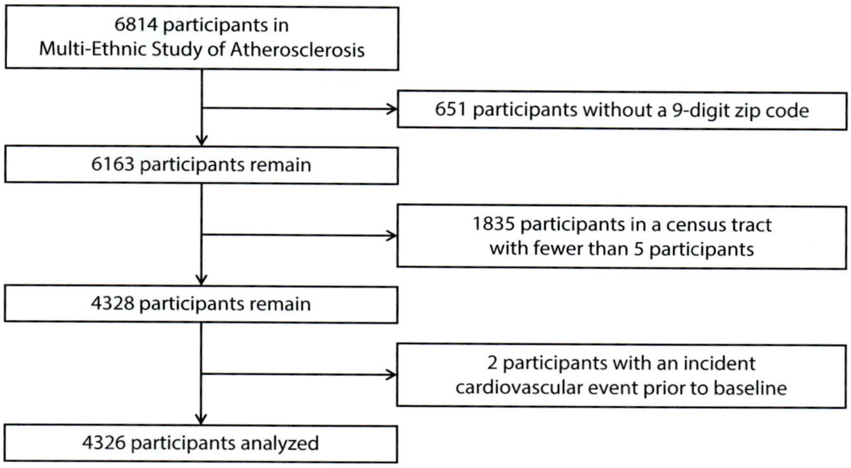

FIGURE 1— Flowchart of Participants Selected for Analysis: Multi-Ethnic Study of Atherosclerosis Cohort, United States, 2000–2019

infarction, angina pectoris, coronary revascularization, peripheral vascular disease, cardiac arrest, stroke, and coronary heart disease. We defined incident CVD as the first instance of any of the included events. Two physician adjudicators independently reviewed events, and the MESA Mortality and Morbidity Review Committee resolved disagreements.

Myocardial infarction was classified based on symptoms, electrocardiogram findings, and biomarkers. Angina pectoris was classified as definite or probable based on symptoms of chest pain, tightness, or shortness of breath produced by myocardial ischemia and evidence of coronary atherosclerosis. Revascularization included coronary artery bypass graft, percutaneous transluminal coronary angioplasty, coronary stent, coronary atherectomy, and other arterial revascularization. We defined peripheral vascular disease using MESA-adjudicated clinical events, which included symptomatic peripheral artery disease confirmed by objective testing or procedures.[11] Cardiac arrest was identified from medical records.[10] We defined stroke using MESA-adjudicated clinical events, which included a rapid onset of neurologic deficit, headache, or meningismus, and neurologic deficits not secondary to brain trauma (closed head injury), tumor, infection (e.g., encephalitis or meningitis), or other nonvascular causes, and clinically relevant lesion on brain imaging or duration greater than 24 hours or death within 24 hours. Coronary heart disease was categorized as definite or probable based on medical records.

We used data from exam 1 for all covariates except daytime sleepiness, which was assessed at exam 2. Sociodemographic covariates were assessed using in-person self-report questionnaires and included age, sex, race/ethnicity, site, education level, and annual income. Standardized questionnaires administered by trained interviewers were used to collect information on covariates, including cigarette use, alcohol use, physical activity, and daytime sleepiness. Additional covariates, including diabetes, hypertension, hypertension medication use, total cholesterol, high-density lipoprotein (HDL) cholesterol, and triglycerides, were measured at MESA exams.

We categorized cigarette use as never, former, or current. We classified any alcohol use as either yes or no. Physical activity was assessed using a questionnaire adapted from the Cross-Cultural Activity Participation Study, which evaluates the frequency and duration of physical activity.[16] We categorized daytime sleepiness into 4 groups: "never or rarely" (1 day/month or less), "sometimes" (2–4 days/month), "often" (5–15 days/month), and "almost always" (16–30 days/month). We defined diabetes as fasting glucose of 126 milligrams per deciliter or greater or hypoglycemic medication use. We defined hypertension as systolic blood pressure of 140 millimeters of mercury or greater, diastolic blood pressure of 90 millimeters of mercury or greater, or antihypertensive medication use. Blood pressure, cholesterol levels, and body mass index were measured using standard protocols. Lipoprotein (LDL) cholesterol was calculated via the Friedewald equation.[17]

Statistical Analysis

We conducted analyses in SAS 9.4 (SAS Institute, Cary, NC). We stratified baseline participant characteristics by quartiles of neighborhood disadvantage and by whether the participant moved between 2000 and 2019. We evaluated trends across quartiles of neighborhood disadvantage using linear regression, the Cochran-Armitage trend test, and the Cochran-Mantel-Haenszel trend test. We assessed differences between participants who moved or did not move using the χ^2 test, the *t*-test, and the Cochran-Armitage trend test.

Multilevel cause-specific Cox proportional hazards regression models with robust error variance generated hazard ratios (HRs) and 95% confidence intervals (CIs) for incident CVD. We assessed linearity using Martingale residuals and the proportional hazards assumption via Schoenfeld residuals. Neither assumption was violated for the exposure (i.e., neighborhood disadvantage) or moderators (i.e., anger and optimism). We handled ties using the Efron method. We specified a shared frailty term with a log-normal distribution[18] at the neighborhood-level to account for similarities among participants in the same census tract. We measured follow-up time from July 2000 until the first documented CVD event and censored participants at study dropout, death, or administrative censoring in December 2019.

All models permitted intersectional subgroup differences by stratifying by sex, race/ethnicity, and site. Models adjusted for baseline measures of age, education, annual income, cigarette use, alcohol use, physical activity, daytime sleepiness, diabetes, hypertension, hypertension medication use, total cholesterol, HDL cholesterol, LDL cholesterol, and triglycerides. We imputed missing baseline measures using multiple imputation by chained equations.[19] The imputation model included all measures previously described. We generated 5 imputed data sets based on a 2-stage analysis,[20] which indicated adequate precision from 2 or more imputations. We partitioned each covariate into a neighborhood-level mean and subject-specific deviation from the neighborhood-level mean. We included neighborhood-level and person-level measures in all models to accurately adjust for within- and between-neighborhood effects.[21] We combined parameter estimates from models fit to imputed data using Rubin's rules.[22]

Initial models estimated independent effects of neighborhood disadvantage and a single psychosocial risk or resilience measure. Subsequent models estimated joint effects by specifying an interaction between neighborhood disadvantage and psychosocial measures. We computed multiplicative interactions as the product of the exposure and moderator. We estimated additive interactions as the relative excess risk owing to interaction, where 0 indicates no interaction, greater than 0 indicates positive interaction, and less than 0 indicates negative interaction. We visualized the conditional effect of a 1 SD increase in neighborhood disadvantage using the Johnson–Neyman technique.[23]

We assessed robustness of the results using 3 sensitivity analyses. The first sensitivity analysis examined whether estimates for multiplicative or additive interactions varied when we included different sets of covariates in the model. The second sensitivity analysis was identical to the first analysis except that the analytic sample excluded 88 participants who developed CVD before optimism was assessed at exam 2 (2002–2004). The third sensitivity analysis incorporated inverse probability of censoring weights to account for competing risks such as death. Exploratory analyses generated estimates of CVD risk in strata defined by race/ethnicity, sex, and change in residence after the baseline assessment.

RESULTS

Among the 4326 participants, the mean ±SD baseline age was 61.9 ±10.2 years; 54% were women, 46% were White, 28% were Black, 16% were Hispanic, and 11% were Chinese American. Participants residing in neighborhoods with higher ADI rankings (meaning at a greater disadvantage) were more likely to be younger, Black or Hispanic, and live in communities with higher levels of collective anger and lower levels of collective optimism (Table A, available as a supplement to the online version of this article at http://www.ajph.org). Participants who changed addresses between July 2000 and December 2019 were more likely to be younger, have a lower annual income, and live in communities with higher levels of anger (data available upon request). The median time to an incident event or censoring was 17.59 years. By the time of administrative censoring in December 2019, 879 instances of incident CVD were documented and 27% of the cohort was deceased.

Full Sample

In fully adjusted models, higher neighborhood disadvantage was associated with an increased risk of incident CVD (Table 1). This association was moderated by psychosocial risk and resilience factors. The multiplicative interaction with neighborhood-level trait anger (HR = 1.21; 95% CI = 1.05, 1.38) and anger reaction (HR = 1.21; 95% CI = 1.04,

TABLE 1— Main Effects and Multiplicative Moderation of Psychosocial Risk and Resilience in the Association Between Neighborhood Disadvantage and Incident Cardiovascular Disease: Multi-Ethnic Study of Atherosclerosis Cohort, United States, 2000–2019

	Model 1: Main Effects, HR (95% CI)	Model 2: Interaction, HR (95% CI)
Model set 1, moderator: trait anger		
Neighborhood disadvantage	1.17 (1.00, 1.36)	1.16 (1.00, 1.35)
Neighborhood-level factor score of moderator	1.04 (0.89, 1.22)	1.04 (0.89, 1.21)
Person-level factor score of moderator	0.98 (0.91, 1.07)	0.98 (0.91, 1.06)
Neighborhood disadvantage × neighborhood-level moderator		1.14 (0.99, 1.30)
Neighborhood disadvantage × person-level moderator		1.00 (0.92, 1.08)
Model set 2, moderator: anger reaction		
Neighborhood disadvantage	1.17 (1.00, 1.36)	1.17 (1.01, 1.36)
Neighborhood-level factor score of moderator	1.01 (0.86, 1.20)	0.98 (0.83, 1.17)
Person-level factor score of moderator	1.04 (0.95, 1.13)	1.03 (0.95, 1.12)
Neighborhood disadvantage × neighborhood-level moderator		1.17 (1.01, 1.35)
Neighborhood disadvantage × person-level moderator		1.04 (0.95, 1.13)
Model set 3, moderator: anger temperament		
Neighborhood disadvantage	1.17 (1.01, 1.36)	1.16 (1.00, 1.35)
Neighborhood-level factor score of moderator	1.11 (0.94, 1.32)	1.12 (0.94, 1.33)
Person-level factor score of moderator	0.93 (0.86, 1.01)	0.93 (0.86, 1.02)
Neighborhood disadvantage × neighborhood-level moderator		0.96 (0.83, 1.10)
Neighborhood disadvantage × person-level moderator		0.94 (0.86, 1.02)
Model set 4, moderator: optimism		
Neighborhood disadvantage	1.19 (1.02, 1.40)	1.23 (1.05, 1.44)
Neighborhood-level factor score of moderator	1.07 (0.93, 1.24)	1.08 (0.93, 1.25)
Person-level factor score of moderator	1.08 (0.99, 1.17)	1.08 (0.99, 1.17)
Neighborhood disadvantage × neighborhood-level moderator		0.87 (0.77, 0.98)
Neighborhood disadvantage × person-level moderator		0.98 (0.91, 1.07)

Note. CI = confidence interval; HR = hazard ratio; MESA = Multi-Ethnic Study of Atherosclerosis. Study population size was n = 4326. We estimated HRs and 95% CIs using cause-specific multilevel Cox proportional hazards regression models with robust error variance and a shared frailty term (log-normal distribution). We computed multiplicative interactions by estimating the product of the exposure and moderators. We employed multiple imputation by chained equations to impute missing covariates. We stratified all models by sex, race/ethnicity, and site and adjusted them for age, education, annual income, cigarette use, alcohol use, physical activity, daytime sleepiness, diabetes, hypertension, hypertension medication use, total cholesterol, high-density lipoprotein cholesterol, low-density lipoprotein cholesterol, and triglycerides. We defined all covariates as time-invariant baseline measures separated into neighborhood-level means and person-level deviations from those means.

1.40) magnified the risk for incident CVD, whereas neighborhood-level optimism (HR = 0.84; 95% CI = 0.74, 0.95) and person-level anger temperament (HR = 0.92; 95% CI = 0.88, 0.96) diminished risk. Additive interactions were in the same direction but had larger point estimates (Table C, available as a supplement to the online version of this article at http://www.ajph.org), suggesting the strongest form of interaction along the interaction continuum.[24] These associations were largely consistent in models that adjusted for different sets of covariates (Tables D and E, available as a supplement to the online version of this article at http://www.ajph.org) or excluded participants who developed CVD before optimism was assessed (Tables F and G, available as a supplement to the online version of this article at http://www.ajph.org). The associations were attenuated and lacked precision in models that accounted for competing risks, such as death (Tables H and I, available as a supplement to the online version of this article at http://www.ajph.org).

Visualizations showed stronger effects above the mean for anger and below the mean for optimism (Figure 2). In the analytic sample, 56.9% of participants resided in neighborhoods with a

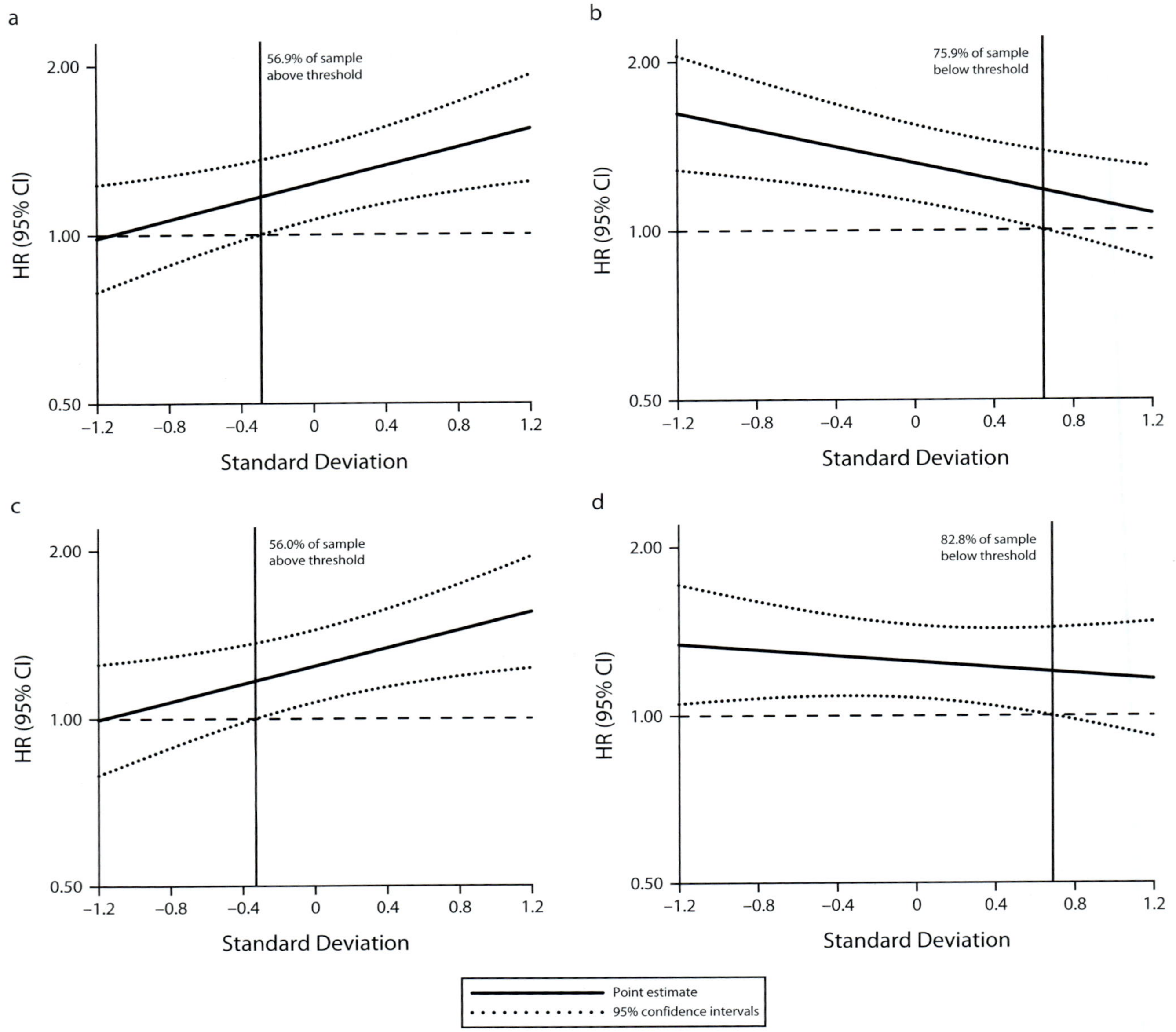

FIGURE 2— Johnson-Neyman Visualization of Conditional Effect of 1 SD Increase in Neighborhood Disadvantage on Incident Cardiovascular Disease by Neighborhood-Level Psychosocial Risk and Resilience: Multi-Ethnic Study of Atherosclerosis Cohort, United States, 2000–2019

Note. CI = confidence interval; HR = hazard ratio. Study population size was n = 4326. We calculated parameter estimates from cause-specific, multilevel Cox proportional hazards regression models with robust error variance and a shared frailty term with a log-normal distribution. Models were fit to imputed data stratified by race/ethnicity. Visualization of multiplicative interaction was based on a hypothetical participant whose characteristics equaled the sample means of the full cohort.

mean level of anger above the statistically significant threshold of −0.29 SD, which implies that interventions that reduce collective anger in these communities may reduce the person-level risk of CVD. Similarly, 75.9% of participants resided in neighborhoods with a mean level of optimism below 0.65 SD. These neighborhoods may benefit from interventions that elevate collective optimism. It is also noteworthy that 48.5% of participants live in a neighborhood where collective anger is above and optimism is below the statistically significant threshold, suggesting these are ideal locations for targeted interventions.

Stratified Samples

Analyses stratified by ethnoracial group offer a more detailed portrait of how psychosocial risk and resilience influence the impact of neighborhood disadvantage on the development of CVD (Figure 3; Tables J and K, available as a supplement to the online version of this article at http://www.ajph.org). Among Chinese American participants, person-level optimism magnified the associations between neighborhood disadvantage and incident CVD (HR = 1.97; 95% CI = 1.14, 3.41). By contrast, among Black participants, neighborhood-level optimism mitigated the association between neighborhood disadvantage and incident CVD (HR = 0.75; 95% CI = 0.58, 0.98). Among Hispanic participants, neighborhood-level trait anger and anger reaction magnified the association between neighborhood disadvantage and incident CVD (HR = 2.22; 95% CI = 1.38, 3.56 and HR = 1.88; 95% CI = 1.12, 3.17, respectively). The interactions between neighborhood disadvantage and neighborhood-level risk and resilience were also more pronounced in men (Tables L and M, available as a supplement to the online version of this article at http://www.ajph.org) and in participants who resided in the same neighborhood for the duration of the study (Tables N and O, available as a supplement to the online version of this article at http://www.ajph.org).

DISCUSSION

Our study affirms that neighborhood disadvantage is associated with a higher risk of incident CVD and offers insights into how psychosocial factors (i.e., optimism and anger) moderate this relationship. Although trait anger—specifically a tendency toward anger reactivity—amplified CVD risk, optimism mitigated the impacts of neighborhood disadvantage, potentially through mechanisms involving chronic stress and stress-related physiological dysregulation.[25] Our study also provides evidence of ethnoracial differences in how specific psychosocial factors influence the impact of social environmental stressors on the development of CVD among a community-based sample of self-identified Black, Chinese American, and Hispanic individuals. Our findings challenge the assumption that social exposures have uniform health effects across social groups. The patterns that emerged revealed the roles of culture and lived experience in shaping health.

Optimism has been shown to reduce CVD risk through indirect pathways,[26] such as fostering healthier coping strategies and behaviors, as well as through direct effects on physiological processes via perception and response to stress.[3,25] Findings among Black persons in our study aligned with this evidence; in this group, residing in a neighborhood with more optimistic residents was associated with a lower risk of CVD related to neighborhood disadvantage.

By contrast, among Chinese American persons, greater optimism was associated with increased CVD risk. This counterintuitive finding may reflect type 1 error. Alternatively, cultural influences on values may shape how optimism is interpreted. Although the LOT-R has been adapted for cross-cultural use, it reflects Western ideals of individualism, whereby optimism is defined as expecting good things to come for oneself.[27] By contrast, some Chinese cultural perspectives may frame optimism as accepting continuous change and navigating present circumstances, rather than expecting stable future positive outcomes.[28] This conceptual difference suggests that the LOT-R may capture a qualitatively different construct in Chinese persons, potentially measuring a characteristic that does not function as psychological resilience in this population.

Although estimates were less precise, a similar pattern was observed among Hispanic persons, many of whom may also come from cultural backgrounds with more emphasis on familial units,[29] conflicting with the individualistic perspective on optimism.

Neighborhood-level optimism mitigated CVD risk exclusively among Black persons. Although this differs from previous findings in a heterogeneous Hispanic US cohort,[9] it aligns with the unique sociocultural experiences of Black persons that may render group-level optimism particularly protective in mitigating chronic social stress. A history of disempowerment through interpersonal and systemic racism in the United States has likely positioned dispositional optimism as an essential resilience tool in Black communities,[30] which may have developed as an adaptive response to a unique form of ongoing racialized adversity.

By modulating the stress response in the limited ways historically available to Black persons,[10] optimism may aid in navigating persistent implicit and explicit anti-Black racism and mitigate its physiological consequences. Additionally, dispositional optimism promotes healthy coping mechanisms.[31] Evidence suggests that Black communities have developed highly effective stress management mechanisms, most notably collective coping strategies that emphasize family and social networks.[32] Our findings that neighborhood-level optimism is more strongly associated with better outcomes for Black persons than for other ethnoracial groups may reflect how shared optimism reinforces these systems and fosters communal resilience specifically in Black communities. Notably, the association between neighborhood-level optimism and outcomes was strongest at lower levels of

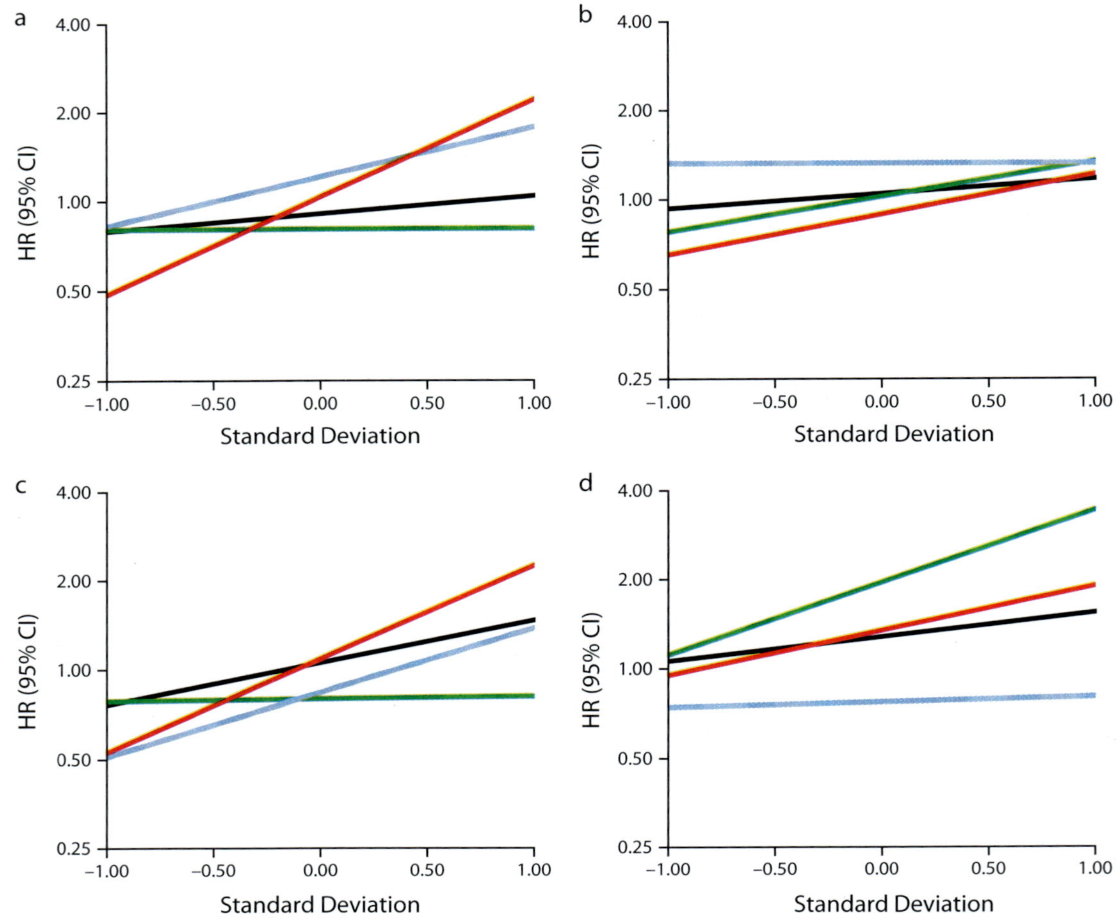

Race/Ethnicity	No.	Parameter	Anger HR (95% CI)	Optimism HR (95% CI)	Anger Reaction HR (95% CI)	Anger Temperament HR (95% CI)
White	1975	Exposure	1.21 (0.92, 1.60)	1.31 (0.97, 1.77)	1.25 (0.94, 1.65)	1.21 (0.92, 1.58)
		Moderator	0.91 (0.65, 1.26)	1.05 (0.82, 1.34)	1.06 (0.75, 1.49)	1.28 (0.93, 1.77)
		Interaction	0.95 (0.73, 1.24)	0.85 (0.68, 1.07)	1.11 (0.84, 1.47)	1.00 (0.77, 1.30)
Chinese	474	Exposure	1.66 (0.71, 3.87)	1.19 (0.58, 2.45)	1.40 (0.61, 3.17)	1.03 (0.56, 1.89)
		Moderator	0.81 (0.52, 1.24)	1.02 (0.54, 1.94)	0.80 (0.48, 1.33)	1.96 (1.04, 3.69)
		Interaction	0.60 (0.32, 1.14)	1.10 (0.58, 2.10)	0.73 (0.36, 1.48)	1.71 (0.99, 2.94)
Black	1200	Exposure	1.12 (0.81, 1.53)	1.32 (0.93, 1.88)	1.19 (0.85, 1.66)	1.07 (0.78, 1.46)
		Moderator	1.21 (0.88, 1.66)	1.33 (0.99, 1.79)	0.84 (0.60, 1.17)	0.78 (0.56, 1.08)
		Interaction	1.32 (0.90, 1.94)	0.75 (0.58, 0.98)	1.39 (0.96, 2.01)	0.98 (0.73, 1.32)
Hispanic/ Latino	677	Exposure	0.96 (0.63, 1.47)	1.35 (0.86, 2.11)	1.10 (0.71, 1.70)	1.33 (0.87, 2.05)
		Moderator	1.03 (0.61, 1.76)	0.89 (0.55, 1.45)	1.09 (0.60, 1.99)	1.35 (0.68, 2.66)
		Interaction	2.22 (1.38, 3.56)	1.01 (0.69, 1.50)	1.88 (1.12, 3.17)	1.06 (0.62, 1.82)

FIGURE 3— Visualization of Multiplicative Interaction of 1 SD Increase in Neighborhood-Level Moderator on the Relationship Between Neighborhood Disadvantage and Incident Cardiovascular Disease Stratified by Race/Ethnicity: Multi-Ethnic Study of Atherosclerosis Cohort, United States, 2000–2019

Note. CI = confidence interval; HR = hazard ratio. Study population size was n = 4326. We calculated parameter estimates from cause-specific, multilevel Cox proportional hazards regression models with robust error variance and a shared frailty term with a log-normal distribution. Models were fit to imputed data. Visualization of multiplicative interaction was based on a hypothetical participant whose characteristics equaled the sample means. Dotted lines represent 95% confidence intervals. Each panel indicates the percentage of the analytic sample for which the interaction is statistically significant and offers insights into targets for interventions. For example, the panel for optimism indicates that 75.9% of the participants reside in neighborhoods with a mean level of optimism below 0.65 SD and that increasing this level would reduce the person-level risk of cardiovascular disease.

optimism (Figure 2), suggesting that efforts to enhance optimism may be particularly impactful in communities with the lowest baseline levels.

Patterns in the moderating role of anger also suggest variations across ethnoracial groups. Overall, neighborhood-level anger reaction moderated the relationship between neighborhood disadvantage and CVD, but stratified analyses revealed that this pattern was driven by a particularly strong association among Hispanic participants. To further assess whether generalized anger or anger in response to perceived injustices differentially moderated the association between neighborhood disadvantage and incident CVD, we examined 2 subscales of trait anger: anger temperament and anger reaction. Our data suggested that anger reaction (i.e., anger in response to perceived injustice) exacerbates the association between neighborhood disadvantage and CVD among Hispanic persons more than other ethnoracial groups. Compared with other marginalized groups, such as Black persons, who have historically channeled anger at injustice into activism, Hispanic persons may perceive fewer avenues to address such injustices. Given that Hispanic persons are more likely to be immigrants than are non-Hispanic persons,[33] individuals in these groups may feel deterred from activism because of concerns about individual or family immigration status, potentially contributing to the internalization and embodiment of anger in response to injustice.

With these psychosocial factors operating at the neighborhood level, collective emotional climates may shape individual emotional states, further intensifying the health impacts of neighborhood disadvantage. Given that neighborhood-level variance accounted for most of the variability in optimism and anger, social environments directly influence CVD risk and may alter individual psychosocial factors in ways that magnify this risk. Further exploration of these pathways will be instrumental in developing more detailed, culturally informed approaches to CVD prevention. Future research should also consider culturally adapted measures of optimism that account for collectivist versus individualist orientations and culture-specific expressions of positive psychological states.

Strengths and Limitations

To the best of our knowledge, this is the first study on how the interplay between social environment, individual psychosocial factors, and cardiovascular disease risk interact across different ethnoracial groups. Our study has several strengths, including the use of high-quality longitudinal data from a community-based cohort, a rigorous methodological design, and a foundation in interdisciplinary theory. However, there are some limitations to consider. Generalizability to the broader US population may be limited because of the specific geographic locations of our sample. Nonetheless, MESA's robust recruitment strategies enhance the representativeness of the cohort. Additionally, although we observed differences in results based on how long individuals remained in their neighborhoods and did not account for this in our main analysis, MESA exhibits high residential stability, and our sensitivity analysis (Tables N and O) showed that associations were weaker but consistent among those who moved.

Furthermore, we measured neighborhood disadvantage only at baseline, which may not reflect changes in neighborhoods over the 19-year follow-up period, particularly after major events such as the Great Recession in 2008, which resulted in a 45% increase in the number of extremely poor neighborhoods nationally.[34] If included neighborhoods experienced substantial deterioration during follow-up, our baseline measures may have misclassified participants' actual cumulative exposure to disadvantage, potentially biasing our estimates. However, misclassification bias is unlikely to explain our findings, as previous studies indicate that neighborhood socioeconomic conditions are moderately stable over time and that baseline deprivation strongly predicts long-term health outcomes.[35] Therefore, our baseline index likely provides a reasonable approximation of participants' cumulative neighborhood context. Lastly, although residual confounding remains a possibility, we mitigated this concern by conducting sensitivity analyses.

Public Health Implications

Our findings reveal the critical role of psychosocial factors (i.e., anger and optimism) in shaping cardiovascular health outcomes across distinct sociocultural contexts. Our results underscore the need to move beyond universal approaches and understand how and why these psychosocial factors function differently within and across communities. The differential effects we observed across ethnoracial groups suggest that structural, historical, and cultural contexts shape both the experience and impact of psychosocial states, with implications for how communities respond to neighborhood stressors. Given that psychosocial factors shape stress responses[5] and are linked to structural inequity, public health efforts should focus on understanding how traits such as optimism and anger serve as either buffers or additional burdens across ethnoracial groups in disadvantaged communities.

Efforts should prioritize identifying representative, identity-based interventions[5] that are developed in collaboration with the communities they are intended to serve. Designing effective interventions will require engaging the communities most affected to ensure cultural relevance and center lived experience in the development and implementation of these strategies. Improved recruitment and representation in intervention studies are essential, as is a more granular understanding of how psychosocial factors interact with place, identity, power, and other facets of structural inequity. Addressing cardiovascular health inequity demands a broader commitment to structural change, community partnership, and contextually grounded public health strategies that reflect the complex interplay between identity, psychosocial resilience, and structural oppression. AJPH

ABOUT THE AUTHORS

Hannah Pleasants and Ganga S. Bey are with the Department of Epidemiology, University of North Carolina at Chapel Hill. James R. Pike is with the Optimal Aging Institute, New York University Grossman School of Medicine, New York. Priya Palta is with the Department of Neurology, University of North Carolina at Chapel Hill. Alain G. Bertoni and Timothy M. Hughes are with Public Health Sciences, Wake Forest University School of Medicine, Winston-Salem, NC. Qian Xiao is with the University of Texas Health Sciences Center, Houston. Jana A. Hirsch is with the Dornsife School of Public Health, Drexel University, Philadelphia, PA.

CORRESPONDENCE

Correspondence should be sent to Ganga Bey, Department of Epidemiology, University of North Carolina at Chapel Hill, 123 W. Franklin St., Chapel Hill, NC 27516 (e-mail: gbeyster@email.unc.edu).

PUBLICATION INFORMATION

Full Citation: Pleasants H, Pike JR, Palta P, et al. Psychosocial risk and resilience as moderators of the association between neighborhood disadvantage and incident cardiovascular disease across ethnoracial groups: Multi-Ethnic Study of Atherosclerosis, United States, 2000–2019. *Am J Public Health*. 2026;116(5):711–721.

Acceptance Date: January 1, 2026.

DOI: https://doi.org/10.2105/AJPH.2025.308407

ORCID iDs:
Hannah Pleasants https://orcid.org/0009-0006-2754-6611

James R. Pike https://orcid.org/0000-0002-6858-620X

Alain G. Bertoni https://orcid.org/0000-0002-7503-6273

Jana A. Hirsch https://orcid.org/0000-0003-3355-5558

CONTRIBUTORS

H. Pleasants made substantial contributions to drafting the article and to data interpretation. J. R. Pike conducted the data analysis and contributed to results interpretation. P. Palta, A. G. Bertoni, T. M. Hughes, Q. Xiao, and J. A. Hirsch, contributed to critically revising the article for important intellectual content. G. S. Bey made substantial contributions to the conceptualization and design of the work, contributed to data interpretation, and assisted with drafting the article. All authors reviewed and approved the final version of the article and agree to be accountable for all aspects of the work.

ACKNOWLEDGMENTS

This research was supported by the National Heart, Lung, and Blood Institute (contracts 75N92025D00022, 75N92020D00001, HHSN268201500003I, N01-HC-95159, 75N92025D00026, 75N92020D00005, N01-HC-95160, 75N92020D00002, N01-HC-95161, 75N92025D00024, 75N92020D00003, N01-HC-95162, 75N92025D00027, 75N92020D00006, N01-HC-95163, 75N92025D00025, 75N92020D00004, N01-HC-95164, 75N92025D00028, 75N92020D00007, N01-HC-95165, N01-HC-95166, N01-HC-95167, N01-HC-95168, and N01-HC-95169) and the National Center for Advancing Translational Sciences (grants UL1-TR-000040, UL1-TR-001079, and UL1-TR-001420).

The authors thank the other investigators, staff, and participants of the MESA study for their valuable contributions. A full list of participating MESA investigators and institutions can be found at https://mesa-nhlbi.org. This article has been reviewed and approved by the MESA Publications and Presentations Committee.

Note. The contents of this article are solely the responsibility of the authors and do not necessarily represent the official views of the funders.

CONFLICTS OF INTEREST

The authors report no conflicts of interest.

HUMAN PARTICIPANT PROTECTION

The Multi-Ethnic Study of Atherosclerosis protocol was approved by the University of Washington institutional review board, with reliance agreements from participating institutions. All participants provided written informed consent. This study is a secondary analysis of data collected under the approved protocol.

REFERENCES

1. Kershaw KN, Magnani JW, Diez Roux AV, et al. Neighborhoods and cardiovascular health: a scientific statement from the American Heart Association. *Circ Cardiovasc Qual Outcomes*. 2024;17(1):e000124. https://doi.org/10.1161/HCQ.0000000000000124
2. Clark CR, Ommerborn MJ, Hickson DA, et al. Neighborhood disadvantage, neighborhood safety and cardiometabolic risk factors in African Americans: biosocial associations in the Jackson Heart Study. *PLoS One*. 2013;8(5):e63254. https://doi.org/10.1371/journal.pone.0063254
3. Rozanski A, Bavishi C, Kubzansky LD, Cohen R. Association of optimism with cardiovascular events and all-cause mortality: a systematic review and meta-analysis. *JAMA Netw Open*. 2019;2(9):e1912200. https://doi.org/10.1001/jamanetworkopen.2019.12200
4. Sims M, Lipford KJ, Patel N, Ford CD, Min YI, Wyatt SB. Psychosocial factors and behaviors in African Americans: the Jackson Heart Study. *Am J Prev Med*. 2017;52(suppl 1):S48–S55. https://doi.org/10.1016/j.amepre.2016.09.020
5. Bey GS. The Identity Vitality–Pathology model: a novel theoretical framework proposing "identity state" as a modulator of the pathways from structural to health inequity. *Soc Sci Med*. 2022;314:115495. https://doi.org/10.1016/j.socscimed.2022.115495
6. Bey GS, Jesdale B, Forrester S, Person SD, Kiefe C. Intersectional effects of racial and gender discrimination on cardiovascular health vary among Black and White women and men in the CARDIA study. *SSM Popul Health*. 2019;8:100446. https://doi.org/10.1016/j.ssmph.2019.100446
7. Roux AVD. Neighborhoods and health: What do we know? What should we do? *Am J Public Health*. 2016;106(3):430–431. https://doi.org/10.2105/AJPH.2016.303064
8. Bey GS, Pike JR, Palta P. Distinct moderating pathways for psychosocial risk and resilience in the association of neighborhood disadvantage with incident heart failure among Black persons. *SSM Popul Health*. 2023;24:101475. https://doi.org/10.1016/j.ssmph.2023.101475
9. Hernandez R, González HM, Tarraf W, et al. Association of dispositional optimism with Life's Simple 7's cardiovascular health index: results from the Hispanic Community Health Study/Study of Latinos (HCHS/SOL) sociocultural ancillary study (SCAS). *BMJ Open*. 2018;8(3):e019434. https://doi.org/10.1136/bmjopen-2017-019434
10. Bey GS, Pike JR, Zannas AS, et al. The relationship of neighborhood disadvantage, biological aging, and psychosocial risk and resilience factors in heart failure incidence among Black persons: a moderated mediation analysis. *J Gerontol B Psychol Sci Soc Sci*. 2024;79(1):gbad121. https://doi.org/10.1093/geronb/gbad121
11. Bild DE, Bluemke DA, Burke GL, et al. Multi-Ethnic Study of Atherosclerosis: objectives and design. *Am J Epidemiol*. 2002;156(9):871–881. https://doi.org/10.1093/aje/kwf113

12. Kind AJH, Buckingham WR. Making neighborhood-disadvantage metrics accessible—the Neighborhood Atlas. *N Engl J Med.* 2018;378(26):2456–2458. https://doi.org/10.1056/NEJMp1802313

13. Scheier MF, Carver CS, Bridges MW. Distinguishing optimism from neuroticism (and trait anxiety, self-mastery, and self-esteem): a reevaluation of the Life Orientation Test. *J Pers Soc Psychol.* 1994;67(6):1063–1078. https://doi.org/10.1037//0022-3514.67.6.1063

14. Spielberger CD, Gorsuch RL, Lushene R, Vagg PR, Jacobs GA. *Manual for the State-Trait Anxiety Inventory (Self-Evaluation Questionnaire).* Palo Alto, CA: Consulting Psychologists Press; 1983.

15. Muthén BO. Multilevel covariance structure analysis. *Sociol Methods Res.* 1994;22(3):376–398. https://doi.org/10.1177/0049124194022003006

16. Ainsworth BE, Irwin ML, Addy CL, Whitt MC, Stolarczyk LM. Moderate physical activity patterns of minority women: the Cross-Cultural Activity Participation Study. *J Womens Health Gend Based Med.* 1999;8(6):805–813. https://doi.org/10.1089/152460999319129

17. Friedewald WT, Levy RI, Fredrickson DS. Estimation of the concentration of low-density lipoprotein cholesterol in plasma, without use of the preparative ultracentrifuge. *Clin Chem.* 1972; 18(6):499–502. https://doi.org/10.1093/clinchem/18.6.499

18. Austin PC, Wagner P, Merlo J. The median hazard ratio: a useful measure of variance and general contextual effects in multilevel survival analysis. *Stat Med.* 2017;36(6):928–938. https://doi.org/10.1002/sim.7188

19. van Buuren S. Multiple imputation of discrete and continuous data by fully conditional specification. *Stat Methods Med Res.* 2007;16(3):219–242. https://doi.org/10.1177/0962280206074463

20. von Hippel PT. How many imputations do you need? A two-stage calculation using a quadratic rule. *Sociol Methods Res.* 2020;49(3):699–718. https://doi.org/10.1177/0049124117747303

21. Yaremych HE, Preacher KJ, Hedeker D. Centering categorical predictors in multilevel models: best practices and interpretation. *Psychol Methods.* 2023; 28(3):613–630. https://doi.org/10.1037/met0000434

22. Rubin DB. *Multiple Imputation for Nonresponse in Surveys.* New York, NY: John Wiley & Sons; 1987.

23. Johnson PO, Fay LC. The Johnson–Neyman technique, its theory and application. *Psychometrika.* 1950;15(4):349–367. https://doi.org/10.1007/BF02288864

24. VanderWeele TJ. The interaction continuum. *Epidemiology.* 2019;30(5):648–658. https://doi.org/10.1097/EDE.0000000000001054

25. Baumgartner JN, Schneider TR, Capiola A. Investigating the relationship between optimism and stress responses: a biopsychosocial perspective. *Pers Individ Differ.* 2018;129:114–118. https://doi.org/10.1016/j.paid.2018.03.021

26. Hernandez R, Kershaw KN, Siddique J, et al. Optimism and cardiovascular health: Multi-Ethnic Study of Atherosclerosis (MESA). *Health Behav Policy Rev.* 2015;2(1):62–73. https://doi.org/10.14485/HBPR.2.1.6

27. Chang EC. *Optimism & Pessimism: Implications for Theory, Research, and Practice.* Washington, DC: American Psychological Association; 2001. https://doi.org/10.1037/10385-000

28. Spencer-Rodgers J, Williams MJ, Peng K. Cultural differences in expectations of change and tolerance for contradiction: a decade of empirical research. *Pers Soc Psychol Rev.* 2010;14(3):296–312. https://doi.org/10.1177/1088868310362982

29. Sabogal F, Marín G, Otero-Sabogal R, Marín BV, Perez-Stable EJ. Hispanic familism and acculturation: what changes and what doesn't? *Hisp J Behav Sci.* 1987;9(4):397–412. https://doi.org/10.1177/07399863870094003

30. Taylor HA, Washington-Plaskett T, Quyyumi AA. Black resilience—broadening the narrative and the science on cardiovascular health and disease disparities. *Ethn Dis.* 2020;30(2):365–368. https://doi.org/10.18865/ed.30.2.365

31. Nes LS, Segerstrom SC. Dispositional optimism and coping: a meta-analytic review. *Pers Soc Psychol Rev.* 2006;10(3):235–251. https://doi.org/10.1207/s15327957pspr1003_3

32. Utsey SO, Bolden MA, Lanier Y, Williams O. Examining the role of culture-specific coping as a predictor of resilient outcomes in African Americans from high-risk urban communities. *J Black Psychol.* 2007;33(1):75–93. https://doi.org/10.1177/0095798406295094

33. Cohn D, Brown A, Lopez MH. Hispanic identity and immigrant generations. May 14, 2021. Available at: https://www.pewresearch.org/race-and-ethnicity/2021/05/14/hispanic-identity-and-immigrant-generations. Accessed February 11, 2025.

34. Brookings Institution. US concentrated poverty in the wake of the Great Recession. Available at: https://www.brookings.edu/articles/u-s-concentrated-poverty-in-the-wake-of-the-great-recession. Accessed October 20, 2025.

35. Xiao Q, Berrigan D, Powell-Wiley TM, Matthews CE. Ten-year change in neighborhood socioeconomic deprivation and rates of total, cardiovascular disease, and cancer mortality in older US adults. *Am J Epidemiol.* 2018;187(12):2642–2650. https://doi.org/10.1093/aje/kwy181

Population-Level Violence as a Whole

Michelle Degli Esposti, PhD, David K. Humphreys, PhD, and Joseph Murray, PhD

Violence is preventable, and the United Nations' Sustainable Development Goals set out violence prevention as a global priority—calling for countries to halve their violent death rates by 2030. Despite action since then, there has been limited progress in reducing violence globally.

In this essay, we argue that current violence prevention efforts are being heavily shaped by reductionism—the now-dominant research paradigm across the sciences. We make the case that this reductionist philosophy has prematurely misguided violence research away from studying populations as a whole. We further argue that the mainstream statistical methods in violence research are reinforcing this reductionist bias by oversimplifying cause–effect relationships.

After revisiting foundational principles in sociology and public health, and drawing on advances in social epidemiology and complexity science, we suggest that violence—at any level—is better understood as an emergent property of a complex system. We call on the field of violence research to return to a holistic lens to maximize gains in explanatory theory and better position the evidence to directly inform effective intervention strategies for reducing violence at scale. (*Am J Public Health*. 2026;116(5):722–731. https://doi.org/10.2105/AJPH.2025.308366)

AJPH May 2026, Vol. 116, No. 5

Interpersonal violence took over 458 000 lives worldwide in 2021 alone.[1] It is therefore not surprising that the 2030 Sustainable Development Goals (SDGs) placed violence center stage, calling for global action to half homicide rates by 2030 (SDG 16.1).[2] "Immediate action and radical changes" are needed if we are to curb population-level violence on a global scale.[2] Current violence prevention efforts, however, have fallen short.

In this analytic essay, we argue that the current shortcomings in violence prevention efforts can be traced back to the evidence used to inform them. The dominant research paradigm used to generate knowledge on the causes of population-level violence is misguided in 2 critical ways. First, although the study of population-level violence originated from disciplines concerned with the population as a whole, violence research has come to be dominated by the reductionist philosophy that population-level violence is best understood by individuals, the individuals' causes, and the link between individuals and populations.[3–5] Second, the ability to identify the causes of population-level violence is being heavily shaped by mainstream statistical methods—such as regression techniques—that assume that independent causal effects are identifiable and cause–effect relationships are unidirectional.[6] By going back to basics and asking what population-level violence is, and what causes it, we make a case for the pragmatic importance and possible autonomy of higher-level population properties that—although they may depend on and emerge from individuals—are not fully explained by, and irreducible to, these individuals. We then draw on lessons learned from other disciplines to suggest that population-level violence is better characterized as an emergent property of a complex system,[7] and call for future research on population-level violence to return to the disciplinary roots of holism to maximize gains in causal explanations and intervention efforts.[8]

DEFINITION OF POPULATION-LEVEL VIOLENCE

Interpersonal violence is an individual's intentional use of force against another individual, which either results in or has a high likelihood of resulting in injury or death.[9] Although some forms of violence (e.g., structural violence) might occur at different levels, interpersonal violence occurs at the individual level via individual cases of violent perpetration or violent victimization; it logically follows that any summary measure of group-level violence, including population-level violence, is simply the aggregate of these individual cases of violence. This is because population counts are the sum of individual cases of violence, and the population rate is the proportion (a special type of ratio) of population counts (numerator) over the population size (denominator).[10]

In a naïve sense—that is, from a mathematical perspective—population-level violence is simply the aggregation of individual cases of violence. It is important to distinguish between population-level violence and its causes. Just because population-level violence is defined as the sum of individual cases of violence does not mean it is caused by the sum of individual causes of cases of violence.

CAUSES OF POPULATION-LEVEL VIOLENCE

There is evidence to suggest that the sum of individual causes of cases of violence alone cannot capture the complete picture. Rather, violence is caused by levels beyond the individual. Seminal socioecological models of human behavior postulate that causes span from more proximal influences (e.g., familial and household dysfunction) to wider influences at the institutional and societal level (e.g., cultural norms, social inequality, and social disorganization),[11,12] while multilevel modeling has provided empirical evidence of the significance of multiple influences—which originate from different levels and yet can each help to explain violence.[13]

These multiple levels of possible causes present the "levels of explanation problem" (micro–macro problem), which lies at the heart of the ecological and atomistic fallacies.[5] Distilled down, the problem can be summarized as, what causes an outcome at one level might not cause the same analogical outcome at another level of analysis. For instance, the percentage of a country's population living in poverty might cause population-level violence, but this does not necessarily mean that being poor causes an individual to be violent. Differences between individual and population causes reflect how exposures are distributed. For example, a national economic recession that equally affects everyone living in that country may cause an increase in population rates of violence, but it is unable to explain differences in individual cases of violence as the economic recession is ubiquitous: every individual experiences the same exposure.[14]

Although the levels of explanation problem is pervasive across research disciplines and topics, it was Geoffrey Rose that placed it center stage for public health research and prevention strategies. Rose showed that the causes of individual cases are not the same as the causes of population incidence.[15] Whereas the former seeks to explain within-population variation in violence to understand why some individuals are more likely to perpetrate (or be a victim of) violence than others, the latter seeks to explain between-population variation in violence, asking questions like (1) why is Brazil more than 30-fold more violent than Japan[16] and (2) why did the United States recently experience an unprecedented rise in lethal violence?[17] Answers to these questions may be critical to understanding the causes of population-level violence yet reveal little about what causes an individual to engage in violence.[14]

A BRIEF HISTORY OF THE STUDY OF POPULATION-LEVEL VIOLENCE

The idea that populations deserve studying in their own right—as *the* unit of analysis—has a long history before Geoffrey Rose. In the 19th century, the observation that populations are predictable and can behave like a collective individual, where some behaviors are universal to all individuals within the group so that the group takes on its own form of behavior, gave birth to a new wave of sciences, including sociology and epidemiology.[18,19] These sciences sought to study populations, propped up by the methodological holistic belief that a population is not just a sum of its individuals (Box 1). Instead, causality operates at the population level (as well as the individual level), and population properties, such as population-level violence, cannot be fully understood, predicted, or reduced to its individuals and their properties.[5,20] The influence of these ideas extended beyond science at the time, as seen in Figure 1, in which French artist Eugène Delacroix depicts a distinct collective persona of the crowd during the 1830 July Revolution, which could not have been predicted by the crowd's individuals.

The Reduction to Individuals

The search for population-level causes of violence has proven elusive. Although epidemiological and sociological studies continue to document a growing list of population-level correlates (e.g., social determinants of health), there has been limited success in establishing population-level causes.[21] In contrast, the search for individual-level causes of

BOX 1— Relevant Concepts From the Philosophy of the Mind and Science

Methodological holism. The belief that causality operates directly at the population level and therefore that population-level phenomena, such as violence, cannot be fully reduced to individuals and individual-level mechanisms. Original thinkers include the sociologists Adolphe Quetelet and Emile Durkheim.

Methodological individualism. The belief that causality only operates at the individual level and therefore population phenomena, such as violence, can only be ultimately explained by individuals and individual-level mechanisms. Methodological individualism is anchored by a reductionist perspective, and original thinkers include the philosopher Karl Popper and the sociologists Max Weber and Carl Menger.

Reductionism. The idea that complex phenomena (e.g., population-level violence) can be fully explained by reducing them to their simplest parts (e.g., individuals). Reductionism has become the dominant research paradigm across the sciences through its great successes in explaining quantum physics and infectious diseases.

Supervenience. Describes a relationship where higher-level properties (e.g., population-level violence) depend on lower ones (e.g., individuals). Thus, there can be no change in the higher-level property without some change in the lower-level property. Although supervenience is a necessary condition for reduction, it is not sufficient.

Multiple realization. Describes a relationship between lower- and higher-level properties, whereby the same higher-level property (e.g., same rate of population-level violence) arises from numerous different lower-level (e.g., individuals) mechanisms.

Wild disjunction. Describes the scenario when an overly broad and heterogenous set of lower-level properties (e.g., individuals) are used to try to explain a higher-level property (e.g., population-level violence). Jerry Fodor argued that a true scientific law cannot have wildly disjunctive components.

Emergence. When a high-level property arises that is not additive and not predicted or fully reducible to lower-level properties. Instead, the emergent property only exists at that higher level.

violence has been more fruitful. For example, poverty has been repeatedly shown to increase the risk of individual violent behavior, even when controlling for confounding.[22]

This asymmetry in causal evidence has shifted research toward individualism.[3–5] There have been attempts to bridge the gap between macro- and microlevel explanations by developing frameworks that link population-level phenomena to individual behaviors.[3,4] These theoretical frameworks, foundational to the subfields of analytical sociology and criminology, have helped integrate different levels of analyses and clarify how population-level causes may work through individual-level mechanisms.[4] Figure 2a shows the original framework of the classic Coleman's boat, depicting the relationships between multiple levels of analyses. Although there have been small variations to Coleman's boat since then,[5] the underlying principle has remained the same: population-level causes can only operate via individuals and individual-level mechanisms (pathways 1–3, Figure 2a).

This move toward methodological individualism is not specific to violence.[23] The idea that population-level phenomena are best explained by individuals is now the dominant research paradigm in the sciences, including those that historically evolved to study populations as wholes (e.g., epidemiology).[24] The rise in methodological individualism is often attributed to the successes of germ theory in epidemiology.[25] Germ theory demonstrated that disease epidemics can be fully explained by specific organisms that are transmitted via individual behavior. This is because each contagious disease depends on individuals being infected with 1 specific organism, and each disease only results from being infected by that specific organism. This singular dependency of the organism (i.e., cause) to the contagious disease (e.g., effect) satisfies the 2 conditions of supervenience and realization—concepts that originate from the philosophy of mind (Box 1). As a result, germ theory was able to showcase the explanatory power of reductionism for disease causation and revolutionize public health interventions, including the advent of vaccines. It is then not surprising that other sciences have been influenced to place individuals at the heart of causal explanations.[24]

When Supervenience Is Not Enough

Supervenience is a concept that originates from the philosophy of mind (Box 1). It describes a relationship where a higher-level property, such as cognition or population-level violence, depends on lower-level properties, such as brain states or individuals.[20] The reduction of population-level phenomena to individual-level explanations has seemed particularly appropriate for violence research because population-level violence clearly supervenes on the number of violent individuals. There can be no change in population-level violence without some change in the number of individual cases of violence. Individuals are the perpetrators, victims, or agents of any act of violence, which researchers are able to directly interrogate by

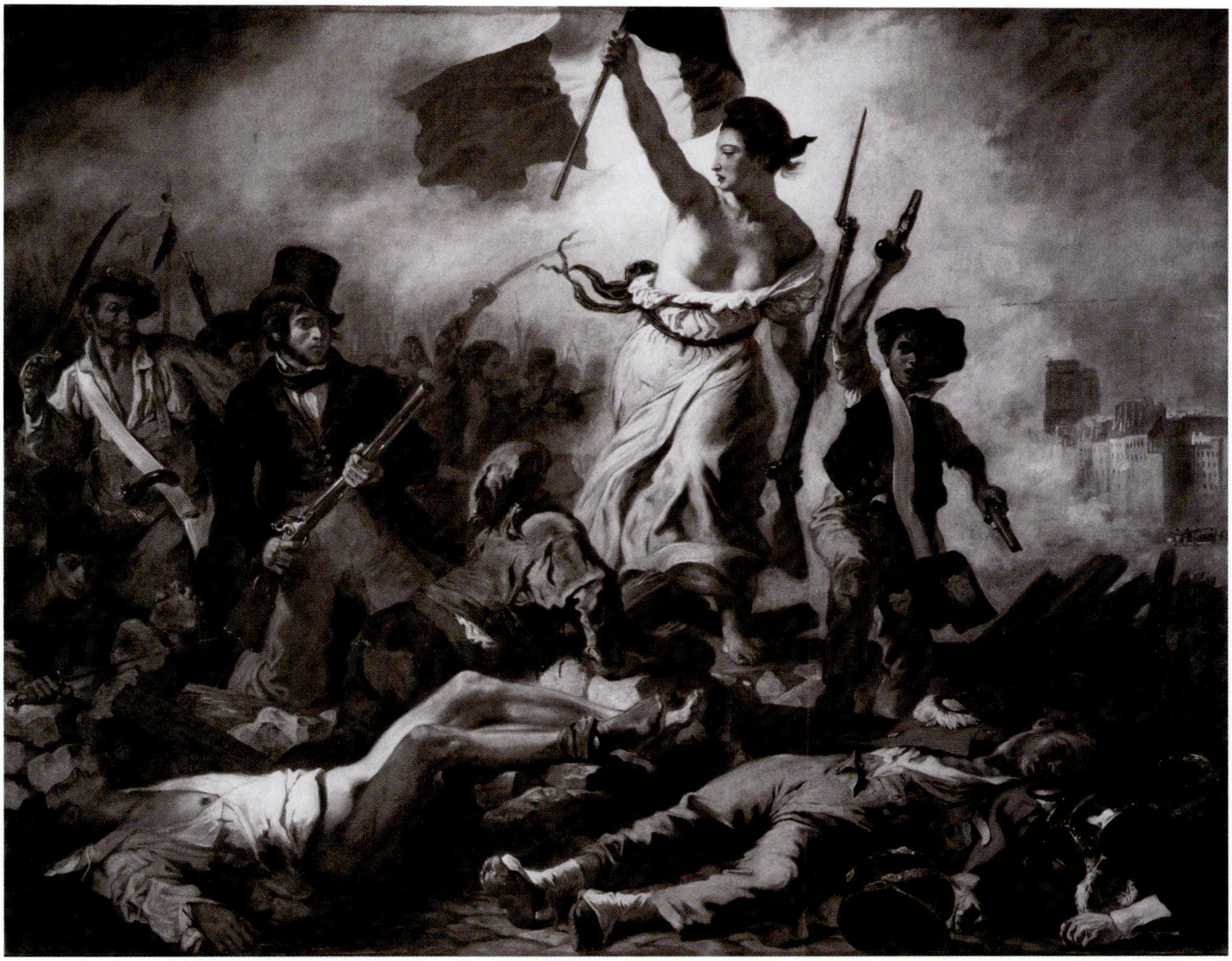

FIGURE 1— *Liberty Leading the People*, Oil on Canvas by Eugène Delacroix, 1830, on Display in the Louvre Museum, Paris

Note. The image is a faithful photographic reproduction of a two-dimensional, public domain work of art obtained from Wikipedia. Permission to reuse is covered by the public domain (common licensing) in the United States because it was published (or registered with the US Copyright Office) before January 1, 1930.

measuring and studying people's intentions, beliefs, and desires.[20] The same cannot be said for populations.

Centuries of debate in the philosophy of mind has shown that supervenience is a necessary condition for reductionism; however, it is not sufficient.[20] Dependency does not equate to causality, much like correlation does not imply causation. Unlike contagious diseases that have the "germ" as a common explanatory basis, population-level violence is a complex phenomenon that can be realized by a very different subset of individuals via very different individual-level mechanisms. For example, in one country with extreme inequality, poor individuals may resort to violence for material gain. In a second country with the same rate of violence, generations of racial discrimination may lead members of the marginalized group to engage in retaliatory violence. In a third country with the same rate of violence, a natural disaster, such as flooding, may result in individuals committing acts of domestic violence because of heightened stress and strain. Each scenario creates the same numeric outcome at the population level but via distinct individual-level mechanisms.

Population-level violence is multiply realized. Multiple realizability alone is not necessarily incompatible with reductionism, especially if there are only a few different individual-level explanations or if those explanations share some common feature. However, the usefulness of reductionism comes into

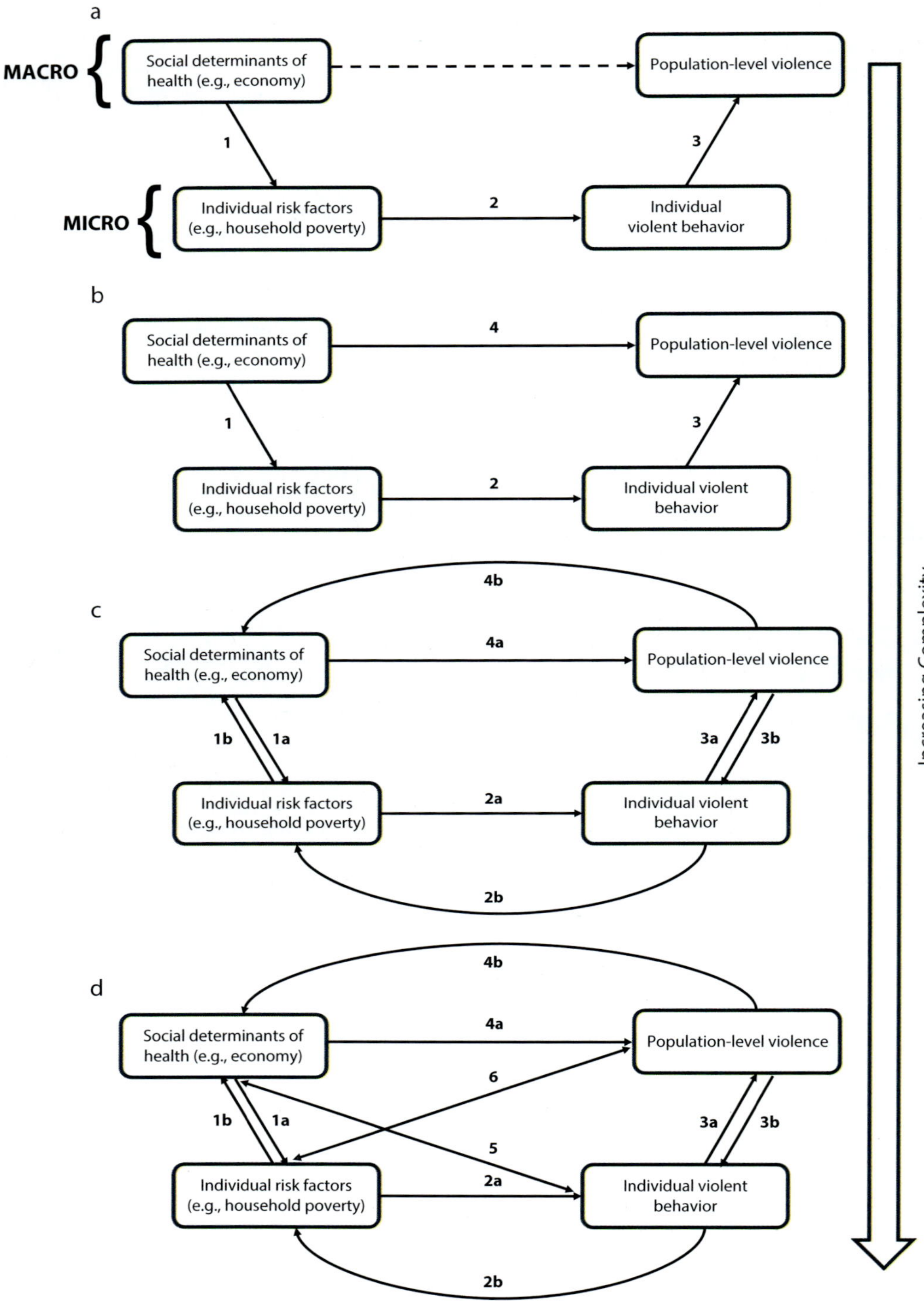

FIGURE 2— Iteratively Building Complexity to Reflect the Functioning of a Complex System, Starting With a Simple Macro- to Micro-Level Framework

Note. Panel a is adapted from Coleman[4] and reflects Coleman's original micro–macro "boat" framework. Panel b extends this framework by incorporating causal influences that operate directly at the macro level. Panel c introduces the complexity of bidirectional relationships within and across levels of analysis, including positive and negative feedback loops. Panel d further adds diagonal bidirectional relationships (e.g., social determinants of health directly constraining individual violent behavior, and vice versa). For illustrative purposes, we include only 2 levels to represent the population (macro, higher level) and individuals (micro, lower level). However, the frameworks should also be used to build in other important ("meso") levels, including families, neighborhoods, and communities.

question when the same population level of violence can arise from an endless combination of wildly disjunctive individual-level properties so that the individual-level explanations become too numerous, heterogenous, and context-dependent to be able to offer a generalizable understanding of population-level violence (Box 1).[20] Even if every population's violence can be ultimately and fully reduced to a different set of individuals (and their causes and mechanisms), such explanations have limited predictive power and are thus poorly placed to identify common leverage points for population-level intervention.

Emergence

Another challenge to the traditional reductionist paradigm is that some population properties are seemingly irreducible to individuals. For instance, population rates of violence are remarkably stable over time, even as individuals join and leave the population.[19] This casts doubt on whether individuals can be the explanatory basis; if individuals were only using free will, rates would fluctuate erratically, yet they remain remarkably stable from one year to the next.[19] They would also change as individuals move in and out of a given population. Yet the predictability of populations over time is so well-established that many quasi-experimental study designs, including interrupted time series analyses, leverage the fact that prior population rates are the strongest predictor of future population rates to control for confounding by design.[26]

The idea that there are some population properties that cannot be predicted by their constituent parts mirrors the philosopher George Henry Lewes's (1875) need to differentiate between effects that are resultant and those that are emergent.[20] An emergent effect is one that is not additive, not predicted by its knowledge of constituent parts, and not fully reducible to its parts (Figure 1). Instead, an emergent property belongs to the whole. In the case of population-level violence, the whole is the population and its emergent properties are those that arise from a large network of individuals continuously interacting over time.[8,20]

Examples of causal emergence go beyond human populations. For example, ants individually have minimal intelligence and, in their near-blindness, limited chances of survival. A collection of 100 ants will walk around in circles until they die of exhaustion. But put half a million ants together and colony behavior emerges, which is collectively organized, intelligent, and can create complex structures that are critical for the survival of the colony. Similar properties emerge when moving from white blood cells to an immune system or from vocabulary (tokens) to large language models, such as ChatGPT.[27] Human populations are just one of many examples in our complex world of when new, unexpected properties emerge that belong to the collective whole.

AN EMERGENT PROPERTY OF A COMPLEX SYSTEM

A complex systems approach offers a different lens.[6,7] Rather than hunting population causes or reducing explanations to individuals, a systems approach recognizes that violence—at any level—emerges from the functioning of a complex system over time (Box 2). This complex system of a human population includes heterogeneous agents at multiple levels (e.g., individuals, communities, populations), interactions between agents (within and across levels), bidirectionality (e.g., feedback loops), and nonlinearity (e.g., leverage points).[28] Hence, a complex systems approach is able to overcome some of the limitations of reductionism while building on

BOX 2— Relevant Concepts From Complex Systems Approaches

Complex systems. A large network of interconnected agents with no central control, only simple rules, and yet as a coherent whole show complex collective behavior, sophisticated information processing, and adaptation via learning or evolution. These collective behaviors are nonlinear, dynamic, and often unpredictable and irreducible to the agents alone.

Agents. Autonomous entities in a system that interact with each other and higher levels of the system according to specific rules. Agents can be individuals, ants, or cells, depending on the system in question, and are the fundamental basis for any agent-based models.

Feedback loops. Circular chains where the results of a cause—effect return as a future input to influence the system. Feedback mechanisms can be positive (reinforcing), amplifying change, or negative (balancing), minimizing change by stabilizing the system. Policy resistance is an example of a stabilizing response of a complex system.

Adaptation. The process by which a system and its agents change behavior in response to learning from feedback mechanisms. For example, adaptative systems can learn to evolve for survival or learn to improve their performance.

Leverage points. Critical places within the system where a small change leads to an amplified effect, thus large overall change in the system. Leverage points are instructive for informing effective interventions and identifying what causes matter most.

the cumulated knowledge in violence research.

The analytical sociology and criminology frameworks that bridge the micro–macro gap are a useful starting point from a complex systems standpoint, such as Coleman's boat (Figure 2a). We show in Figure 2 how these existing frameworks can be iteratively developed to capture the complexity needed to reflect how a population ("the system") functions over time. We also draw on empirical findings to support each addition of complexity in this section.

The first addition of complexity is recognizing that causality can operate at the macro level (pathway 4, Figure 2b). Although population-level properties might have originally arisen from individuals and their interactions, the dynamic complexity of human populations means that some emergent properties can no longer be meaningfully traced back to the individuals and take on causal power in their own right.[29] For example, studies have found that people living in neighborhoods that were historically racially segregated via redlining are more at risk for violence, irrespective of the person's race or ethnicity.[30] This demonstrates that the legacy of structural racism in the United States, a population-level property, continues to shape rates of violence in these communities (pathway 4, Figure 2b). More recent analyses of multicohort studies have pointed to the independent influence of social change on criminal behavior, which can be in part explained by changes in the collective efficacy of communities, bolstering mechanisms of social control and alleviating social disorganization.[31] Regardless of how these factors shape population rates of violence, controlling for many possible individual-level risk factors and mechanisms has not yet proved sufficient to knock out these higher-level statistical relationships.[31]

The second addition of complexity is embedding bidirectional relationships to account for reciprocity, feedback loops, and adaptation over time (pathways 1b–4b, Figure 2c; Box 2). At the individual level, a well-documented reciprocal relationship is that poverty increases the risk of violent perpetration, and violent perpetration increases the risk of poverty (pathways 2a–2b, Figure 2c).[22] Across levels of analysis, it has been shown that some properties have a bidirectional relationship, where there is the "objective" population-level measure, such as social inequality or institutional trustworthiness, and the "subjective" perception of social inequality or institutional trust by the individual. The former exerts influence that flows from the population-level measure to the individual-level risk factor poverty (pathway 1a, Figure 2c), whereas the latter starts at the individual level and flows to the population-level measure as it is the individual's perception (pathway 1b, Figure 2c).

There are also clear examples of positive and negative feedback mechanisms in system responses to violence interventions (pathways 4a–b, Figure 2c). Positive feedback mechanisms can explain the presence of leverage points, where small changes result in large amplified (and sometimes delayed) effects. For instance, the public health intervention of urban greening and installing public lighting changes the environment, constraining opportunities for violence and improving perceptions of public safety, which, in turn, promote the presence of people on the streets and further constrain opportunities for violence.[32] Conversely, there is also evidence of negative feedback mechanisms. Since the 1970s, the United States has implemented "tough on crime policies," leading to mass incarceration. Instead of successfully reducing population rates of crime and violence, the complex system has seemingly resisted the intended effects of these policies and has had the unintended impact of disrupting family life and fragmenting communities, thus reinforcing the cycle of violence and intergenerational transmission of offending.[33]

A third, related addition of complexity is the interconnectedness of the whole system. A systems approach expands and places emphasis on the interdependencies and interactions among all individuals and across all levels of analysis (pathways 5–6, Figure 2d). A growing number of studies underline the interconnectedness of violence between individuals, from classical works on the cycle of violence[34] to more recent studies showing that violence has contagion-like features, spreading through networks via social interactions.[35] Violence prevention efforts have also highlighted these interdependencies via interference.[36] Hotspot policing is a commonly cited example of interference, where intensifying policing in one area creates spillover effects, such as displacing or diffusing crime in nearby areas. Real-life violence prevention efforts have thus demonstrated the importance of considering the interconnectedness of the system when intervention planning.

METHODOLOGICAL MYOPIA: THE HIDDEN INFLUENCE OF STATISTICS

Traditional statistical methods in the social sciences, including regression techniques, have also contributed to the current shortcomings in violence research. Common statistical models excel when there is variation in the variables of interest. With more data points comes more power. Collecting big data on violence at the individual level is much more attainable than collecting big data at the population level. If the research question is "Why is Brazil more than 30-fold more violent than Japan?" then analyses are limited to 2 data points.[16] If, on the other hand, the research question is "Why did the United States recently experience an unprecedented rise in lethal violence?"[17] then analyses are restricted to the data that have been historically and consistently collected over time. These challenges in obtaining sufficient population-level data have nudged violence research toward analyses that focus on individual, rather than population, differences.[14]

Regression and related models also require a researcher to select a "cause" and "effect," and in their simplest—and most used—form, they assume a simple unidirectional cause–effect relationship. As the dose of the cause is amplified, there is a proportional increase in the effect. There have been important advances in regression modeling, which allow researchers to incorporate multiple levels of analysis within the same model (i.e., multilevel modeling).[13] Analytical coding software has also facilitated the use of more generalized applications of regression models to capture more complex nonlinear relationships between variables, such as penalized generalized linear models and generalized additive models. Nevertheless, regression techniques are still predicated on 2 fundamental assumptions: (1) there is a unidirectional cause–effect relationship, and (2) causal effects are mathematically identifiable (i.e., they can be isolated).

These assumptions are likely contributing to the lack of success in identifying population causes because if populations do function as a dynamic, interactive multilevel system, then population-level violence is the end result of a multiplicity of processes across different levels. Violence as an emergent property of a complex system cannot be captured by simple linear, logistic, or polynomial relationships. In addition, teasing apart one causal effect from another may be mathematically impossible and nonsensical. When explaining changes in population violence over time, for example, researchers have repeatedly attempted to attribute explanations to changes either to age, period, or cohort effects. However, age-period-cohort effects are perfectly colinear, making it mathematically impossible to identify their effects in a single regression model.[37] Similarly, it may not make sense to statistically control for one variable, such as poverty rates, in an effort to artificially isolate the causal effect of another, such as income inequality. In reality, these characteristics are intrinsically entwined, interacting to shape population properties. The traditional analytical techniques that are commonplace in violence research may thus be poorly placed to uncover the causes and mechanisms that give rise to population-level violence.

TOWARD A HOLISTIC RESEARCH AGENDA

Progress in violence prevention depends on asking—and prioritizing—questions most relevant to populations.[15] To avoid answering the wrong questions (type III error), researchers must not conflate individual causes of violence with population causes, even when data and analytic challenges make individual-level analyses more appealing.[14] Research questions should instead be grounded in conceptual and theoretical relevance, with explicit recognition that population causes may be ubiquitous across individuals and that such interventions may yield only modest benefits for any 1 person. These paradoxes underscore the importance of designing the "right" research questions to generate the "right" answers for population-level violence prevention efforts going forward.[14]

Although traditional statistical methods have contributed to type III errors in the field, promising analytic tools are emerging that are better suited to answer population-level questions. Systems modeling approaches, including social network analysis, agent-based models, and system dynamics modeling, can be used to operationalize violence as an emergent property of a complex system. By simulating dynamic interactions among, within, and across levels of analysis, these approaches move beyond simple cause–effect frameworks. These methods have been used to explain the unintended consequences of interventions and policy resistance,[33] and to identify leverage points for reducing urban violence[38]—embracing a consequentialist perspective of asking "what matters most."[39]

Other advances include the application of machine learning and Bayesian methods to violence research. For example, least absolute shrinkage and selection operator (LASSO) regression addresses multicollinearity by penalizing coefficients and has been incorporated into structured life course modeling approaches to formally test competing life-course hypotheses. This approach has clarified that the effects of poverty on violence primarily reflect cumulative exposure rather than a critical development period.[22] Bayesian statistics, on the other hand, can help to overcome data challenges in population-level analyses. By formally incorporating prior knowledge, Bayesian methods, such as Bayesian hierarchical modeling, can achieve efficient model estimation with smaller data sets and more sparse data than previously required by frequentist frameworks.[40] Together, these methodological advances broaden the toolkit, enabling the field to pursue conceptually grounded questions that capture complexity and are better positioned to directly inform population-level prevention strategies.

CONCLUSIONS

The limited success in the hunt for population-level causes of violence has misguided efforts away from holism, and reductionism has now become the dominant paradigm in violence research. The ontological truth about whether population-level violence can be fully explained and reduced to individuals and individual-level mechanisms will likely remain a lively debate for centuries. We have suggested some reasons why the position of reductionism may not be appropriate for understanding population-level violence. Regardless of the ultimate truth, we argue that a holistic philosophy is most practically relevant for understanding and preventing population-level violence, in the same way that air pressure rather than individual air molecules is used in weather forecasting. We advocate for studying population-level violence as a whole, as this approach offers the greatest gains for explanatory theory and intervention, which is perhaps why the holistic disciplines of sociology, epidemiology, and public health emerged in the first place. By reframing violence an emergent property of a system, building complexity into the existing theoretical frameworks, and coupling the "right" theoretical questions with the "right" methodological tools, the field will be better equipped to inform population-level interventions. Through this holistic lens that crosscuts levels of analysis, the hope is that violence research can identify those intervention strategies that are capable of radically reducing population rates of violence on a global scale. AJPH

ABOUT THE AUTHORS

At the time of the study, Michelle Degli Esposti and Joseph Murray were with the Human Development and Violence (DOVE) Research Centre, Federal University of Pelotas, Pelotas, Brazil. David K. Humphreys is with the Department of Social Policy and Intervention, University of Oxford, Oxford, UK.

CORRESPONDENCE

Correspondence should be sent to Michelle Degli Esposti, Department of Social Policy & Intervention, University of Oxford, Barnett House, 32 Wellington Square, Oxford, OX1 2ER, UK (e-mail: michelle.degliesposti@spi.ox.ac.uk). Reprints can be ordered at https://www.ajph.org by clicking the "Reprints" link.

PUBLICATION INFORMATION

Full Citation: Degli Esposti M, Humphreys DK, Murray J. Population-level violence as a whole. *Am J Public Health.* 2026;116(5):722–731.

Acceptance Date: November 15, 2025.

DOI: https://doi.org/10.2105/AJPH.2025.308366

ORCID iDs:
Michelle Degli Esposti https://orcid.org/0000-0002-0068-5754

CONTRIBUTORS

M. Degli Esposti conceptualized and designed the work and drafted the essay; she is accountable for all aspects of the work. D. K. Humphreys provided critical revisions to the draft. J. Murray contributed to the conceptualization of the work and provided critical revisions to the draft.

CONFLICTS OF INTEREST

The authors declare no potential or actual conflicts of interest.

HUMAN PARTICIPANT PROTECTION

No institutional review board approval was required because the study did not involve human participants.

REFERENCES

1. United Nations Office on Drugs and Crime. Global study on homicide 2023. United Nations. 2023. Available at: www.unodc.org/unodc/en/data-and-analysis/global-study-on-homicide.html. Accessed July 7, 2025.
2. United Nations Development Programme. 2nd global progress report on SDG 16 indicators. Available at: https://www.undp.org/publications/2nd-global-progress-report-sdg-16-indicators. Accessed March 10, 2025.
3. Hedstrom P. *Dissecting the Social: On the Principles of Analytical Sociology.* Cambridge, UK: Cambridge University Press; 2005.
4. Coleman JS. *Foundations of Social Theory.* Cambridge, MA: Harvard University Press; 1994.
5. Matsueda RL. Toward an analytical criminology: the micro–macro problem, causal mechanisms, and public policy. *Criminology.* 2017;55(3):493–519. https://doi.org/10.1111/1745-9125.12149
6. Lemke MK, Wolf DA, Drake SA. A call for complex systems and syndemic theory in firearm violence research. *Am J Prev Med.* 2022;62(3):459–465. https://doi.org/10.1016/j.amepre.2021.08.026
7. Galea S, Hall C, Kaplan GA. Social epidemiology and complex system dynamic modelling as applied to health behaviour and drug use research. *Int J Drug Policy.* 2009;20(3):209–216. https://doi.org/10.1016/j.drugpo.2008.08.005
8. Hoel EP, Albantakis L, Tononi G. Quantifying causal emergence shows that macro can beat micro. *Proc Natl Acad Sci U S A.* 2013;110(49):19790–19795. https://doi.org/10.1073/pnas.1314922110
9. Rosenberg ML, O'Carroll PW, Powell KE. Let's be clear: violence is a public health problem. *JAMA.* 1992;267(22):3071–3072. https://doi.org/10.1001/jama.1992.03480220089034
10. Elandt-Johnson RC. Definition of rates: some remarks on their use and misuse. *Am J Epidemiol.* 1975;102(4):267–271. https://doi.org/10.1093/oxfordjournals.aje.a112160
11. Shaw CR, McKay HD. *Juvenile Delinquency and Urban Areas.* Chicago, IL: University of Chicago Press; 1942.
12. Bronfenbrenner U. Ecological models of human development. In: *International Encyclopedia of Education.* Vol. 3, 2nd ed. Oxford, UK: Elsevier; 1994:37–43.
13. Kaplan GA, Everson SA, Lynch JW. The contribution of social and behavioral research to an understanding of the distribution of disease: a multilevel approach. *Promot Health.* 2000:37–80.
14. Schwartz S, Carpenter KM. The right answer for the wrong question: consequences of type III error for public health research. *Am J Public Health.* 1999;89(8):1175–1180. https://doi.org/10.2105/ajph.89.8.1175
15. Rose G. Sick individuals and sick populations. *Int J Epidemiol.* 2001;30(3):427–432. https://doi.org/10.1093/ije/30.3.427

16. Murray J, Cerqueira DRC, Kahn T. Crime and violence in Brazil: systematic review of time trends, prevalence rates and risk factors. *Aggress Violent Behav.* 2013;18(5):471–483. https://doi.org/10.1016/j.avb.2013.07.003
17. Degli Esposti M, Schell TL, Smart R. The recent rise in homicide: an analysis of weekly mortality data, United States, 2018–2022. *Epidemiology.* 2025;36(2):174–182. https://doi.org/10.1097/EDE.0000000000001815
18. Merton RK. *Social Theory and Social Structure.* New York, NY: Simon and Schuster; 1968.
19. Morabia A. *Enigmas of Health and Disease: How Epidemiology Helps Unravel Scientific Mysteries.* New York, NY: Columbia University Press; 2014.
20. Sawyer RK. Emergence in sociology: contemporary philosophy of mind and some implications for sociological theory. *Am J Sociol.* 2001;107(3):551–585. https://doi.org/10.1086/338780
21. Eisner M, Nivette A, Murray AL, Krisch M. Achieving population-level violence declines: implications of the international crime drop for prevention programming. *J Public Health Policy.* 2016;37(suppl 1):66–80. https://doi.org/10.1057/s41271-016-0004-5
22. Murray J, Degli Esposti M, Loret de Mola C, et al. Life-course influences of poverty on violence and homicide: 30-year Brazilian birth cohort study. *Int J Epidemiol.* 2024;53(4):dyae103. https://doi.org/10.1093/ije/dyae103
23. Anderson PW. More is different: broken symmetry and the nature of the hierarchical structure of science. *Science.* 1972;177(4047):393–396. https://doi.org/10.1126/science.177.4047.393
24. Kincaid H. *Individualism and the Unity of Science: Essays on Reduction, Explanation, and the Special Sciences.* Lanham, MD: Rowman & Littlefield; 1997.
25. Loomis D, Wing S. Is molecular epidemiology a germ theory for the end of the twentieth century? *Int J Epidemiol.* 1990;19(1):1–3. https://doi.org/10.1093/ije/19.1.1
26. Degli Esposti M, Spreckelsen T, Gasparrini A, et al. Can synthetic controls improve causal inference in interrupted time series evaluations of public health interventions? *Int J Epidemiol.* 2021;49(6):2010–2020. https://doi.org/10.1093/ije/dyaa152
27. Mitchell M. *Complexity: A Guided Tour.* Oxford, UK: Oxford University Press; 2009.
28. Diez Roux AV. Complex systems thinking and current impasses in health disparities research. *Am J Public Health.* 2011;101(9):1627–1634. https://doi.org/10.2105/AJPH.2011.300149
29. Elder-Vass D. *The Causal Power of Social Structures: Emergence, Structure and Agency.* Cambridge, UK: Cambridge University Press; 2010.
30. Poulson M, Neufeld MY, Dechert T, Allee L, Kenzik KM. Historic redlining, structural racism, and firearm violence: a structural equation modeling approach. *Lancet Reg Health Am.* 2021;3:100052. https://doi.org/10.1016/j.lana.2021.100052
31. Neil R, Sampson RJ. The birth lottery of history: arrest over the life course of multiple cohorts coming of age, 1995–2018. *Am J Sociol.* 2021;126(5):1127–1178.
32. Kaplan J, Chalfin A. Ambient lighting, use of outdoor spaces and perceptions of public safety: evidence from a survey experiment. *Secur J.* 2022;35(3):694–724. https://doi.org/10.1057/s41284-021-00296-0
33. Sterman JD. Learning from evidence in a complex world. *Am J Public Health.* 2006;96(3):505–514. https://doi.org/10.2105/AJPH.2005.066043
34. Widom CS. The cycle of violence. *Science.* 1989;244(4901):160–166. https://doi.org/10.1126/science.2704995
35. Green B, Horel T, Papachristos AV. Modeling contagion through social networks to explain and predict gunshot violence in Chicago, 2006 to 2014. *JAMA Intern Med.* 2017;177(3):326–333. https://doi.org/10.1001/jamainternmed.2016.8245
36. Nagin DS, Sampson RJ. The real gold standard: measuring counterfactual worlds that matter most to social science and policy. *Annu Rev Criminol.* 2019;2(1):123–145. https://doi.org/10.1146/annurev-criminol-011518-024838
37. Bell A. Age period cohort analysis: a review of what we should and shouldn't do. *Ann Hum Biol.* 2020;47(2):208–217. https://doi.org/10.1080/03014460.2019.1707872
38. Cerdá M, Tracy M, Keyes KM. Reducing urban violence: a contrast of public health and criminal justice approaches. *Epidemiology.* 2018;29(1):142–150. https://doi.org/10.1097/EDE.0000000000000756
39. Galea S. An argument for a consequentialist epidemiology. *Am J Epidemiol.* 2013;178(8):1185–1191. https://doi.org/10.1093/aje/kwt172
40. Degli Esposti M, Gravel J, Kaufman EJ, Delgado MK, Richmond TS, Wiebe DJ. County-level variation in changes in firearm mortality rates across the US, 1989 to 1993 vs 2015 to 2019. *JAMA Netw Open.* 2022;5(6):e2215557. https://doi.org/10.1001/jamanetworkopen.2022.15557

Projected Increase in HIV Incidence in 11 States if Ryan White Ends: A Simulation Study

Melissa Schnure, PhD, ScM, Ryan Forster, PhD, Joyce L. Jones, MD, MS, Catherine R. Lesko, PhD, D. Scott Batey, PhD, MSW, Isolde Butler, MD, MPH, Dafina Ward, JD, Karen Musgrove, PhD, MEd, Keri N. Althoff, PhD, MPH, Mamta K. Jain, MD, MPH, Kelly A. Gebo, MD, MPH, David W. Dowdy, MD, PhD, Maunank Shah, MD, PhD, Parastu Kasaie, PhD, MS, and Anthony T. Fojo, MD, MHS

Objectives. To estimate the increase in HIV infections in 11 US states if Ryan White services are interrupted or ended.

Methods. We applied a population-level model of HIV transmission to 11 states. We represented the proportion of people with HIV receiving Ryan White AIDS drug assistance, outpatient health services, or support services, and simulated a loss of suppression in each category if services permanently end or return after delays of 1.5 or 3.5 years.

Results. Cessation of Ryan White services in 2025 was projected to result in 69 695 additional infections from 2025 to 2030 (95% credible interval [CrI] = 18 943, 123 628), 68% more (95% CrI = 18%, 118%) than if Ryan White were continued. Temporary interruptions of 1.5 and 3.5 years resulted in 26 951 (95% CrI = 7341, 47 534) and 53 594 (95% CrI = 14 645, 94 860) additional infections, respectively. Excess infections varied across states, from a 45% increase in Texas to 126% in Missouri.

Conclusions. Projected increases in HIV infections because of disruptions of Ryan White services threaten the progress made in curtailing the US HIV epidemic, illustrating the critical role Ryan White plays in preventing HIV transmission. (*Am J Public Health*. 2026;116(5):732–735. https://doi.org/10.2105/AJPH.2025.308409)

AJPH May 2026, Vol. 116, No. 5

The Ryan White HIV/AIDS Program provides comprehensive services for over half of the 1.2 million people with HIV (PWH) in the United States, often functioning as a "payer of last resort" for those who would otherwise be unable to access care.[1] The program provides assistance through several mechanisms: payment for antiretroviral therapy through the AIDS Drug Assistance Program, organizational funding for routine outpatient ambulatory health services, and nonmedical support including case management and transportation.[2] Consequently, Ryan White clients have higher rates of viral suppression, rendering clients unlikely to transmit HIV.[2–4]

The Ryan White Program is administered by the Health Resources and Services Administration and operates under annual budgetary approval from Congress.[1] Ryan White funds ($2.5 billion in fiscal year 2025) are distributed through grants to local jurisdictions and HIV care organizations.[1] Disruptions to Ryan White services could substantially increase HIV transmission in the United States. We sought to estimate the increase in HIV infections in 11 states if Ryan White services were interrupted or discontinued.

METHODS

The Johns Hopkins Epidemiologic and Economic Model is a dynamic, compartmental model of HIV transmission that stratifies the adult population by age, race/ethnicity, sex, and HIV status[5] (Figure A, available as a supplement to the online version of this article at http://www.ajph.org). Model calibration has been described previously[5]; we simulated state-level HIV epidemics using a similar process (see online Appendix; Github Repository: https://github.com/tfojo1/jheem_analyses.git).

We simulated HIV epidemics from January 2025 to December 2030 in 11 states, in which 63% of people diagnosed with HIV in the United States reside: Alabama, California, Florida, Georgia, Illinois, Louisiana, Mississippi, Missouri, New York, Texas, and Wisconsin. These states were chosen via author consensus to represent varied geographic regions, Medicaid expansion status, and prioritization within the national Ending the HIV Epidemic initiative.[6]

A prior analysis examining the impact of Ryan White Program cessation at the city level describes our methodology for representing program services.[7] We simulated the proportion of PWH receiving services in 3 mutually exclusive categories: (1) AIDS drug assistance (regardless of whether clients also received other services), (2) outpatient ambulatory health services at HIV care facilities (excluding those receiving drug assistance), and (3) other Ryan White support services (but not drug assistance or outpatient ambulatory health services; online Figure B).[2] Calibration targets for Ryan White service utilization included the number of clients accessing each service type and the proportion of clients who were virally suppressed in each state (Table B and Figure C).

Based on a survey of Ryan White clinic directors, administrators, and public health officials who estimated the proportion of clients who would lose viral suppression if services stopped, we assumed a mean 65% (interquartile range [IQR] = 40%–90%) loss of viral suppression among recipients of AIDS drug assistance, 49% (IQR = 25%–70%) among other outpatient health services recipients, and 37% (IQR = 10%–60%) among Ryan White clients receiving other services[7] (Table A). We ran 1000 simulations in each state, sampling the effects of ending services from the range of survey responses, conditional on Medicaid expansion status. Because survey respondents might overestimate the impact of disruptions, we performed a "conservative" secondary analysis in which we also incorporated data from 2 published studies on the association between Ryan White services and viral suppression.[7–9]

We modeled 3 scenarios in which services stopped in July 2025 and viral suppression falls: (1) "cessation," in which suppression never recovers; (2) "brief" (1.5-year) interruption, where suppression recovers from January to December 2027; and (3) "prolonged" (3.5-year) interruption, where suppression recovers from January to December 2029.

RESULTS

Assuming Ryan White services continue, we projected 103 101 new HIV infections (95% credible interval [CrI] = 97 773, 109 048) from 2025 to 2030 across all 11 states. If Ryan White services end permanently in 2025 ("cessation"), we projected 69 695 additional infections (95% CrI = 18 943, 123 628) from 2025 to 2030, an excess of 68% (95% CrI = 18%, 118%; Figure 1 and Figures D and E). In the "brief" (1.5-year) interruption scenario, we projected 26 951 (95% CrI = 7341, 47 534) additional infections, an excess of 26% (95% CrI = 7%, 46%). In the "prolonged" (3.5-year) interruption scenario, we projected 53 594 (95% CrI = 14 645, 94 860) additional infections, an excess of 52% (95% CrI = 14%, 90%). In the "conservative" analysis, additional infections were approximately half of those from the primary analysis for all scenarios (Figures F and G). Infections increased most among adults aged younger than 35 years and men who have sex with men, without large differences by race (Table D).

Projected excess HIV infections varied across states (Figure 1), from 45% (95% CrI = 10%, 88%) in Texas to 126% (95% CrI = 25%, 246%) in Missouri (for individual states, see https://jheem.org/ryan-white-state-level). New infections would more than double in 4 states: Missouri, Alabama, Wisconsin, and Illinois. States with a greater proportion of PWH receiving Ryan White services in 2025 had more excess HIV infections (Figure H). In the 5 modeled Medicaid expansion states, fewer clients lost viral suppression, but because clients in those states had higher baseline suppression rates than in the 6 nonexpansion states, the relative increase in the number of unsuppressed PWH was similar, leading to similar increases in infections (Figure 1).

DISCUSSION

We used a validated HIV transmission model, informed by Centers for Disease Control and Prevention surveillance data and Ryan White Program reports, to project the impact of disruptions to the US Ryan White HIV/AIDS Program in 11 US states from 2025 to 2030. Permanently ending these services would lead to nearly 70 000 additional HIV infections in the next 5 years. Even temporary interruptions could result in a rise of over 26 000 additional infections. Impacts are expected to vary substantially at the state level, with the largest increases in new HIV infections in Missouri, Alabama, Wisconsin, and Illinois.

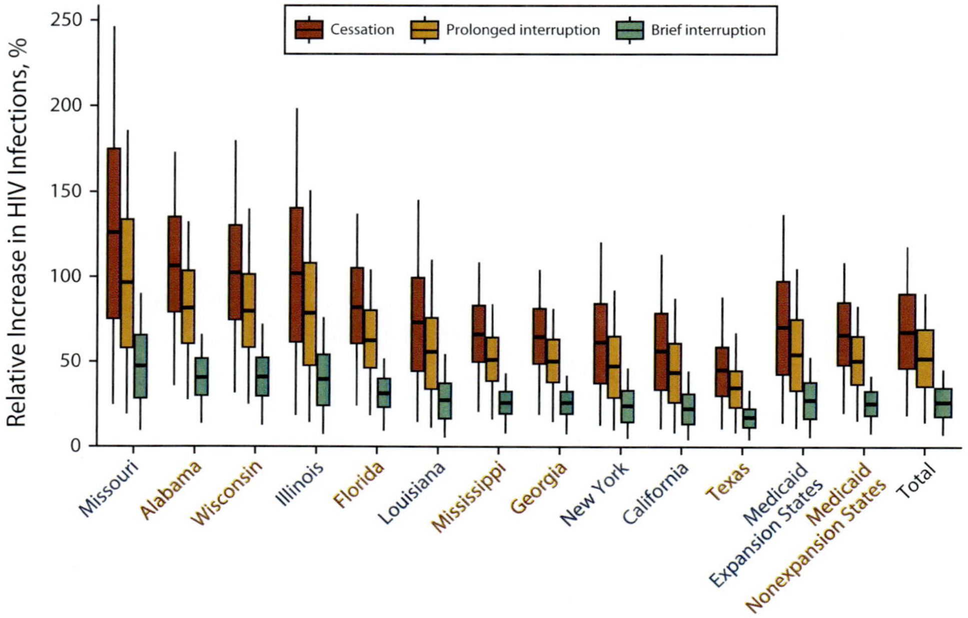

FIGURE 1— State-Level Relative Excess HIV Infections From 2025 to 2030 if Ryan White Programs Are Stopped or Interrupted

Note. Boxplots display the projected percentage increase in new HIV infections under 3 scenarios in which all Ryan White services stop in July 2025: "Cessation" (red)—viral suppression among Ryan White clients never recovers; "Prolonged [3.5-year] Interruption" (orange)—viral suppression among Ryan White clients recovers from January to December 2029; "Brief [1.5-year] Interruption" (green)—viral suppression among Ryan White clients recovers from January to December 2027. The value along the y-axis represents the relative increase in cases versus a scenario in which Ryan White services continue uninterrupted. The dark horizontal lines indicate the median projection across 1000 simulations, the boxes indicate interquartile ranges (IQR), and whiskers cover the 95% credible interval. Medicaid nonexpansion states are denoted by orange labels; expansion states are indicated by purple ones.

AJPH May 2026, Vol. 116, No. 5

Our analysis is subject to limitations, especially as the individual-level effects of ending Ryan White services are uncertain. Without empirical evidence on these effects, we relied on estimates from those with expertise in Ryan White programming. We captured the uncertainty around these estimates by simulating effects across the range of survey responses. The wide credible intervals around our projections reflect the variation in these responses, which ranged from almost no effect of Ryan White cessation to nearly 100% losses in viral suppression. Our secondary, "conservative" analysis avoids potential bias in survey responses, but likely understates the causal effect of widespread cessation of Ryan White services. Second, we assume that cessation or interruption of programming will only affect individuals accessing services. However, the implications of funding cuts to clinics (such as reducing staff or limiting services) will likely also affect the non–Ryan White clients who receive care at these locations. From this perspective, our estimates may underestimate the true impacts of reducing Ryan White funding. Finally, although we limited the scope of our analysis to estimate impacts on future transmission, interrupting Ryan White services would also affect both quality of life and mortality for those currently living with HIV.

The modeling approach used here has several strengths. Our Bayesian calibration process is a rigorous approach to handling unknown variables and missing data in HIV epidemiology. Furthermore, by calibrating to stratified epidemiological data at the state level, we can compare across settings and capture local differences in HIV epidemics.

In summary, projected increases in new HIV infections threaten progress made in curtailing the US HIV epidemic, should Ryan White services be interrupted or discontinued. These findings illustrate the critical role that Ryan White services play in preventing the transmission of HIV and the importance of maintaining these programs at the state level. AJPH

ABOUT THE AUTHORS

At the time of the study, Melissa Schnure, Joyce L. Jones, Kelly A. Gebo, Maunank Shah, and Anthony T. Fojo were with the Johns Hopkins University School of Medicine, Baltimore, MD. Ryan Forster, Catherine R. Lesko, Keri N. Althoff, David W. Dowdy, and Parastu Kasaie are with the Johns Hopkins Bloomberg School of Public Health, Baltimore, MD. D. Scott Batey is with the Tulane School of Social Work, New Orleans, LA. Isolde

Butler is with Crescent Care, New Orleans, LA. At the time of this study, Dafina Ward was with the Southern AIDS Coalition, Birmingham, AL. Karen Musgrove is with Birmingham AIDS Outreach, Birmingham, AL. Mamta K. Jain is with UT Southwestern Medical Center, Dallas, TX.

CORRESPONDENCE

Correspondence should be sent to Melissa Schnure, 1830 East Monument St, Office 8047a, Baltimore, MD 21287 (e-mail: mschnur3@jhmi.edu). Reprints can be ordered at https://www.ajph.org by clicking the "Reprints" link.

PUBLICATION INFORMATION

Full Citation: Schnure M, Forster R, Jones JL, et al. Projected increase in HIV incidence could rise by 68% in 11 states if Ryan White ends: a simulation study. *Am J Public Health*. 2026;116(5):732–735.

Acceptance Date: December 14, 2025

DOI: https://doi.org/10.2105/AJPH.2025.308409

ORCID iDs:

Melissa Schnure https://orcid.org/0000-0003-2745-3715

Ryan Forster https://orcid.org/0009-0007-7099-4660

Catherine R. Lesko https://orcid.org/0000-0002-1717-2592

D. Scott Batey https://orcid.org/0000-0002-2422-5787

Mamta K. Jain https://orcid.org/0000-0003-2292-6544

Kelly A. Gebo https://orcid.org/0000-0003-4010-398X

Maunank Shah https://orcid.org/0000-0002-0979-2388

CONTRIBUTORS

M. Schnure made substantial contributions to study conceptualization and design, conducted the formal analyses, and led interpretation of results; she drafted the initial manuscript and integrated critical revisions from all coauthors. R. Forster made substantial contributions to study conceptualization and design, analytic approach, and interpretation of findings as a core member of the analytic team; he provided critical revisions that shaped the intellectual content of the manuscript. J. L. Jones contributed to study question development and contributed clinical and public health expertise that informed interpretation of findings and their implications for practice; she critically revised the manuscript. C. R. Lesko contributed to refinement of the study question, methodological considerations, and epidemiological interpretation of results; she critically revised the manuscript. D. S. Batey contributed substantial expertise related to HIV service delivery and policy implementation, informing interpretation of findings; he critically revised the manuscript. I. Butler contributed clinical and implementation expertise relevant to HIV care delivery, informing interpretation of the results; she critically revised the manuscript. D. Ward contributed policy expertise related to HIV programs and systems, informing interpretation and policy relevance of the findings; she critically revised the manuscript. K. Musgrove contributed community-based and programmatic expertise that informed interpretation of results and real-world relevance; she critically revised the manuscript. K. N. Althoff contributed to study design, interpretation of findings within the broader HIV epidemiology literature, and conceptual framing; she critically revised the manuscript. M. K. Jain contributed clinical and public health expertise that informed interpretation of findings and their implications for practice; she critically revised the manuscript. K. A. Gebo contributed to study question development and contributed clinical and public health expertise that informed interpretation of findings and their implications for practice; she critically revised the manuscript. D. W. Dowdy contributed to conceptual framing, interpretation of modeling results, and methodological considerations; he critically revised the manuscript. M. Shah contributed to conceptual framing, interpretation of modeling results, and methodological considerations; he critically revised the manuscript. P. Kasaie made substantial contributions to study design, modeling methodology, and interpretation of results as a core member of the analytic team; she critically revised the manuscript. A. T. Fojo served as senior author and developed the underlying simulation model; he co-conceived the analysis, contributed to study design and interpretation of findings, and provided substantial intellectual guidance and critical revisions. All authors approved the final version of the manuscript.

ACKNOWLEDGMENTS

This research was supported by the National Institutes of Health (grant no. R01MD018539).

We thank Youngjee Choi for her assistance in developing the survey, Andrew Zalesak for his contributions to model development, Zoe Dansky for her work curating input data, and Nicholas Sizemore and Kendall Reid for developing the Web tool. We thank the 180 Ryan White clinic directors, administrators, and public health officials who responded to the survey.

CONFLICTS OF INTEREST

The authors have no conflicts of interest to declare.

HUMAN PARTICIPANT PROTECTION

This study consisted solely of mathematical modeling using publicly available data and did not involve interaction with human participants; therefore, institutional review board approval was not required.

REFERENCES

1. KFF. The Ryan White HIV/AIDS Program: the basics. 2022. Available at: https://www.kff.org/hivaids/fact-sheet/the-ryan-white-hivaids-program-the-basics. Accessed May 6, 2025.
2. Bradley H, Viall AH, Wortley PM, Dempsey A, Hauck H, Skarbinski J. Ryan White HIV/AIDS program assistance and HIV treatment outcomes. *Clin Infect Dis.* 2016;62(1):90–98. https://doi.org/10.1093/cid/civ708
3. Cohen MS, Chen YQ, McCauley M, et al. Antiretroviral therapy for the prevention of HIV-1 transmission. *N Engl J Med.* 2016;375(9):830–839. https://doi.org/10.1056/NEJMoa1600693
4. Rodger AJ, Cambiano V, Bruun T, et al. Risk of HIV transmission through condomless sex in serodifferent gay couples with the HIV-positive partner taking suppressive antiretroviral therapy (PARTNER): final results of a multicentre, prospective, observational study. *Lancet.* 2019;393(10189):2428–2438. https://doi.org/10.1016/S0140-6736(19)30418-0
5. Fojo AT, Schnure M, Kasaie P, Dowdy DW, Shah M. What will it take to end HIV in the United States? A comprehensive, local-level modeling study. *Ann Intern Med.* 2021;174(11):1542–1553. https://doi.org/10.7326/M21-1501
6. HIV.gov. Ending the HIV epidemic: plan for America. 2023. Available at: https://www.hiv.gov/federal-response/ending-the-hiv-epidemic/overview. Accessed November 10, 2020.
7. Forster R, Schnure M, Jones J, et al. The potential impact of ending the Ryan White HIV/AIDS Program on HIV Incidence: a simulation study in 31 US cities. *Ann Intern Med.* 2025;178(11):1580–1590. https://doi.org/10.7326/ANNALS-25-01737
8. Erly SJ, Khosropour CM, Hajat A, Sharma M, Reuer JR, Dombrowski JC. AIDS Drug Assistance Program disenrollment is associated with loss of viral suppression beyond differences in homelessness, mental health, and substance use disorders: an evaluation in Washington State 2017–2019. *PLoS One.* 2023;18(5):e0285326. https://doi.org/10.1371/journal.pone.0285326
9. Diepstra KL, Rhodes AG, Bono RS, Patel S, Yerkes LE, Kimmel AD. Comprehensive Ryan White assistance and human immunodeficiency virus clinical outcomes: retention in care and viral suppression in a Medicaid nonexpansion state. *Clin Infect Dis.* 2017;65(4):619–625. https://doi.org/10.1093/cid/cix380

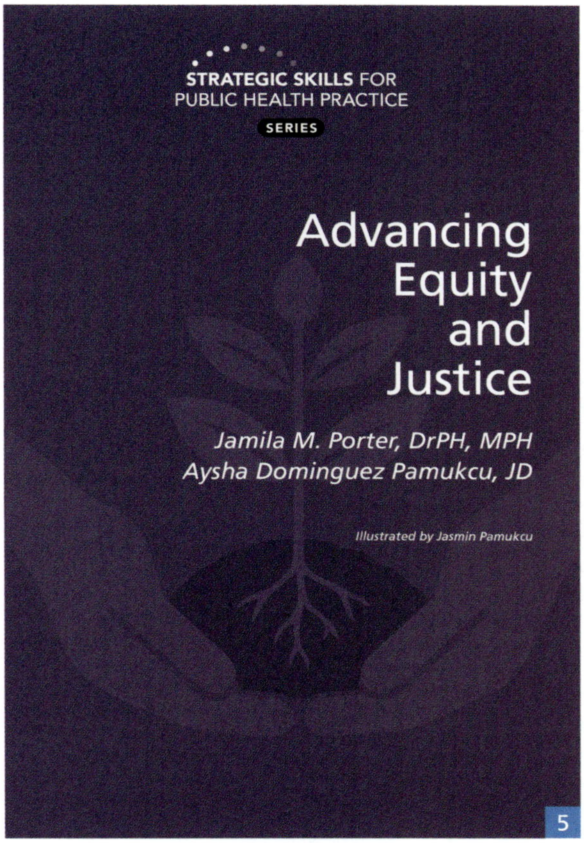

ISBN 978-0-87553-3599, 220 PP., 2026,
SOFTCOVER, PRINT ON DEMAND

Strategic Skills for Public Health Practice: Advancing Equity and Justice

Jamila M. Porter, DrPH, MPH, and Aysha Dominguez Pamukcu, JD

Strategic Skills for Public Health Practice: Advancing Equity and Justice is a call to reimagine public health as a dynamic social movement rooted in community leadership. Grounded in bold vision and practical application, this book confronts the root causes of health inequities — powerful systems that determine how long and how well we live. *Advancing Equity and Justice* challenges practitioners to move beyond limited technical fixes to embrace the moral clarity and collective action necessary to improve health for all.

APHA
Policy Action Institute

June 9-10, 2026
Optional Hill Day on June 11
Arlington, VA and Digitally

Registration opens April 6.
Space is limited.

APHA.org/PAI

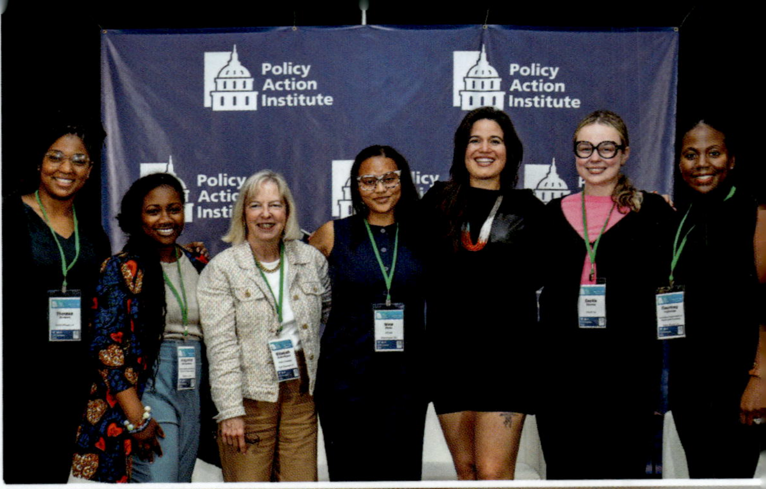

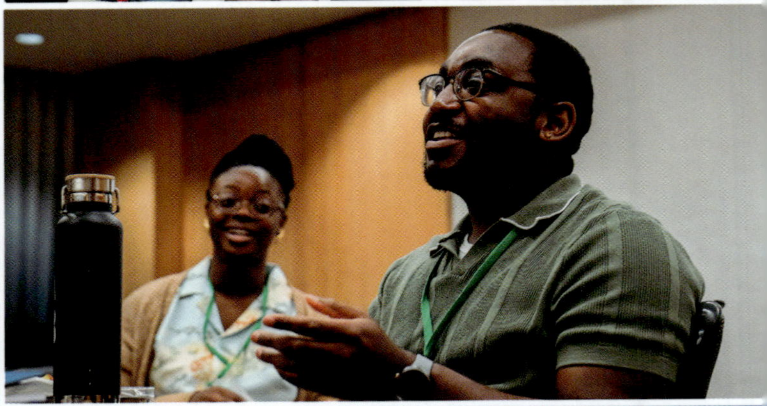

APHA 2026
ANNUAL MEETING & EXPO

Save the Date

Nov. 1-4, 2026
San Antonio, TX
Registration and housing open in June.

APHA.org/AnnualMeeting

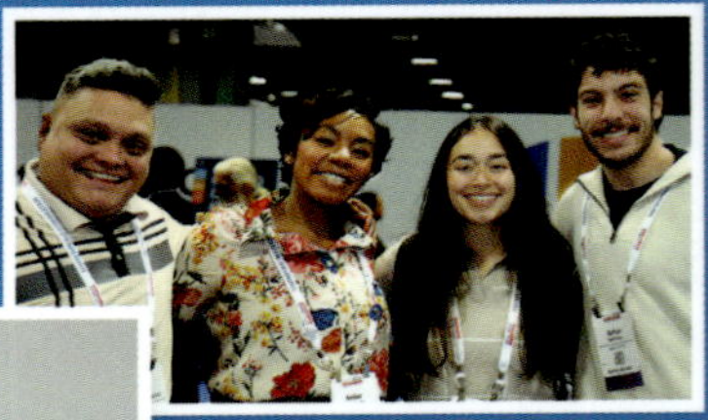

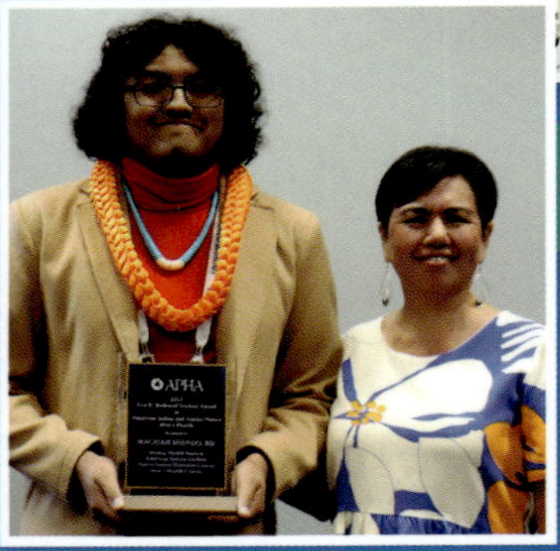

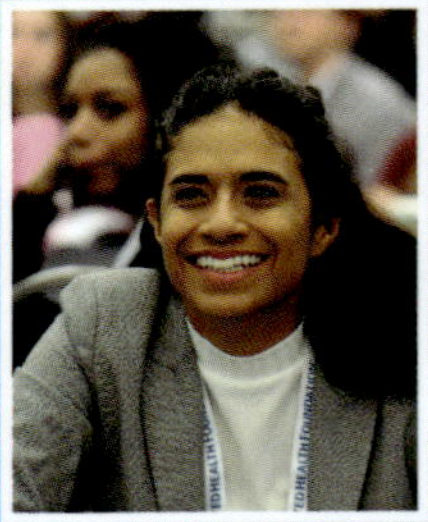

APHA
AMERICAN PUBLIC HEALTH ASSOCIATION
For science. For action. For health.

Learn more about our events at
APHA.org/Calendar